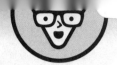

Self-Care

ALL-IN-ONE

by Shamash Alidina; Allen Elkin, PhD;
David N. Greenfield, PhD, MS;
Steven Hickman, PsyD;
Linda Larsen, BS, BA; Liz Neporent;
Suzanne Schlosberg; Eva Selhub, MD;
and Jonathan Wright, MD

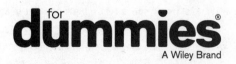

A Wiley Brand

Self-Care All-in-One For Dummies®

Published by: **John Wiley & Sons, Inc.,** 111 River Street, Hoboken, NJ 07030-5774, www.wiley.com

Copyright © 2022 by John Wiley & Sons, Inc., Hoboken, New Jersey

Published simultaneously in Canada

No part of this publication may be reproduced, stored in a retrieval system or transmitted in any form or by any means, electronic, mechanical, photocopying, recording, scanning or otherwise, except as permitted under Sections 107 or 108 of the 1976 United States Copyright Act, without the prior written permission of the Publisher. Requests to the Publisher for permission should be addressed to the Permissions Department, John Wiley & Sons, Inc., 111 River Street, Hoboken, NJ 07030, (201) 748-6011, fax (201) 748-6008, or online at http://www.wiley.com/go/permissions.

Trademarks: Wiley, For Dummies, the Dummies Man logo, Dummies.com, Making Everything Easier, and related trade dress are trademarks or registered trademarks of John Wiley & Sons, Inc., and may not be used without written permission. All other trademarks are the property of their respective owners. John Wiley & Sons, Inc., is not associated with any product or vendor mentioned in this book.

LIMIT OF LIABILITY/DISCLAIMER OF WARRANTY: WHILE THE PUBLISHER AND AUTHORS HAVE USED THEIR BEST EFFORTS IN PREPARING THIS WORK, THEY MAKE NO REPRESENTATIONS OR WARRANTIES WITH RESPECT TO THE ACCURACY OR COMPLETENESS OF THE CONTENTS OF THIS WORK AND SPECIFICALLY DISCLAIM ALL WARRANTIES, INCLUDING WITHOUT LIMITATION ANY IMPLIED WARRANTIES OF MERCHANTABILITY OR FITNESS FOR A PARTICULAR PURPOSE. NO WARRANTY MAY BE CREATED OR EXTENDED BY SALES REPRESENTATIVES, WRITTEN SALES MATERIALS OR PROMOTIONAL STATEMENTS FOR THIS WORK. THE FACT THAT AN ORGANIZATION, WEBSITE, OR PRODUCT IS REFERRED TO IN THIS WORK AS A CITATION AND/OR POTENTIAL SOURCE OF FURTHER INFORMATION DOES NOT MEAN THAT THE PUBLISHER AND AUTHORS ENDORSE THE INFORMATION OR SERVICES THE ORGANIZATION, WEBSITE, OR PRODUCT MAY PROVIDE OR RECOMMENDATIONS IT MAY MAKE. THIS WORK IS SOLD WITH THE UNDERSTANDING THAT THE PUBLISHER IS NOT ENGAGED IN RENDERING PROFESSIONAL SERVICES. THE ADVICE AND STRATEGIES CONTAINED HEREIN MAY NOT BE SUITABLE FOR YOUR SITUATION. YOU SHOULD CONSULT WITH A SPECIALIST WHERE APPROPRIATE. FURTHER, READERS SHOULD BE AWARE THAT WEBSITES LISTED IN THIS WORK MAY HAVE CHANGED OR DISAPPEARED BETWEEN WHEN THIS WORK WAS WRITTEN AND WHEN IT IS READ. NEITHER THE PUBLISHER NOR AUTHORS SHALL BE LIABLE FOR ANY LOSS OF PROFIT OR ANY OTHER COMMERCIAL DAMAGES, INCLUDING BUT NOT LIMITED TO SPECIAL, INCIDENTAL, CONSEQUENTIAL, OR OTHER DAMAGES.

For general information on our other products and services, please contact our Customer Care Department within the U.S. at 877-762-2974, outside the U.S. at 317-572-3993, or fax 317-572-4002. For technical support, please visit https://hub.wiley.com/community/support/dummies.

Wiley publishes in a variety of print and electronic formats and by print-on-demand. Some material included with standard print versions of this book may not be included in e-books or in print-on-demand. If this book refers to media such as a CD or DVD that is not included in the version you purchased, you may download this material at http://booksupport.wiley.com. For more information about Wiley products, visit www.wiley.com.

Library of Congress Control Number: 2022934345

ISBN 978-1-119-87505-5 (pbk); ISBN 978-1-119-87506-2 (ebk); ISBN 978-1-119-87507-9 (ebk)

SKY10033766_032522

Contents at a Glance

Introduction 1

Book 1: Being Present through Mindfulness 5

CHAPTER 1: Discovering Mindfulness 7

CHAPTER 2: Enjoying the Benefits of Mindfulness 19

CHAPTER 3: Making Mindfulness a Daily Habit 33

CHAPTER 4: Humans Being Versus Humans Doing 47

CHAPTER 5: Using Mindfulness for Yourself 61

CHAPTER 6: Using Mindfulness in Your Daily Life 73

Book 2: Treating Yourself with Compassion 91

CHAPTER 1: Exploring Self-Compassion 93

CHAPTER 2: The Self-Compassion Road Ahead 109

CHAPTER 3: Common Humanity: Connection and Belonging 129

CHAPTER 4: Cultivating Your Innate Kindness 149

CHAPTER 5: Discovering Core Values: Your Inner Compass 159

Book 3: Facing Challenges with Resilience 173

CHAPTER 1: Embarking on the Journey to Resilience 175

CHAPTER 2: The Basis of Resilience: Harmony Versus Stress 187

CHAPTER 3: Developing Mental Toughness and Clarity 199

CHAPTER 4: Achieving Emotional Equilibrium 211

CHAPTER 5: Improving Your Relationship with Yourself 221

Book 4: Feeling Better with a Bit of Fitness 241

CHAPTER 1: Cardio Crash Course: Getting the Right Intensity .. 243

CHAPTER 2: Exercising Outdoors 255

CHAPTER 3: Strengthening and Lengthening Your Muscles 269

CHAPTER 4: All about Yoga 289

CHAPTER 5: Choosing an Exercise Class or Virtual Workout 303

Book 5: Providing Your Body with Top-Notch Nutrition ... 315

CHAPTER 1: Eating Clean for a Healthier Body, Mind, and Soul . 317

CHAPTER 2: Applying Eating Clean Principles to Daily Living .. 331

CHAPTER 3: Nutrition Basics: You Really Are What You Eat 345

CHAPTER 4: Eat More, Eat Often 375

Book 6: Scaling Back the Stress in Your Life 387

CHAPTER 1: Getting a Handle on the Causes and Effects of Stress.............389

CHAPTER 2: Relaxing Your Body 403

CHAPTER 3: Finding More Time...425

CHAPTER 4: Stress-Reducing Organizational Skills..........................447

CHAPTER 5: De-Stressing at Work 467

Book 7: Reining In Online Activities 485

CHAPTER 1: Defining and Overcoming Internet Addiction in a Nutshell 487

CHAPTER 2: Discovering What Makes the Internet and Smartphones
So Addictive...499

CHAPTER 3: Examining the Addictive Nature of Social Media 511

CHAPTER 4: The Endless Stream: Binge Watching TV and Online
Entertainment...523

CHAPTER 5: Adopting Self-Help Strategies..................................533

Index 549

Table of Contents

INTRODUCTION 1

About This Book. 1

Foolish Assumptions. 1

Icons Used in This Book 2

Beyond the Book 2

Where to Go from Here 3

BOOK 1: BEING PRESENT THROUGH MINDFULNESS 5

CHAPTER 1: Discovering Mindfulness 7

Understanding the Meaning of Mindfulness. 8

Looking at Mindfulness Meditation 9

Using Mindfulness to Help You 10

Allowing space to heal 11

Enjoying greater relaxation 12

Improving focus and feeling happier 13

Developing greater wisdom. 14

Discovering your true self 15

CHAPTER 2: Enjoying the Benefits of Mindfulness 19

Relaxing the Body 20

Getting back in touch 20

Boosting your immune system 21

Reducing pain. 22

Calming the Mind 22

Listening to your thoughts. 23

Making better decisions 24

Coming to your senses. 24

Creating an attentive mind 25

Soothing Your Emotions. 27

Understanding your emotions 27

Managing feelings differently 28

Uplifting Your Spirit. 28

Knowing Thyself: Discovering Your Observer Self 29

CHAPTER 3: Making Mindfulness a Daily Habit 33

Discovering the Secret to Change. 33

Designing your life for mindfulness 34

Starting small: The secret to creating new habits. 35

Being playful with your new habit...........................39
Watering the seeds of your mindful habits...................39
Scattering seeds of mindfulness throughout the day..........40
Exploring Your Intentions.................................41
Clarifying intention in mindfulness........................41
Finding what you're looking for...........................43
Developing a vision....................................44

CHAPTER 4: **Humans Being Versus Humans Doing**...............47
Delving into the Doing Mode of Mind.......................47
Embracing the Being Mode of Mind.........................49
Combining Being and Doing...............................50
Being in the Zone: The Psychology of Flow..................52
Understanding the factors of mindful flow..................52
Discovering your flow experiences........................53
Encouraging a Being Mode of Mind.........................54
Dealing with emotions using being mode....................56
Finding time to just be................................57
Living in the moment..................................58

CHAPTER 5: **Using Mindfulness for Yourself**....................61
Using a Mini Mindful Exercise............................62
Introducing the breathing space..........................62
Practicing the breathing space...........................63
Using the breathing space between activities...............66
Using Mindfulness to Look After Yourself...................67
Exercising mindfully...................................67
Preparing for sleep with mindfulness......................68
Looking at a mindful work–life balance....................70
Building a better relationship with yourself................70

CHAPTER 6: **Using Mindfulness in Your Daily Life**...............73
Using Mindfulness at Work...............................74
Beginning the day mindfully.............................74
Dropping in with mini meditations........................75
Going from reacting to responding........................76
Solving problems creatively.............................78
Practicing mindful working..............................79
Trying single-tasking..................................81
Finishing by letting go.................................81
Using Mindfulness on the Move...........................82
Walking mindfully.....................................82
Driving mindfully.....................................83

Traveling mindfully on public transport. 84

Using Mindfulness in the Home 85

Waking up mindfully. 85

Doing everyday tasks with awareness 85

Second hunger: Overcoming problem eating. 88

BOOK 2: TREATING YOURSELF WITH COMPASSION. 91

CHAPTER 1: **Exploring Self-Compassion**. 93

Befriending Yourself: A Splendid New Relationship. 94

Understanding Self-Compassion. 95

Compassion at the core 96

Mindfulness 98

Common humanity 98

Self-kindness 99

Looking at the Yin and Yang of Self-Compassion 100

Asking the Fundamental Question of Self-Compassion 102

Activating Your Secret Weapon for Safety, Warmth, and

Connection. 103

Discovering which form of touch works for you. 103

Knowing that sometimes it's all in the tone. 104

Introducing the Mindful Self-Compassion Program. 105

Practice: The Self-Compassion Break. .106

Inquiring: What arose for you when you took a

Self-Compassion Break?. 107

CHAPTER 2: **The Self-Compassion Road Ahead** 109

Why Self-Compassion Isn't Always Easy. 110

Getting the Most Out of a Self-Compassion Practice. 112

Having the spirit of an adventurer 113

Being a self-compassion scientist. 114

Being willing to be a slow learner and your own best teacher. . .116

If it's a struggle, it's not self-compassion 116

The Four Noble Truths: A Buddhist Perspective on Being Human. . .118

First noble truth: Suffering exists 118

Second noble truth: The cause of suffering. 119

Third noble truth: The end of suffering 119

Fourth noble truth: The path to relief of suffering. 120

Finding What You Need to Feel Safe and Courageous. 120

Opening and closing to adjust your "dosage" 121

Finding your sweet spot of tolerance. .124

The experience of belonging and deserving 126

CHAPTER 3: **Common Humanity: Connection and Belonging**..129

The Inescapable Truth: We Need Each Other.....................130
Acknowledging Our Universal Human Need.....................133
Survival equals love...134
What arises if we feel unloved . . . or unlovable? 135
Three common blocks to embracing your common humanity ...137
Starting small with common humanity 141
Two Tasks to Embrace Common Humanity 142
Claiming your human birthrights 143
Avoiding the perils of perfection.............................144
Practice: Just Like Me 145
Just Like Me meditation 145
Inquiring: What was it like to see how others are just like you?...147

CHAPTER 4: **Cultivating Your Innate Kindness**........................149

We All Just Want to Be Happy 150
Investing in Your Capacity to Be Kind...........................152
Practice: Lovingkindness for a Loved One 153
Inquiring: What was it like to cultivate kindness?..............154
What if you practiced and felt absolutely nothing? 157
What if you practiced lovingkindness and felt great?..........158

CHAPTER 5: **Discovering Core Values: Your Inner Compass**....159

Core Values Guide Us and "Re-Mind" Us 160
Finding meaning through core values 161
Your core values determine your experience.................162
The relationship between core values and suffering...........163
Practice: Uncovering your core values 163
Inquiring: What was it like to discover your core values? 166
Translating values into action 167
Dark Nights and Dark Clouds: Wisdom Gleaned from
Life's Challenges 168
Seasoning in the stew.......................................169
How failure and hardship teach us...........................169
Exercise: Silver linings and golden gifts 170
Inquiring: Were you able to identify a silver lining? 171

BOOK 3: FACING CHALLENGES WITH RESILIENCE........173

CHAPTER 1: **Embarking on the Journey to Resilience** 175

Noting That Resilience Is for Everyone............................175
Figuring Out the Factors That Determine Resilience 176
Your genes 177
Childhood development.......................................177

Culture. 178
Psychological outlook 178
Coping habits 179
Social support 179
Humor. 180
Spirituality. 180
Understanding What Resilience Is Not. 180
The victim mindset 181
Learned helplessness 182
Hopelessness 184
Breaking the Victim Cycle 185

CHAPTER 2: **The Basis of Resilience: Harmony Versus Stress**. . .187
Understanding the Perpetual Quest for Harmony. 188
Examining the Stress Response Feedback Loop. 189
Fight-or-flight 189
The feedback loop. 190
Living in Disharmony: The Real Stress 191
Expecting a Good Outcome Is the Key 192
Coping to Adapt, or Not 193
Maladaptive coping. 194
Adaptive coping 194
Harmonizing Stress and Becoming Resilient. 195
Quieting the stress response. 196
Being open to learn and understand 196
Building and restoring 197

CHAPTER 3: **Developing Mental Toughness and Clarity**. 199
What Kind of Mindset Do Resilient People Have?. 200
Fixed Versus Growth Mindsets When It Comes to Resilience. 201
Developing Mental Toughness 202
Getting in control. 203
Making a commitment 205
Embracing challenges. 206
Being confident 207
Accessing Mental Clarity. 208

CHAPTER 4: **Achieving Emotional Equilibrium**. 211
Emotions Exist for a Very Good Reason. 211
How Emotions Influence Perception and Coping. 213
Evaluating Your Feelings. 214
Choosing to Manage Your Emotions 215
Calming Your Emotions By Calming the Stress Response. 217
Shifting to Positive Detachment and Reappraisal 218

Enhancing Your Self-Awareness and Willingness to Grow 219
Always Choosing Love. 220

CHAPTER 5: **Improving Your Relationship with Yourself** 221
Connecting Resilience with Self-Worth. 222
Believing in Your Worth 223
Noting Self-Criticism 224
Evaluating Your Self-Value 225
Starting to Take Action 227
Practicing self-awareness. 227
Making a conscious choice. 228
Celebrating yourself 229
Keeping an inventory 229
Accepting and being your unique self .230
Holding on to your vision. 231
Being loving toward yourself. 232
Taking Care of YOU 233
Nourish yourself with nutrient-rich food. 233
Exercise and stay active 233
Connect with support. 234
Quiet your mind. 234
Heal through your negative emotions .235
Have fun!. 235
Appreciate all that you have and all that you are. 236
It's okay to rest. 236
Allowing Love In. 237

BOOK 4: FEELING BETTER WITH A BIT OF FITNESS 241

CHAPTER 1: **Cardio Crash Course: Getting the
Right Intensity** 243
Comparing Aerobic and Anaerobic Exercise. 244
Understanding the Importance of Warming Up and
Cooling Down. 245
Warming up 245
Cooling down 246
Using Simple Methods to Gauge Your Level of Effort 246
The talk test 247
Perceived exertion. 247
Measuring Your Heart Rate 248
Looking at what heart rate tells you. 248
Understanding your target zone. 250
Finding your maximum and target heart rates. 250
Measuring your pulse. 252

CHAPTER 2: Exercising Outdoors 255

Walking for Fitness 256

Essential walking gear 256

Walking with good form 257

Walking tips for rookies 257

Running: Get Up and Go 258

Essential running gear 258

Running with good form 260

Running tips for rookies 260

Bicycling Around 261

Essential cycling gear 261

Cycling with good form 262

Cycling tips for rookies 263

Exercising in Water 263

Essential water exercise gear 264

Swimming with good form 265

Swimming tips for rookies 265

CHAPTER 3: Strengthening and Lengthening Your Muscles 269

Why You've Gotta Lift Weights 270

Staying strong for everyday life 270

Keeping your bones healthy 271

Preventing injuries 271

Looking better 272

Speeding up your metabolism 272

Flexibility Training: Getting the Scoop on Stretching 273

Understanding why you need to stretch 274

Deciding when to stretch 276

Exploring Stretching Techniques 276

Still Life: Doing Static Stretching 278

Following a few rules of static stretching 278

Trying a simple static stretching routine 279

CHAPTER 4: All about Yoga 289

Looking at What Yoga Can Do for Your Body 289

Finding a Yoga Style That's Right for You 290

Getting Started 292

Taking yoga classes 292

Looking at yoga equipment and clothing 293

Following yoga tips for beginners 293

Trying a Yoga Routine 294

Downward-Facing Dog 294

Forward Bend 295

Child's Pose 296

Modified Sage Twist 297
Cat Pose 298
Triangle Pose 299
Sun Salutation 300

CHAPTER 5: **Choosing an Exercise Class or Virtual Workout** . . . 303
Getting Through When You Haven't a Clue: Taking an
Exercise Class. 304
Signing up. 304
Knowing what to expect from a live instructor 304
Getting the most out of your classes .305
Considering popular classes 306
Working Out with an Onscreen Instructor. 311

**BOOK 5: PROVIDING YOUR BODY WITH
TOP-NOTCH NUTRITION** 315

CHAPTER 1: **Eating Clean for a Healthier Body, Mind,
and Soul** 317
What Clean Eating Really Is 318
Eating clean doesn't mean cleaning your food before
eating it 318
Comparing whole versus processed foods 319
Gaining control with six degrees of clean eating 320
Considering the Dangers in Processed Foods. 322
Preservatives and additives 322
Label claims (also known as marketing hype). 324
Junk food addiction 325
Surveying the Benefits of Eating Clean. 326
Overall good health. 326
Weight loss and disease prevention. 328
A longer, more active life 329

CHAPTER 2: **Applying Eating Clean Principles to
Daily Living**. 331
The Principles of Clean Eating 332
Getting your footing on the eating clean platform. 332
Making clean changes in your life. 334
Discovering real flavor 335
Managing Cravings and Feelings of Deprivation 339
Understanding cravings 339
Dealing with deprivation 341
Living with lapses and backsliding 342

CHAPTER 3: **Nutrition Basics: You Really Are What You Eat**.... 345

Figuring Out What Your Body Needs (And What It Doesn't Need)...346

How your body uses food 346

What happens to additives and chemicals 348

What happens to excess macronutrients and calories 351

What happens if you don't get the micronutrients you need....355

Considering the Roles of Proteins, Carbs, and Fats 356

Clean proteins: Amino acids, the building blocks of life 356

Carbohydrates: Energy for your body 357

Essential and clean fats 359

Getting the Vitamins and Minerals You Need to Stay Healthy 362

Recommended daily allowances and reference intakes 363

The role of vitamins. 364

The role of minerals 366

Protecting Your Health with Fiber. 371

Surveying the different types of clean fiber 371

Bulking up your fiber intake. 372

Chew on this: Connecting fiber and weight loss. 372

Water: The Essential Nutrient 373

CHAPTER 4: **Eat More, Eat Often** 375

Listening to Your Body 376

Decoding hunger cues 376

Identifying thirst cues 378

Understanding satiety. 379

Getting Started with Good Food Choices. 381

Knowing what (and what not) to eat. 382

Eating mini meals to combat hunger 384

Combining clean eating with your daily routine. 386

BOOK 6: SCALING BACK THE STRESS IN YOUR LIFE 387

CHAPTER 1: **Getting a Handle on the Causes and Effects
of Stress** 389

Experiencing a Stress Epidemic?. 389

Understanding Where All This Stress Is Coming From 390

Coping with the pandemic. 390

Our politics is stressing us out. 391

Struggling in a struggling economy. 391

Getting frazzled at work 392

Feeling frazzled at home 392

Piling on new stresses with technology 394

Dealing with daily hassles (the little things add up) 395

Looking at the Signs and Symptoms of Stress 396
Understanding How Stress Can Make You Sick 397
Understanding how stress can be a pain in the neck
(and other places) 398
Taking stress to heart 398
Hitting below the belt 399
Compromising your immune system 400
The cold facts: Connecting stress and the sniffles 401
"Not tonight, dear. I have a (stress) headache." 401

CHAPTER 2: **Relaxing Your Body** 403
Stress Can Be a Pain in the Neck (And That's Just for Starters) 403
Funny, I don't feel tense 404
Invasion of the body scan 405
Breathing Away Your Tension 406
Your breath is fine; it's your breathing that's bad 406
"Why change now? I've been breathing for years." 406
Evaluating your breathing 408
Cutting yourself some slack 408
Changing the way you breathe, changing the way you feel 409
The yawn that refreshes 412
Tensing Your Way to Relaxation 413
Exploring how progressive relaxation works 413
Scrunching up like a pretzel 416
Mind over Body: Using the Power of Suggestion 417
Stretching Away Your Stress 419
Massage? Ah, There's the Rub! 420
Massaging yourself 420
Becoming the massage-er or massage-ee 422
Taking a Three-Minute Energy Burst 422
More Ways to Relax 423

CHAPTER 3: **Finding More Time** 425
Determining Whether You Struggle with Time Management 426
Being Mindful of Your Time 426
Knowing where your time goes 427
Figuring out what you want more time for 428
Knowing what you want to spend *less* time doing 429
Minding your time with cues and prompts 429
Questioning your choices and changing behaviors 430
Becoming a List Maker 431
Starting with a master to-do list 431
Creating a will-do-today list 432

Having a will-do-later list 434
Keeping some tips in mind as you make your lists 434
Minimizing Your Distractions and Interruptions. 436
Managing electronic interruptions 436
Losing the visitors 437
Lowering the volume 437
Limiting your breaks 438
Shifting your time 438
Turning it into a positive. 438
Minimizing your TV time. 439
Winning the waiting game 439
Getting around Psychological Roadblocks to Time Management . . .440
Getting over your desire to be perfect. 440
Overcoming procrastination 441
Letting Go: Discovering the Joys of Delegating 443
The fine art of delegating. 444
Delegating begins at home 444
Buying Time 445
Avoid paying top dollar. 445
Strive for deliverance 446

CHAPTER 4: **Stress-Reducing Organizational Skills** 447
Figuring Out Why Your Life Is So Disorganized. 448
Are you organizationally challenged?. 448
Identifying your personal disorganization. 449
Clearing Away the Clutter. 450
Bust those clutter excuses. 450
Get yourself motivated. 452
Draw yourself a clutter roadmap 452
Get your feet wet. 453
Stop kidding yourself 453
Avoid discouragement 454
Get down to the nitty-gritty 454
Organizing Your Space 456
Organizing Information 458
Losing the paper trail 458
Organizing the papers you do need to keep. 459
Organizing electronically 463
Managing your email 464
Keeping Your Life Organized 465
Being proactive 465
Buying less 466

CHAPTER 5: De-Stressing at Work.................................467
Reading the Signs of Workplace Stress 467
Knowing What's Triggering Your Work Stress....................468
Making Positive Changes to Control Your Workplace Stress 469
Overcoming SNS (Sunday night stress) 470
Starting your workday unstressed 470
Calming your daily commute...............................471
Minimizing your travel stress.............................472
De-stressing during your workday 473
Stretching and reaching for the sky 474
Creating a stress-resistant workspace 476
Managing your work time 480
Nourishing your body (and spirit).........................480
Taking Advantage of Company Perks............................482
Gyms and health clubs....................................482
Flextime...482
Working from home 483
Employee assistance programs.............................483
Coming Home More Relaxed (And Staying That Way)............483

BOOK 7: REINING IN ONLINE ACTIVITIES 485

CHAPTER 1: Defining and Overcoming Internet Addiction in a Nutshell 487
Defining Behavioral Addiction.................................488
Understanding How and Why People Get Addicted to
Screens and the Internet 489
Digging into Digital Devices and the Internet 491
Recognizing the Threats......................................492
Social media...492
Streaming audio and video 493
Video games...493
Identifying the Signs and Symptoms of Internet and Screen
Addiction..494
Recovering from Internet and Screen Addiction................496
Exploring self-help options 497
Getting professional help.................................497
Balancing Technology with Real-Time Living..................498

CHAPTER 2: Discovering What Makes the Internet and Smartphones So Addictive 499
Eyes on the Prize: Factors Involving Focus on a Screen..........500
Examining ease of access and near-constant availability 501
Talking about time distortion 501
Giving you the world online: The illusion of online productivity....502

The Good (or Bad) Stuff: Factors Involving Content...............502
 Finding out about content intoxication 503
 Mixing stimulating content and digital devices................503
 Understanding instant gratification 504
 Defining infotainment......................................505

This Must Be the Place: The Internet as the Car, Map, and
Destination..505
 Getting the word in and out: Broadcast intoxication..........506
 Weaving a web: A story without an end......................506
 Apprehending the myth of multi-tasking.....................507
 Telling a social story: The net effect on people...............507

The Human Factor: The Internet as a Digital Drug.............508
 Grasping the power of "maybe" 509
 Seeing how dynamic interaction keeps people coming
 back for more..510

CHAPTER 3: **Examining the Addictive Nature
of Social Media**...511
A Social Network: A Rose by Any Other Name 512
Recognizing What Makes You Come Back to Social Media
for More 513
 Looking at social validation looping 514
 Understanding the big deal about variable reinforcement......515
Seeking Communication and Self-Esteem — But at a Price 517
Seeing Why Social Media Can Be Counter-Social 519
 Broadcast intoxication on social media......................519
 Cyberbullying 520
 Cyberstalking and trolling 521
Finding Relief: Life beyond Social Media 522

CHAPTER 4: **The Endless Stream: Binge Watching TV
and Online Entertainment**................................523
Missing Your Life While Being Entertained: The Ease of the Binge ...524
 Understanding the allure of endless choice 525
 Finding the power of instant access.........................526
 Recognizing the pitfalls of effortless starting 526
 Unpacking user experience engineering 527
 Seeing the influence of social media 528
Looking at Other Problems of Watching TV All the Time...........529
 Intensity is addictive 530
 TV acts as your social companion...........................531
 One form of screen use is almost as good as another 531
It's a Choice: Screening the Stream...........................532

CHAPTER 5: **Adopting Self-Help Strategies** 533

    Remembering That Life Isn't Lived on a Screen 534

        Recognizing that it's tough to limit tech use 534

        Striving for lower-tech (not no-tech) living. 535

        Decreasing your stress with less tech 536

    Disrupting Your Tech Habits with a Digital Detox. 537

        Defining a "digital detox" 537

        Getting set for success 538

    Monitoring and Limiting Your Time and Content on Screens. 539

        Turning off Internet access at a specified time. 539

        Limiting specific content. 540

    Establishing Values-Based Tech Use. 541

        Introducing a values map. 542

        Deciding where your eyes go. 542

    Removing Notifications and Addictive Apps 544

        Knowing that notifications invite you to waste time 544

        Getting rid of apps, websites, and software 544

    Filling Your Life with Real-Time Activities. .545

INDEX 549

Introduction

L ife in the 21st century is hectic and stressful — which is why taking care of yourself is more important than ever. You can't care for others if you don't take care of yourself! *Self-Care All-in-One For Dummies* is here to help you build and consistently use healthy, uplifting, and fulfilling habits.

About This Book

Self-Care All-in-One For Dummies provides guidance, tools, and resources for incorporating self-care practices into your busy everyday life. Here, you get tips on practicing mindfulness, building self-compassion and resilience, starting a fitness routine, eating clean, managing stress, and living a lower-tech life.

A quick note: Sidebars (shaded boxes of text) dig into the details of a given self-care technique or topic, but they aren't crucial to understanding it. Feel free to read them or skip them. You can pass over the text accompanied by the Technical Stuff icon, too. The text marked with this icon gives some interesting but nonessential information about a particular self-care method.

One last thing: Within this book, you may note that some web addresses break across two lines of text. If you're reading this book in print and want to visit one of these web pages, simply key in the web address exactly as it's noted in the text, pretending as though the line break doesn't exist. If you're reading this as an e-book, you've got it easy — just click the web address to be taken directly to the web page.

Foolish Assumptions

Here are some assumptions about why you're picking up this book:

>> You're looking for small yet meaningful steps to improve your overall wellbeing.

>> You want to manage stress and remain resilient in the face of daily challenges.

>> You want to develop the ability to quiet your inner critic and give yourself compassion.

>> You're interested in starting (or restarting) a fitness routine and clean eating habits.

>> You wonder whether you're spending too much time online and want proven methods for reducing your Internet activity.

Icons Used in This Book

Like all *For Dummies* books, this book features icons to help you navigate the information. Here's what they mean.

 REMEMBER If you take away anything from this book, it should be the information marked with this icon.

 TECHNICAL STUFF This icon flags information that digs a little deeper than usual into a given self-care practice.

 TIP This icon highlights especially helpful advice about starting or continuing a self-care practice.

 WARNING This icon points out situations and actions to avoid as you start taking better care of yourself.

Beyond the Book

In addition to the material in the print or e-book you're reading right now, this product comes with some access-anywhere goodies on the web. Check out the free Cheat Sheet for information on mindfulness, self-compassion, resilience, fitness, clean eating, stress management, and reducing online activity. To get this Cheat Sheet, simply go to www.dummies.com and search for "*Self-Care All-in-One For Dummies* Cheat Sheet" in the Search box.

Where to Go from Here

You don't have to read this book from cover to cover, but you can if you like! If you just want to find specific information on a type of self-care practice, take a look at the table of contents or the index, and then dive into the chapter or section that interests you.

For example, if you want the basics of mindfulness, go to Book 1. If you want to explore self-compassion and resilience, check out Books 2 and 3. If you prefer to find out more about fitness and clean eating, head to Books 4 and 5. Stress getting you down? Flip to Book 6. Or if you want the scoop on living a lower-tech life, Book 7 is the place to be.

No matter where you start, you'll find the information you need to take better care of yourself every day. Good luck!

1

Being Present through Mindfulness

Contents at a Glance

CHAPTER 1: Discovering Mindfulness 7

Understanding the Meaning of Mindfulness. 8

Looking at Mindfulness Meditation 9

Using Mindfulness to Help You 10

CHAPTER 2: Enjoying the Benefits of Mindfulness 19

Relaxing the Body 20

Calming the Mind 22

Soothing Your Emotions. 27

Uplifting Your Spirit. 28

Knowing Thyself: Discovering Your Observer Self 29

CHAPTER 3: Making Mindfulness a Daily Habit 33

Discovering the Secret to Change. 33

Exploring Your Intentions. 41

CHAPTER 4: Humans Being Versus Humans Doing 47

Delving into the Doing Mode of Mind 47

Embracing the Being Mode of Mind. 49

Combining Being and Doing 50

Being in the Zone: The Psychology of Flow 52

Encouraging a Being Mode of Mind 54

CHAPTER 5: Using Mindfulness for Yourself 61

Using a Mini Mindful Exercise 62

Using Mindfulness to Look After Yourself 67

CHAPTER 6: Using Mindfulness in Your Daily Life 73

Using Mindfulness at Work 74

Using Mindfulness on the Move 82

Using Mindfulness in the Home 85

Chapter **1**

Discovering Mindfulness

Mindfulness means flexibly paying attention on purpose, in the present moment, infused with qualities such as kindness, curiosity, acceptance, and openness.

Through being mindful, you discover how to live in the present moment in an enjoyable way rather than worrying about the past or being concerned about the future. The past has already gone and can't be changed. The future is yet to arrive and is completely unknown. The present moment, this very moment now, is ultimately the only moment you have. Mindfulness shows you how to live in this moment in a harmonious way. You find out how to make the present moment a more wonderful moment to be in — the only place in which you can create, decide, listen, think, smile, act, or live.

You can develop and deepen mindfulness through doing mindfulness meditation on a daily basis, from a few minutes to as long as you want. This chapter introduces you to mindfulness and mindfulness meditation and welcomes you aboard a fascinating journey.

Understanding the Meaning of Mindfulness

REMEMBER

Mindfulness was originally developed in ancient times, and can be found in Eastern and Western cultures. Mindfulness is a translation of the ancient Indian word *Sati*, which means awareness, attention, and remembering.

>> **Awareness:** This is an aspect of being human that makes you conscious of your experiences. Without awareness, nothing would exist for you.

>> **Attention:** Attention is a focused awareness; mindfulness training develops your ability to move and sustain your attention wherever and however you choose.

>> **Remembering:** This aspect of mindfulness is about remembering to pay attention to your experience from moment to moment. Being mindful is easy to forget. The word "remember" originally comes from the Latin *re* ("again") and *memorari* ("be mindful of").

Say that you want to practice mindfulness to help you cope with stress. At work, you think about your forthcoming presentation and begin to feel stressed and nervous. By becoming *aware* of this, you *remember* to focus your mindful *attention* to your own breathing rather than constantly worrying. Feeling your breath with a sense of warmth and gentleness helps slowly to calm you down.

Dr. Jon Kabat-Zinn, who first developed mindfulness in a therapeutic setting, says: "Mindfulness can be cultivated by paying attention in a specific way, that is, in the present moment, and as non-reactively, non-judgmentally and openheartedly as possible."

REMEMBER

You can break down the meaning even further:

>> **Paying attention:** To be mindful, you need to pay attention, whatever you choose to attend to.

>> **Present moment:** The reality of being in the here and now means you just need to be aware of the way things are, *as they are now*. Your experience is valid and correct just as it is.

>> **Non-reactively:** Normally, when you experience something, you automatically react to that experience according to your past conditioning. For example, if you think, "I still haven't finished my work," you react with thoughts, words, and actions in some shape or form.

Mindfulness encourages you to *respond* to your experience rather than *react* to thoughts. A reaction is automatic and gives you no choice; a response is deliberate and considered action.

>> **Non-judgmentally:** The temptation is to judge experience as good or bad, something you like or dislike. You want to feel bliss; you don't like feeling afraid. Letting go of judgments helps you to see things as they are rather than through the filter of your personal judgments based on past conditioning.

>> **Openheartedly:** Mindfulness isn't just an aspect of mind. Mindfulness is of the heart as well. To be open-hearted is to bring a quality of kindness, compassion, warmth, and friendliness to your experience. For example, if you notice yourself thinking, "I'm useless at meditation," you discover how to let go of this critical thought and gently turn your attention back to the focus of your meditation, whatever that may be.

REMEMBER

World-renowned monk Ajahn Brahm says the word *mindfulness* doesn't capture the importance of kindness in the practice. So what word does he recommend? *Kindfulness.* This term can help remind you to bring a warm, friendly awareness when practicing mindfulness — and it just may make you smile too! Be sure to practice being kindful, not just mindful.

Looking at Mindfulness Meditation

Mindfulness meditation is a particular type of meditation that's been well researched and tested in clinical settings.

REMEMBER

Meditation isn't thinking about nothing. Meditation is kindly paying attention in a systematic way to whatever you decide to focus on, which can include awareness of your thoughts. By listening to your thoughts, you discover their habitual patterns. Your thoughts have a massive impact on your emotions and the decisions you make, so being more aware of them is helpful.

In mindfulness meditation, you typically focus on one, or a combination, of the following:

>> The feeling of your own breathing

>> Any one of your senses

>> Your body

>> Your thoughts or emotions

>> Your intentions

>> Whatever is most predominant in your awareness

Mindfulness meditation comes in two distinct types:

>> **Formal meditation:** This meditation is where you intentionally take time in your day to embark on a meditative practice. Time gives you an opportunity to deepen your mindfulness practice and understand more about your mind, its habitual tendencies, and how to be mindful for a sustained period of time, with a sense of kindness and curiosity toward yourself and your experience. Formal meditation is mind training.

>> **Informal meditation:** This is where you go into a focused and meditative state of mind as you go about your daily activities such as cooking, cleaning, walking to work, talking to a friend, driving — anything at all. Think of it as everyday mindfulness. In this way, you continue to deepen your ability to be mindful, and train your mind to stay in the present moment more often rather than habitually straying into the past or future. Informal mindfulness meditation means you can rest in a mindful awareness at any time of day, whatever you're doing. See Chapter 6 in Book 1 for more ways to be mindful informally.

REMEMBER

To practice meditation means to engage in the meditation exercise — not practicing in the sense of aiming one day to get the meditation perfect. You don't need to judge your meditation or perfect it in any way. Your experience is your experience. In this instance, practice doesn't mean rehearsal.

WARNING

Mindfulness is not just about having your attention caught — it's about cultivating a flexible attention. Flexible attention means you can choose where to focus your attention. For example, when a child (or adult!) is playing a computer game, they may have their full attention on the game, but the attention is usually not flexible. Their attention is caught by the game. That's not mindfulness. As you become more mindful, you're able to move your attention from one place to the other more in a flexible way.

Using Mindfulness to Help You

You know how you get lost in thought? Most of the day, as you go about your daily activities, your mind is left to think whatever it wants. You're operating on "automatic pilot" (explained more fully in Chapter 4 of Book 1). But some of your automatic thoughts may be unhelpful to you, or perhaps you're so stuck in those thoughts that you don't actually experience the world around you. For example, you go for a walk in the park to relax, but your mind is lost in thoughts about your next project. First, you're not really living in the present moment, and second, you're making yourself more stressed, anxious, or depressed if your thoughts are unhelpful.

Mindfulness isn't focused on fixing problems. Mindfulness emphasizes acceptance first, and change may or may not come later. So if you suffer from anxiety, mindfulness shows you how to accept the feeling of anxiety rather than denying or fighting the feeling, and through this approach change naturally comes about. Consider this idea: "What you resist, persists. What you accept, transforms."

This section explores the many ways in which mindfulness can help you.

WARNING

In mindfulness, acceptance means to *acknowledge* your present-moment experience, whether pleasant or unpleasant, is already here. You're discovering how to "make peace" with your present-moment experience rather than fighting it. Acceptance doesn't mean resignation or giving up. Acceptance is an active and empowering state of mind.

Allowing space to heal

When you have a physical illness, it can be a distressing time. Your condition may be painful or even life-threatening. Perhaps your illness means you're no longer able to do the simple things in life you took for granted before, such as run up the stairs or look after yourself in an independent way. Illness can shake you to your very core. How can you cope with this? How can you build your inner strength to manage the changes that take place, without being overwhelmed and losing all hope?

High levels of stress, particularly over a long period of time, have been clearly shown to reduce the strength of your immune system. Perhaps you went down with the flu after a period of high stress. The scientific evidence strongly agrees. For example, research on care-givers who experience high levels of stress for long periods of time shows that they have a weaker immune system in response to diseases like the flu.

Mindfulness reduces stress, and for this reason is one way of managing illness. By reducing your stress you improve the effectiveness of your immune system, and this may help increase the rate of healing from the illness you suffer, especially if the illness is stress-related.

REMEMBER

Mindfulness can reduce stress, anxiety, pain, and depression, and boost energy, creativity, the quality of relationships, and your overall sense of wellbeing. The more you engage in mindfulness, the better: monks who've practiced mindfulness all their lives have levels of wellbeing, measured in their brains, way above anything scientists thought was possible. Sometimes their happiness levels are so high, they think there's something wrong with their brain scanners!

Enjoying greater relaxation

Mindfulness can be a very relaxing experience. As you discover how to rest with an awareness of your breathing or the sounds around you, you may begin to feel calmer.

However, *the aim of mindfulness is not relaxation*. Relaxation is one of the welcome by-products. In clinical studies comparing the benefits of mindfulness and relaxation, there's often little beneficial effect in the relaxation exercises but significant benefits in practicing mindfulness. This shows how different they are.

Mindfulness is the development of awareness of your inner and outer experiences, whatever they are, with a sense of kindness, curiosity, and acceptance. You may experience very deep states of relaxation when practicing mindfulness, or you may not. If you don't, this certainly doesn't mean you're practicing mindfulness incorrectly.

Why are relaxation and mindfulness so different? Mindfulness is about cultivating greater awareness of what's going on within or around you. It's a state of wakefulness. Whereas relaxation is associated with falling asleep, letting go, and reducing your level of awareness. Mindfulness is about moving toward challenging experiences to help you learn from difficult thoughts, feelings, urges, and sensations. Relaxation is often about moving away from such challenges — which means you can't learn from them.

REMEMBER

When you first begin practicing mindfulness, you may not find it relaxing at all. This is totally normal and nothing to worry about. Try shortening your practices and take a break whenever you wish. Be kind to yourself and let the process of mindfulness be unforced and gentle.

Table 1-1 shows the difference between relaxation and mindfulness exercises.

TABLE 1-1

Relaxation versus Mindfulness

Exercise	Aim	Method
Mindfulness	To pay attention to your experience from moment to moment, as best you can, with kindness, curiosity, acceptance, and openness	To observe your experience and shift your attention back to its focus if you drift into thought, without self-criticism if you can
Relaxation	To make muscles relaxed and to feel calm	Various, such as tightening and letting go of muscles

Improving focus and feeling happier

To be mindful, you usually need to do one thing at a time. When walking, you just walk. When listening, you just listen. When writing, you just write. By practicing formal and informal mindfulness meditation, you're training your brain, with mindful attitudes such as kindness, curiosity, and acceptance.

So, if you're writing a report, you focus on that activity as much as you can, without overly straining yourself. Each time your mind wanders off to another thought, you notice what you were thinking about (curiosity), and then without criticizing (remember you're being kind to yourself), you guide your attention back to the writing. So, you finish your report sooner (less time spent thinking about other stuff) and the work is probably of better quality (because you gave the report your full attention). The more you can focus on what you're doing, the more you can get done. So mindfulness can help you finish your work early — yippee!

REMEMBER

You can't suddenly decide to focus on your work and then become focused. The power of attention isn't just a snap decision you make. You can train attention, just as you can train your biceps in a gym. Mindfulness is gym for the mind. However, you don't need to make a huge effort as you do when working out. When training the mind to be attentive, you need to be gentle or the mind becomes less attentive. This is why mindfulness requires kindness. If you're too harsh with yourself, your mind rebels. Be mindful with your mind, not against your mind.

Your work also becomes more enjoyable if you're mindful, and when you're enjoying something, you're more creative and focused. If you're training your mind to be curious about experience rather than bored, you can be curious about whatever you engage in.

Eventually, through experience, you begin to notice that work flows through you, rather than you doing the work. You find yourself feeding the children or making that presentation. You lose the sense of "me" doing this and become more relaxed and at ease. When this happens, the work is effortless, often of a very high quality, and thoroughly enjoyable — which sounds like a nice kind of focus, don't you think? In psychology, this is called being in a state of flow, and it is strongly associated with greater wellbeing and happiness — yay! (More on going with the flow is in Chapter 4 of Book 1.)

Developing greater wisdom

Wisdom is regarded highly in Eastern and Western traditions. Socrates and Plato considered philosophy as literally the love of wisdom (*philo-sophia*). According to Eastern traditions, wisdom is your essential nature and leads to a deep happiness for yourself and to helping others to find that happiness within themselves too.

You can access greater wisdom. Mindfulness leads to wisdom, because you learn to handle your own thoughts and emotions skillfully. Just because you have a negative thought, you don't believe the thought to be true. And when you experience tricky emotions such as sadness, anxiety, or frustration, you're able to process them using mindfulness rather than being overwhelmed by them.

With your greater emotional balance, you're able to listen deeply to others and create fulfilling, lasting relationships. With your clear mind, you're able to make better decisions. With your open heart, you can be happier and healthier.

Mindfulness leads to wisdom because of your greater level of awareness. You become aware of how you relate to yourself, others, and the world around you. With this heightened awareness, you're in a much better place to make informed choices. Rather than living automatically like a robot, you're consciously awake and you take action based on reflection and what's in the best interest of everyone, including yourself.

The Dalai Lama is an example of a wise person. He's kind and compassionate, and thinks about the welfare of others. He seeks to reduce suffering and increase happiness in humanity as a whole. He isn't egocentric, laughs a lot, and doesn't seem overwhelmed with all his duties and the significant losses he's experienced. People seem to thoroughly enjoy spending time with him. He certainly seems to live in a mindful way.

Think about who you consider to be wise people. What are their qualities? You may find them to be conscious and aware of their actions, rather than habitual and lost in their own thoughts — in other words, they're mindful!

Discovering
Mindfulness

REACHING THE OTHER SIDE

One day, a young man was going for a walk when he reached a wide river. He spent a long time wondering how he would cross such a gushing current. Just when he was about to give up his journey, he saw his teacher on the other side. The young man shouted from the bank: "Can you tell me how to get to the other side of this river?"

The teacher smiled and replied: "My friend, you *are* on the other side."

You may feel that you have to change, when actually you just have to realize that perhaps you're fine just the way you are. You're running to achieve goals so that you can be peaceful and happy, but actually you're running away from the peace and happiness. Mindfulness is an invitation to stop running and rest. You're already on the other side.

Discovering your true self

Mindfulness can lead to an interesting journey of personal discovery. The word *person* comes from the Latin word *persona*, originally meaning a character in a drama, or a mask. The word *discovery* means to discover or to uncover. So in this sense, personal discovery is about uncovering your mask.

As Shakespeare said: "All the world's a stage, and all the men and women merely players." Through mindfulness practice, you begin to see your roles, your persona or mask(s) as part of what it means to be you. You still do everything you did before: you can keep helping people or making money or whatever you like doing, but you know that this is only one way of seeing things, one dimension of your being.

You probably wear all sorts of different masks for different roles that you play. You may be a parent, daughter or son, partner, employee. Each of these roles asks you to fulfill certain obligations. You may not be aware that it's possible to put all the masks down through mindfulness practice.

REMEMBER

Mindfulness is an opportunity to just be yourself. When practicing mindfulness meditation, you sometimes have clear experiences of a sense of being. You may feel a deep, undivided sense of peace, of stillness and calm. Your physical body, which usually feels so solid, sometimes fades into the background of your awareness or may feel like it disappears altogether, and you can have a deep sense of connection and oneness with your surroundings.

Some people become very attached to these positive experiences in meditation and try hard to repeat them, as if they're "getting closer" to something. However, over time you come to realize that even these seemingly blissful experiences also come and go. Enjoy them when they come, and then let them go.

Through the practice of mindfulness, you may come to discover that you're a witness to life's experiences. Thoughts, emotions, and bodily sensations come and go in your mindfulness practice, and yet a part of you is just observing this all happening — awareness itself. This is something very simple that everyone can see and experience. In fact, being naturally yourself is so simple, you easily overlook it.

In research into the latest form of mindfulness therapy called Acceptance and Commitment Therapy (ACT), becoming aware of this sense of self that is beyond your thoughts, emotions, sensations, and urges is a key part of mindfulness. Through identifying with this "Observer Self" you become more psychologically flexible and resilient against the challenges of life.

According to Eastern philosophy, as this witness, you're perfect, whole, and complete just as you are. You may not feel as if you're perfect, because you identify with your thoughts, emotions, and body, which are changing over time. Ultimately you don't need to do anything to attain this natural state, because you are this natural state all the time — right here and right now.

For these reasons, mindfulness is not about self-improvement. At the core of your being, you're perfect just the way you are! Mindfulness exercises and meditations are just to help gently train your brain to be more focused and calm, and your heart to be warm and open. Mindfulness is not about changing you: It's about realizing that you're perfectly beautiful within, just the way you are.

Consider what Eckhart Tolle, author of *A New Earth: Create a Better Life*, says: "What a liberation to realize that the 'voice in my head' is not who I am. Who am I then? The one who sees that."

Once you spend more time being the witness of your internal experiences, you're less disturbed by the ups and downs of life. This understanding offers you a way to a happier life. It's that little bit easier to go with the flow and see life as an adventure rather than just a series of struggles.

A TASTE OF MINDFULNESS: MINDFULNESS OF SENSES

You may like to experience a little mindfulness. You could read endlessly about what a coconut tastes like, but you won't really know till you taste it yourself. The same goes for mindfulness.

The beauty of this simple mindfulness exercise is that it covers everything you need to know about mindfulness. The exercise is adapted from a technique taught at a "school of practical philosophy."

Find a comfortable posture for you. You can sit in a chair, sit on a couch, or lie down on a mat — whatever you prefer. Begin by noticing the colors entering your eyes. Notice the tones, shades, and hues. Enjoy the miracle of sight that some people don't have. Then, gently close your eyes and be aware of the sense of touch. The sensations of your body. The feeling of your body naturally and automatically breathing. Feel areas of tension and relaxation. Next, be aware of scent. Then move on to any taste in your mouth. Next, become aware of sounds. Sounds near and far. Listen to the sound itself, not so much your thoughts about the sounds. Let go of all effort when listening — allow the sounds to come to you. Finally drop into your observer self — the awareness that lights up all your senses. Rest in that background awareness, whatever that means for you. The feeling of "being." The feeling of "I am" that everyone has. Just let go of all effort to do something, and just be . . . and when you're ready, bring this mindful exercise to a close and stretch your body if you wish.

Consider these questions: What effect did that exercise have on your body and mind? What did you discover?

If you want to become more mindful, you could simply practice this exercise a few times a day. The exercise is simple but powerful and transformative when practiced regularly.

Chapter **2**

Enjoying the Benefits of Mindfulness

The enjoyment that comes from mindfulness is a bit like the enjoyment that comes from dancing. Yes, it's only the second chapter and you are already hitting the dance floor! Do you dance just because of the cardiovascular benefits or for boosting your brain by following a tricky dance routine? When you dance but are overfixated on a goal or motive, it kind of spoils it a bit, right? Dancing for the sake of dancing is far more fun. But of course, dancing for the sheer pleasure of it doesn't reduce the benefits on your mind and body of dancing — they're just the icing on the cake. Yummy!

In the same way, be mindful for the sake of being mindful. Mindfulness is about connecting with your senses, being curious, and exploring the inner workings of the human mind. If you're too concerned about reaping the benefits of mindfulness, you spoil the fun of it. The journey of mindfulness isn't to reach a certain destination: the journey *is* the destination. Keep this in mind as you read about the various benefits of mindfulness described in this chapter, and let the dance of mindfulness unfold within you. The benefits of mindfulness — relaxation, better mental and emotional health, and an improved relationship with yourself and others — are just the added bonuses along the way. Read on to discover how mindfulness can help you.

Relaxing the Body

The body and mind are almost one entity. If your mind is tense with anxious thoughts, your body automatically tenses as well. They go together, hand in hand.

Why does your body become tense when you experience high levels of stress? The reason is mechanical and wired in the human body. When you experience stress, a chain reaction starts in your body, and your whole being prepares to fight or flee the situation. This is very helpful in dangerous situations when you need to fight or run away, but not so useful when chatting to your boss. So a lot of energy surges through your body; because your body doesn't know what to do with this energy, you tense up.

REMEMBER

The aim of mindfulness isn't to make you more relaxed. Mindfulness goes far deeper than that. Mindfulness — a mindful awareness — is about becoming aware and exploring your moment-by-moment experience, in a joyful way if at all possible.

So if you're tense, mindfulness means becoming aware of that tension. Which part of your body feels tense? Does the tension have an associated shape, color, and texture? What's your reaction to the tension; what are your thoughts? Mindfulness is about bringing curiosity to your experience. Then you can begin breathing into the tense part of your body, bringing kindness and accepting your present moment experience — again, not trying to change or get rid of the tension. And that's it. Rest assured, doing this often leads to relaxation — just don't make that your aim.

Getting back in touch

As a baby, you were probably very much in touch with your body. You noticed subtle sensations, and may have enjoyed feeling different textures in the world around you. As you grew up, you learned to use your head more and your body less. You probably aren't as in touch with your body as you were as a young child. You may not notice subtle messages that the body gives you through the mind. I'm sure that some people see the body as simply a vehicle for carrying the brain from one meeting to another!

In fact, the messages between your mind and body are a two-way process. Your mind gives signals to your body, and your body gives signals to your mind. You think, "I fancy reading that mindfulness book," and your body picks it up. You feel hungry, and your body signals to your mind that it's time to eat. What about the feeling of stress? If you notice the tension in your shoulders, the twitch in your eye, or the rapid beating of your heart, again your body is sending signals to your mind.

WARNING

What if your mind is so busy with its own thoughts that it doesn't even notice the signals from your body? When this happens, you're no longer in touch with or looking after your body. Hunger and thirst, tiredness and stress — you're no longer hearing clearly your instinctual messages. This leads to a further disconnection between bodily signals and your mind, so things can get worse. Stress can spiral out of control through this lack of awareness.

Mindfulness emphasizes awareness of your body. An important mindfulness meditation is the body scan. In this meditation, you spend 10–30 minutes simply being guided to pay attention to different parts of your body, from the tips of your toes to the top of your head. Some people's reaction is, "Wow, I've never paid so much attention to my body; that was interesting!" or "I now feel I'm moving back into my body." One person even said: "That was like have a massage from the inside out!"

REMEMBER

The body scan meditation can offer a healing experience. Emotions you experienced in the past but weren't ready to feel, perhaps because you were too young, can be suppressed and trapped in the body. Sometimes, people suffer for years from a particular physical ailment, but doctors are unable to explain the cause of it. Then, through counseling or meditation, the suppressed emotion arises into consciousness, which releases the emotion. The tightness in the body or the unexplained "disease" sometimes disappears with the release of the emotion. This is another example of how interconnected mind and body really are, and of the benefits of getting back in touch with the body.

Boosting your immune system

If something's wrong with your body, normally your immune system fights it. Unfortunately, one aspect of the stress response is your immune system not working as hard. When threatened, your body puts all its resources into surviving that threat; energy required for digestion or immunity is turned off temporarily.

REMEMBER

Stress isn't necessarily bad for you. If your stress levels are too low, you're unable to perform effectively and get bored easily. However, if you're stressed for sustained periods of time at high levels, your body's natural immune system is going to stop working properly.

The latest research has found that if you have a positive attitude toward stress, seeing stress as energizing and uplifting, the stress seems to have no negative effect on your body. So even your attitude toward stress has a huge effect on your wellbeing.

Mindfulness enables you to notice subtle changes in your body. At the first sign of excessive stress, you can bring a mindful awareness to the situation and discover how to dissipate the stress rather than exacerbate it. By being mindful, you can also remember to see the positive, energizing benefits of stress rather than just its negatives. In this way, mindfulness can really benefit your immune system.

Reducing pain

Amazingly, mindfulness has been proven to actually reduce the level of pain experienced by people practicing it over a period of eight weeks. Some people couldn't find anything to help them manage and cope with their pain until they began using mindfulness meditation.

When you experience pain, you quite naturally want to block out that pain. You tighten your muscles around the region and make an effort to distract yourself. Another approach is that you want the pain to stop, so you react toward the pain in an angry way. This creates greater tension, not only in the painful region but in other areas of the body. Sometimes you may feel like fighting the pain. This creates a duality between you and your pain, and you burn energy to battle with it. Or perhaps you react with resignation: the pain has got the better of you and you feel helpless.

TIP

Mindfulness takes a radically different approach. In mindfulness, you're encouraged to pay attention to the sensation of pain, as far as you can. So, if your knee is hurting, rather than distracting yourself or reacting in any other way, you actually focus on the area of physical pain with a mindful awareness. This means you bring attitudes such as kindness, curiosity, and acknowledgment toward the area of pain, as best you can. This isn't easy at first, but you can get better with practice. You can then consider the difference between the sensation of the physical pain itself and all the other stuff you bring to the pain. You begin to understand the difference between *physical* pain and *psychological* pain. The physical pain is the actual raw sensation of pain in the body, whereas the psychological pain is the stress, anxiety, and frustration generated. Through mindfulness, you begin to let go of the psychological pain so that only the physical pain is left. When the psychological pain begins to dissolve, the muscle tension around the physical pain begins to loosen, further reducing the perception of pain. You begin to be able to accept the pain as it is in this present moment.

Calming the Mind

Your mind is like the ocean: occasionally wild, and at other times calm. Sometimes your mind goes from thought to thought without stopping to rest. At other times, your thoughts come more slowly and have more space between them.

Mindfulness isn't so much about changing the rate of your thoughts, but about noticing the thoughts arising in the first place. By taking a step back from thoughts, you can hover above the waves. The waves are still there, but you have more possibility of watching the show rather than being controlled by the thoughts themselves.

REMEMBER

Think of your mind like a good friend. If you invited your friend to your home, how do you treat her? Should you force her to drink coffee, eat three chocolate cookies, and listen to you talk about your day even if she doesn't want to? She may prefer tea and sugar cookies, and want to talk about her day too. You *ask* her what she'd like, in a kind and friendly manner. In the same way, treat your mind like a friend. Invite your mind to pay attention to your breath or the work you're doing. When you notice that your mind is restless, acknowledge this. Smile and gently ask your mind to re-focus. The gentle approach is the only way. If you currently treat your mind like your enemy, this shift in attitude could make a significant difference.

Listening to your thoughts

Everything man-made around you was originally a thought in someone's head. Many people consider thought to be all-powerful. All your words, all your actions and activities — everything is motivated by thought. So, being aware of the kind of thoughts going through your mind makes sense.

Have you ever noticed how you have the same sort of thoughts going around and around in your head? The brain easily gets into habitual patterns as your thoughts travel their paths within your brain. *Neurons that fire together, wire together.* Each time you have a particular thought or carry out a particular action, you slightly increase the chance of having the same thought again. Through repeated thinking or action, the connection between neurons strengthens. If you aren't mindful of these thoughts or actions, you may have all sorts of negative, untrue, unhelpful thoughts or behaviors that influence your life without you even being aware of them or questioning the truth or validity of them.

For example, say that a client gives you negative feedback for some work you did. The thought "I'm not good enough for this job" or "That person is so stupid" may keep going around and around your head. You feel rough, your sleep is impacted, and you can't properly focus on today's tasks. That's not a great help. But fret not: mindfulness to the rescue!

Mindfulness encourages you to watch your thoughts, emotions, and actions; then you're better able to notice unhelpful thoughts and question their truth. Additionally, just being mindful of thoughts and emotions with a sense of warmth seems to naturally dissipate them. They become far less of a problem.

Making better decisions

Every moment of every day you make decisions, whether you're aware of them or not. You made a decision to read this chapter. At some point, you'll decide to stop and do something else. Even if you decide to make no decisions, that's a decision too! More significant decisions you have to make have a bigger impact, and a "good" decision is highly desirable. All you do and have at the moment is mostly due to the decisions you made in the past.

REMEMBER

Awareness of your body can help you make better decisions: A gut feeling, sometimes called *intuition*, is a signal from your belly telling you what to do, and has been found in some experiments to be faster and more accurate than logical thinking, especially for more complex decisions involving lots of factors. Research shows that there's a mass of nerves in the gut, and some euphemistically call it the gut brain. Tapping into intuition is routinely used by top entrepreneurs and CEOs of corporations to make critical decisions with great success. Other research has found people who tend to be luckier often practice mindfulness and use their intuition to make decisions about work, home, or their relationships. So be more mindful and make luckier choices in your life.

Why is gut feeling so effective? Your unconscious mind has far more information than your conscious mind can handle. Making decisions just based on conscious logical thought misses out on the huge capacity of the unconscious brain. Mindfulness helps to deepen your level of awareness and helps you to begin to tap into your intuitive side.

Coming to your senses

One of the key ways of becoming more mindful and of calming the mind is to connect with your senses: sight, sound, touch, smell, and taste. Consider the expressions, "That was *sens*ible," "I *sense* something's wrong," and "She's come to her *senses*." People's use of the word "sense" shows we appreciate and value being in touch with our organs of perception. You know innately the value of connecting to your senses if you want to make a *sens*ible decision.

What's the benefit of purposefully connecting with your senses? Well, if you aren't paying attention to the stimulation coming through your five senses, you're only paying attention to your thoughts and emotions. You're not aware of anything else. Your thoughts are mainly based on your experiences from the past — from memory. You may imagine something new, but on the whole your mind reworks past experiences or projects ideas into the future based on your past experiences. Emotions are also influenced by your thoughts. So, without paying attention to your senses, you're stuck with your own thoughts and emotions based on the past instead of the present.

By purposefully connecting with one of your senses — say, touch — you begin naturally to calm your mind a little. In mindfulness you can begin by focusing on your breathing. Focus on your belly stretching or your chest expanding, or perhaps the movement of the air as it enters and leaves your body. By focusing on a particular sense — in this case the sense of touch — you're focusing your attention. Rather than your mind wandering wherever it pleases, you're gently training it to stay on one object, namely your breathing. And in the same way as you train a puppy to walk along a path and not keep running off, each time your attention strays, you bring it back, just as you would gently pull the puppy back to the path. You're discovering how to be gentle with yourself, as well as finding out how to focus your attention.

By coming to your senses mindfully, you are doing the following:

>> Training your attention to focus

>> Being kind to yourself when your mind wanders off

>> Realizing that you have a certain amount of choice about what you pay attention to

>> Understanding that you can deliberately choose to shift attention away from thinking and into the senses

>> Calming your mind and developing a sense of clarity

Creating an attentive mind

Attention is essential in achieving anything. If you can't pay attention, you can't get the job done, whatever the job is. Mindfulness trains your attention by sustaining your attention on one thing, or by switching the type of attention from time to time.

Daniel Goleman, author of the book *Emotional Intelligence: Why It Can Matter More Than IQ*, published a book called *Focus: The Hidden Driver of Excellence*. He explains just how important focus is in every domain of our lives. He also identified a research study that imaged the brains of people practicing mindfulness of breath. Researchers found four different stages while the brain went through the following mental workout:

1. **Focus on your breathing.** The part of the brain that deals with focus is activated.

2. **Notice that your brain is on a train of thought.** The part of the brain that notices that your attention has drifted off into a train of thought is activated.

3. **Let go of that train of thought.** The part of the brain that enables you to let go of your thoughts is activated.

4. **Refocus on your breathing.** The part of the brain used to re-focus on the object you wish to focus on is re-activated.

The parts of the brain dedicated to each of these processes were strengthened through repeated mindfulness practice. If you do this exercise regularly, you become more adept at focusing on whatever you need to pay attention to — whether it's writing an email, listening to a loved one, or watching a sunset.

Your attention can be focused in different ways (shown in Figure 2-1):

>> Narrow attention is focused and sharp, like the beam of a laser. You may use this type of attention when chopping vegetables or writing a letter.

>> Wide attention is more open and spacious, like a floodlight. When you're driving, ideally your attention is open so you notice if a car moves closer to you from the side, or if children are playing farther ahead.

>> Outer attention is attention to the outer world through your senses.

>> Inner attention is an awareness of your thoughts and feelings.

>> Observer or witness awareness is your capacity to know what type of attention you're using. For example, if you're drawing a picture, you're aware that your attention is narrow. If you're walking through the countryside, you're aware that your attention is wide. For more on witness awareness, see the later section "Knowing Thyself: Discovering Your Observer Self."

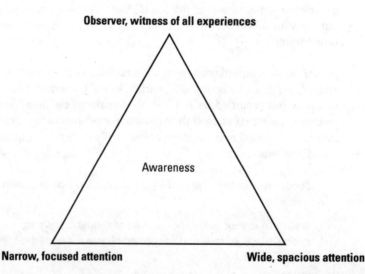

FIGURE 2-1: The different types of attention.

© John Wiley & Sons, Inc.

REMEMBER

Mindfulness is about cultivating a *flexible* attention — not just a focused attention on one thing. So try to practice different mindful exercises so that you're training your mind to be able to both focus narrowly, widely and move attention from one place to another at will.

All the different mindfulness exercises you read about in Book 1 train your mind to be able to sustain attention in the various different ways mentioned in the preceding list.

Soothing Your Emotions

Emotions are tremendously influential on your behavior and thoughts. If you're feeling low, you're probably far more reluctant to go out with friends, or laugh at a joke, or work with zest. If you're feeling great, you're on top of things; everything feels easy, and life flows easily.

How do you deal with emotions? Are you swept up by them, and do you just hope for the best? Mindfulness offers the opportunity to soothe yourself and step back from emotional ups and downs.

Understanding your emotions

What's an emotion, a feeling, or mood?

You experience emotion partly from a survival point of view. If you don't feel scared when faced with a raging bull, you'll find yourself in lots of trouble. Other emotions, such as happiness, help to create social ties with those around you, increasing your security. Even depression is thought to have evolved for your protection, reducing motivation and therefore the chance of experiencing harm or wasting energy through pursuing an unattainable goal.

REMEMBER

Emotion comes from a Latin word meaning "to move out." If you observe emotions, you can discover certain important characteristics:

>> Emotions are always changing. You aren't stuck with one emotion all your life, at the same intensity.

>> Emotions are a very physical experience. If you're feeling anxious, you may feel a tingling in your stomach. If you're feeling angry, you may feel your breathing and heart rate go up.

>> You can observe your own emotions. You can sense the difference between yourself and your emotions. You're not your emotions; you're the observer of your emotions.

>> Emotions make a huge impact on your thoughts. When you're feeling down, you're likely to predict negative things about yourself or other people. When you're feeling happy, you're more likely to think positive thoughts, predict positive outcomes, and look upon the past in a positive light too.

>> You tend to perceive emotions as pleasant, unpleasant, or neutral.

Managing feelings differently

Take a few minutes to consider the following emotions and how you deal with them:

>> Anger

>> Anxiety

>> Fear

>> Depression

Your approach may be to either avoid the emotion and pretend it isn't there, or to express your feelings to whoever is nearby. Mindfulness offers an alternative — a way of meeting emotions that enables you to see them in a different light. The idea is to acknowledge and give mindful attention to difficult feelings, rather than avoid or react to them. Surprisingly, this tends to dissipate the strength and the pain of the emotion.

Uplifting Your Spirit

You may wish to practice mindfulness just for your body or mind — and that's totally fine. But you may be interested in how mindfulness offers a greater sense of purpose in your life, or how it relates to spirituality, whatever that means to you. If that sounds worthwhile, this section is for you.

Everyone defines spirituality differently. For some people, to be spiritual means to value a deeper sense of connection between yourself and something bigger. And that could be your connection with nature, your love for your friends or family, the Universe, or even your love for God, if that's your belief.

Mindfulness offers you a way to deepen your connection with yourself and whatever is most meaningful for you — a connection that comes from both your head and heart. And having a deeper sense of meaning is really important — vital, in fact.

Victor Frankl, in his incredibly moving book *Man's Search for Meaning*, showed how having a deeper sense of meaning helped him survive the hellish conditions of a concentration camp. He was a psychotherapist and observed that others in the concentration camp also survived if they had something deeper worth living for, whether that was a loved one or belief in something greater than themselves. He ended up creating a whole new therapy based on helping people find greater meaning in their lives.

TIP

Take a few moments to reflect or write down what's most important for you. Is it your friends, family, or a loved one? Do you love nature and yearn to spend time with her? Do you have certain values that are most meaningful for you? Perhaps you believe in a God? Or maybe you're a fan of the *Star Wars* movies and want to be one with "The Force." (Sorry, no lightsabers are included with this book!)

Whatever you find most meaningful in your life, once you start practicing mindfulness, your connection may deepen. And as your sense of meaning and connection grows, you're likely to have a greater resilience and stability from the challenges that life throws at you.

Knowing Thyself: Discovering Your Observer Self

Mindfulness helps you to see things from a more holistic perspective. Having a sense of a deeper dimension and connection with the world around you puts the waves of life's challenges into a much bigger context. If you feel interconnected with other people, nature, or even the Universe, you're part of something bigger. If you're the ocean, what trouble do waves give you?

This journey begins with a deeper connection with yourself. Inscribed above the ancient Greek temple of Apollo at Delphi is the phrase "Know thyself," a vitally important concept for Greek philosophers such as Socrates. But self-reflection isn't advocated so much in the 21st century!

Who are you? What is this incredible thing called life? Mindfulness helps you to put things in perspective. If you go from place to place, rushing to finish all that stuff on your to-do list, and when you're done are so exhausted that you just collapse in front of the television, you may have a bit of a problem discovering who you truly are in the meantime. By taking some time to be mindful, you're giving yourself the opportunity to stop and look at all these incessant thoughts and emotions that come and go, and discover the sense of being that's behind the mind chatter. A part of yourself that's peaceful, joyous, and whole.

This book describes one approach to discovering your sense of self that you may find immensely liberating and fascinating. Self-discovery is a personal journey, so you may have a totally different way of understanding your deep, inner being.

TIP

Here's one interesting way to explore your sense of self and awareness: Read each of these paragraphs as slowly as you can. Notice your judgments and desire to agree or disagree with the statements. Try doing neither, and instead just read and reflect.

>> **Are you just your body?** Your body is made up of hundreds of millions of cells. Cells are dying and re-forming all the time. Every few years, pretty much all the cells in your body are replaced with new ones — so your body is completely different to the one you had as a baby. Right now, you're digesting food, your nails and hair are growing, and your immune system is fighting any diseases within you. It's all just happening — you're not doing it. Even if your body becomes totally paralyzed, the sense of you being here will still be present. The very fact that you say "my body" suggests that the body is something you *have*, rather than your core self.

>> **Are you just your thoughts?** Thoughts keep coming, no matter how mindful you are. The fact that you can be aware of your thoughts means that you are separate from them. If you were your thoughts, you wouldn't be able to notice them. The fact that you can observe your thoughts means they're separate and a space lies between you and what you think. In mindfulness practice, you can step back from your thoughts from time to time, but you can't control thoughts. Do you even know what you're going to think in the next few minutes? No. But can you be *aware* of your thoughts? Yes.

>> **Are you just your emotions?** Just as you can observe thoughts, you can also observe your emotions. Doesn't this mean you're separate from your emotions? Emotions arise and eventually pass away. If you were your emotions, then your emotions would never pose any problem at all. You would be able to control emotions and wouldn't choose to have negative feelings.

REMEMBER

So what are you? What's left? You can call it the observer self. There's no specific word in the English language for this. If you're the observer, you can't be that which you observe. In this sense you can say *you are awareness*. Thoughts and ideas, emotions and images, desires, fears, and actions arise *in you* but you're aware of them all. Everything arises *in awareness*, in being. That's what you are. You aren't just the thought "I'm John" or "I'm Jane"; you're that sense of presence that underlies experience.

These are some of the attributes of awareness or the observer self:

>> **You're always aware.** Sometimes that awareness is lost in thoughts and dreams; sometimes it's connected with the senses.

>> **Awareness happens by itself.** Awareness is different from attention. Attention or *mindful* awareness is something to be cultivated and trained, but *pure* awareness is your inner self. To be aware takes no effort. You don't need to *do* awareness. Awareness is effortlessly operating right now as you read. You can't turn off or run away from awareness!

>> **Awareness comes before thought.** As a baby, you had awareness without words and ideas. Thoughts and concepts come after awareness.

>> **In terms of awareness, you're both 'no-thing' and everything.** Without awareness, nothing would exist for you. With awareness, you're a part of every experience you have. This sounds contradictory, but look into these concepts yourself. Ask yourself what your daily experience would be like without awareness.

Having read all these attributes of awareness, what's your reaction? Whether you believe these ideas or not isn't important; what *is* important is examining and exploring these ideas for yourself. As Socrates said, "The unexamined life is not worth living." You may find looking deeper into your identity to be completely transformative and liberating!

TIP

Spend a few minutes resting as an observer of your moment-to-moment experience. This can turn out to be an incredibly peaceful experience. That's a meditation in itself. No need to react to your thoughts, emotions, or any other sensations. Just watch the experiences arise and fall again. Be the observer self. And if you find yourself trying too hard, don't forget to smile! That reminds you that this is a non-doing process — not just another thing that requires a lot of effort.

Chapter **3**

Making Mindfulness a Daily Habit

One of the best ways of boosting your capacity to be mindful is to practice mindfulness every day. Establishing a daily habit of mindfulness isn't always easy, but it's well worth the effort. With a clear understanding of how behavior change works, you can engage in practicing mindfulness regularly. Once the habit of daily mindfulness is created, the routine becomes as natural as having a shower — you now have a way of training and "cleansing" your mind every day, not just your body.

This chapter explores how best to change your behavior effectively, discover the science of habits, and find out what your intentions of mindfulness are.

Discovering the Secret to Change

Every year millions of people make new year resolutions. "I will go to the gym several times a week." "I'll stop eating chocolate cake." And you'll even hear "I'll practice mindfulness every day this year." And yet within just a couple of weeks, most people fail to stick to their resolutions and give up. Have you had that experience too?

New year resolutions are attempts to change behavior. You may not have been successful because you haven't learned *how* to change your behavior. Behavior change is actually a skill — not an innate talent. The good news is you can learn how to change. And with that skill, you can make lots of positive changes in your life, including daily mindfulness!

Although most people consider changing their daily habits to be hard, it's actually not as difficult as you think — once you know how. Learning to change your behavior is like learning to swim — it looks really difficult at first, but it's easy once you know how! And then it gets really exciting to put your new skills to work.

In this section, you're going to learn how to change your behavior so that you're able to make time to practice mindfulness in some form or another every day — however you choose.

Designing your life for mindfulness

As you've picked up this book, you're probably curious about the power of mindfulness and you wish to apply it in your daily life.

REMEMBER

If you dive in without a well-designed plan, you're unlikely to succeed in practicing mindfulness long term. Why? Because you're relying on your motivation. And your motivation doesn't stay high all the time: It goes up and down as shown in Figure 3-1.

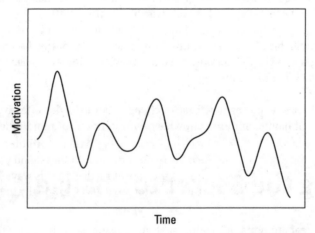

FIGURE 3-1:
The ups and downs of motivation.

© *John Wiley & Sons, Inc.*

For example, after reading some chapters of this book, you may feel highly motivated to practice mindfulness every day. You may say to yourself, "This is brilliant stuff. I'm going to do some mindfulness meditation for half an hour every day. This is going to be my new habit. I can do this!"

This is an example of what most people do. They use determination and sheer will-power to try to drive change into their life. The first few days go fine: You remember to do your mindful meditation and are pleased with yourself. Then a few days in and you wake up with a headache. No way do you feel like practicing mindfulness. That's out of the question! You're not motivated to be mindful. You'd rather stay in bed and sleep. The next day you wake up late. Motivation is still down. Then the next day you forget. A few days pass and you realize you haven't practiced mindfulness, so you give up.

How do you think you'd feel? Probably not that great. Perhaps you may even think of yourself as a failure — someone who can't stick to new habits. Next time you realize you need to create a new habit, you'll be less likely to have a go because you don't want to fail again and think of yourself as a failure.

Most people, at this point, blame themselves. You may think, "If only I tried harder" or "If only I was more disciplined."

Blaming yourself doesn't help you; nor does just giving up. So what's the solution?

Starting small: The secret to creating new habits

As motivation goes up and down in humans, rather than starting habits with a big commitment and requiring lots of willpower, why not start small — *really small*? What if you just began with a mindfulness practice that takes less than 30 seconds?

TIP

If you start small, you don't need lots of motivation to stick to the new habit. Even if you wake up with a headache, or oversleep or whatever other excuse you may have, you always have 30 seconds to do some mindfulness. And you get that sense of success each time you manage the short practice. In this way, you have a much better chance of success. After a week or so, you can gradually increase the length of time you practice mindfulness.

Over time, you don't need to worry about motivation because your mindfulness practice becomes a habit. Once an action becomes a habit in your daily life, high levels of motivation are no longer necessary. The new activity becomes almost automatic — such as brushing your teeth or having a shower. You've cleverly side-stepped the need for motivation.

Mindfulness is about living more consciously, not automatically. So making mindfulness into an automatic habit may sound counterintuitive. But actually, the opposite is true. If you don't put mindfulness practice as part of your routine, you're much less likely to remember to be mindful, and your whole day could pass by automatically. So make the practice of mindfulness a daily habit and look forward to a more mindful life!

To create a new habit, in this case the habit of practicing mindfulness every day, use these three steps:

1. Decide what your daily mindfulness practice will be, which shouldn't take more than 30 seconds.

2. Find a suitable spot in your daily schedule to do your short mindfulness practice.

3. Celebrate your success!

The following subsections go through each of these important steps in turn.

Deciding on your daily mindfulness practice

You can do any mindfulness practice you wish. To help you decide, here are a few options:

>> Mindfulness of breath

>> Mindfully feeling your feet on the floor

>> Drinking a cup of tea or coffee mindfully

>> Mindfully stretching

>> Reflecting on three things you're grateful for

These are just some suggestions. You can pick one of these practices, or if you have some other practice that you'd like to try, go for it!

A short mindfulness practice every day is recommended, rather than once every few days or once a week, because that way it's much easier to make it a habit. Habits generally don't form if they are practiced every few days, and short daily practice is far more powerful than long practices done haphazardly.

Don't think about it too much. Just pick one, have a go, and see what happens. You're experimenting. If it works, great. If not, no problem at all. That's feedback. Try a different one. If you have the attitude of an experimenter trying new things, you won't fear failure so much. You'll see that as part and parcel of your process of learning something new about yourself. Keep the following in mind:

>> Pick something you *want* to do, not something you feel you *have* to do.

>> Keep the mindfulness practice to approximately 30 seconds. This is the hard bit as you may feel that's not enough and want to do more. We humans are over-ambitious at the beginning and then end up giving up. Slow and steady wins the race. Just stick to roughly 30 seconds for now. There's a reason for it. And it doesn't matter if it's a bit more or less. You don't need to use a timer.

Choosing a suitable spot for your daily mindfulness practice

Okay, you've hopefully chosen a *short* mindfulness practice you *want* to experiment with trying every single day. The next step is to find a suitable spot for your mindfulness practice to grow.

Why do you need a suitable spot rather than just randomly practicing whenever you have time? To understand why, you need to learn how habits work. To form a habit, you need to start with a cue — a trigger to tell your brain to carry out the habit.

For example, if you see some chocolate, that can be a cue for you to grab the chocolate bar. An alarm clock going off can be a cue for you to get out of bed (or hit the snooze button). Feelings can also be cues. Feeling tired can be a cue for you to go to bed, or perhaps reach for another cup of coffee. Your life is filled with cues for your habits, so look out for them.

THE POWER OF SMALL STEPS — LITERALLY!

This an amazing experiment has been repeated from the United States to Ireland. Researchers pick two random groups of people in an office who don't exercise regularly. With one group, they give them gift vouchers to buy gym shoes and clothes and offer them free access to a gym for six months. They get everything they need to get started at the gym. With the other group, they just say "On Monday, walk up one flight of stairs. On Tuesday, do the same but add just one extra step. On Wednesday, one more step again. In the same way, keep adding an extra step every single day."

Which group do you think were fitter, happier, and had healthier blood pressure three years later? The walking group.

This experiment shows you the power of taking small steps — literally! Big change happens through taking small, consistent steps every day.

In the same way, if you wish to create the habit of mindfulness every day, you need a reliable cue. The ideal cue for a new daily habit would be a part of your routine that you already have. You sit up in your bed every day. Sitting up in your bed can be your cue to do your mindfulness practice. Or if you start your day with a shower in the morning, you can do your mindfulness practice after getting dressed.

Giving yourself a reward for practicing mindfulness

REMEMBER

To complete your habit loop, you need to have a reward. Without a reward, you don't create a habit. The reward tells your brain that you had a pleasant experience that's worth having again. So here are the three steps required for a habit to form:

1. **Cue:** A prompt to remind you to practice mindfulness. For example, your alarm clock in the morning or when you sit on your bed after getting dressed.

2. **Action:** The practice of mindfulness itself. For example, feeling 10 mindful breaths or mindful listening to the sounds in your surroundings.

3. **Reward:** A positive experience. For example, the feeling of being grounded or saying something positive in your mind.

You can remember the acronym CAR to remind you of these three steps in habit formation shown in Figure 3-2.

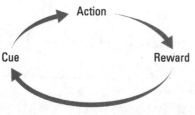

FIGURE 3-2:
To create a habit you need a cue, the action, and a sense of reward.

© John Wiley & Sons, Inc.

Going back to the example of chocolate, the reward is obviously the delicious taste. The reward for, say, checking your mobile phone is a sense of satisfaction that someone has contacted you.

So what's the reward for practicing mindfulness? There are three ways of rewarding yourself, to increase your chance of the mindfulness action becoming a regular habit:

>> Enjoy your practice of mindfulness if you can.

>> Smile during and at the end of your mindfulness practice.

>> Celebrate at the end of your mindfulness practice by saying something positive, fun, or uplifting to yourself such as "Yes!" or "Yippee!" or "Go me!" or even "Yes, I managed to practice 30 seconds of mindfulness yet again. I'm doing so well!"

The more you're able to celebrate your success at completing the short new mindfulness exercise, the higher the likelihood that you'll practice again, resulting in the activity turning into a habit and becoming part of your new daily routine.

Being playful with your new habit

Your new habit will probably not take root straight away. And that's okay! In fact, that's normal. The idea is to experiment with trying to be mindful in different spots to find the right place for you.

For example, you may try a mindful exercise straight after your alarm goes off, but you're too sleepy. So then you may try after coming home from work, but find you're distracted by your kids. Then you experiment with a mindful meditation after getting dressed in the morning, and that's perfect. You feel refreshed and love being mindful then.

Of course, your mindfulness habit doesn't have to be meditation. It could be an everyday mindful practice such as mindful tea drinking, or taking ten mindful breaths as you smile, or noticing five new things you can see, hear, smell, taste, or touch. Experiment with any activity that unlocks you from your automatic thoughts and brings you into the moment.

Watering the seeds of your mindful habits

How do you grow your mindfulness habit? The secret is not to rush to grow it.

Consider a story of a little child who planted a seed. Every day the child watered the seed and watched the soil intensely, waiting for a shoot to come out. After two days, the child decided to dig out the seed to see how it was doing. Of course, the child damaged the tiny seedling that was growing. If the child was a bit more patient, they would have been rewarded with a beautiful new plant.

In the same way, once you find your spot to do your daily mindfulness practice, stick with it for a bit. No need to lengthen the practice. Just stick with the 30 seconds or so until it becomes a habitual part of your day.

After a week or so, increase the length of the habit gradually — maybe 45 seconds or one minute. Keep practicing consistently and increase the length of the habit in such a way that it seems almost too easy. If you do this, you'll find forming your new habit happens with almost no effort. After a month or two, you may find yourself up to 10 minutes or more of daily practice, if that's your aim. You decide what's right for your lifestyle.

Scattering seeds of mindfulness throughout the day

After you have played around with your first habit of mindfulness, perhaps a short mindfulness meditation, you can use cues throughout the day to remind you to practice mindfulness. Here are some ideas for cues that you can use throughout the day:

>> The sound of a phone ringing or a text message

>> Sitting down on some form of public transport

>> Stepping outside in the morning

>> The sound of your doorbell

>> Opening your journal

These are all examples of cues you can use to do short mindfulness practices:

>> Taking a few deep, conscious breaths

>> Holding a gentle smile on your face

>> Checking in with how your body or mind feels

>> Noticing what thoughts are arising in your head and imagining placing them on clouds in the sky of awareness

>> Asking yourself: "How can I best take care of myself right now?"

Each time you practice mindfulness, you increase the chance of being mindful again on another day because any new activity you take on, whether physical or mental, creates a new pathway in the brain. It's a bit like creating a new pathway through a forest. At first, walking through all the overgrowth is a bit difficult. You need to push the overhanging branches out of the way and tread on the long grass under your feet. However, if you keep walking on that path, it becomes easier and easier. Soon enough, you don't need to work hard any more or think about which way to go next. The path is clear. It's the same with pathways in the brain. In fact, that's what a new activity creates in the brain: a pathway to greater mindfulness, awareness and "aliveness."

Exploring Your Intentions

The word *intention* comes from the Latin *intendere*, meaning to direct attention. Intention is purpose — what you hope to achieve from a certain action. If you're driving to work and your intention is to get there on time no matter what happens, you may drive recklessly and dangerously. If you're driving to work and your intention is to get there safely, you try to drive with a more focused attention, and at a safe and reasonable speed. Here's a more startling example. Imagine someone cutting you with a knife — such as a surgeon who has to insert a blade and cut you open. Because the intention of the surgeon is to help restore your health, you're probably willing to undergo this seemingly horrendous procedure. However, a murderer may also use a blade, but with a far less positive intention and you're unlikely to be so willing!

Intention shapes the nature of the whole action itself. Although the action may be the same (as with the example of cutting someone open), the intention itself strongly influences your moment-by-moment experience and state of mind. For this reason, the right intention is vitally important in mindfulness meditation. You may even say that the nature of the intention itself strongly influences the quality of your mindful practice.

Clarifying intention in mindfulness

REMEMBER

Dr. Shauna Shapiro of Santa Clara University, together with several colleagues, came up with a helpful model to suggest how mindfulness works. The researchers identified three key components: *intention*, *attention*, and *attitude*. The components are required together and feed into each other when you engage in mindfulness. The components link in well with the often-used definition of mindfulness, which is *paying attention in a particular way: on purpose, in the present moment, and non-judgmentally*. It's time to break down this definition:

>> Paying attention — *attention*

>> On purpose — *intention*

>> In a particular way — *attitude*

These three components work together seamlessly to create the moment-to-moment experience that is mindfulness. Figure 3-3 shows the components of mindfulness working together.

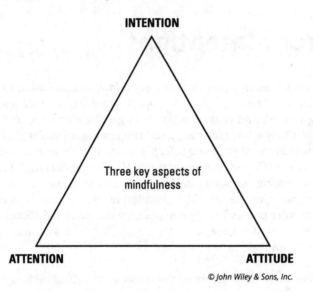

INTENTION

Three key aspects of
mindfulness

ATTENTION   **ATTITUDE**

© John Wiley & Sons, Inc.

FIGURE 3-3:
The three
components of
mindfulness.

Intention is a component that often gets lost when people consider mindfulness, and yet it's vitally important. Intention sets the scene for what unfolds in the practice itself.

Intention evolves. One study has shown that people's intention in mindfulness is usually stress reduction, and moves on to greater understanding of their thoughts and emotions, and finally toward greater compassion. For example, you may begin practicing mindfulness to reduce your anxiety and when that subsides, you practice to attain greater control over your emotions and eventually to be a more compassionate and kind person to your family and friends. What's *your* intention?

REMEMBER

Mindfulness is being developed to relieve the suffering caused by a whole host of different conditions, from eating disorders to anxiety in pregnancy, from reducing students' stress to speeding up the healing process for psoriasis. These are all a wonderful flowering of applications of mindfulness, but keep in mind the original purpose and vision of mindfulness as a way of relieving *all* suffering, both yours and others', and developing a greater sense of compassion. Such a large and positive vision enlarges the practice of mindfulness for those who share those possibilities.

Finding what you're looking for

The following exercise — a "mindful visualization" — can give you great insight into your true and deep intentions in practicing mindfulness. Afterwards, do the writing exercise described in the next section.

Discovering your intention: Mindful visualization

TIP

Find a comfortable position: seated in a chair or sofa, or lying down. Choose a position in which you feel cozy and comfortable. Close your eyes.

> Imagine that you're sitting by the side of a beautiful lake. The place can be somewhere you've been before or seen before, or may be completely created in your imagination — it doesn't matter which. Find a place where you feel calm and relaxed. The lake may have majestic trees around one side and stunning mountains in the distance. The temperature is just about perfect for you, and a gentle breeze ensures that you feel refreshed. A flock of birds are flying across the horizon, and you can sense a freshness in the air. Your body feels relaxed and at ease.
>
> You look down and notice a pebble. You pick it up and look at it. It has a question engraved on it. The question is: "What do I hope to get from mindfulness?" You look carefully at the question as you hold the pebble gently in your hand.
>
> You throw the pebble into the lake. You watch the pebble as it soars through the air in an arc, almost in slow motion, and eventually makes contact with the surface of the water. You see the circular ripples radiate out. As the pebble contacts with the water, you continue to reflect on the question: "What do I hope to get from mindfulness?"
>
> The pebble moves down into the water. You're able to see the pebble as it sinks deeper and deeper into the water. As it continues to smoothly fall downwards in the deep water, you continue to watch it, and you continue to reflect on the question: "What do I hope to get from mindfulness?" You keep watching as the pebble falls, and you keep reflecting on the question.
>
> Eventually, the pebble softly makes contact with the bottom and settles there. The question "What do I hope to get from mindfulness?" is still visible. Reflect on that question for a few more moments.

Bring the exercise to a close, noticing the physical sensations of your body, taking a slightly deeper breath and, when you're ready, slowly opening your eyes. If you keep a journal, record what you discovered in it. This may help to reveal further insights as you write.

No right or wrong answers exist for this "intention" meditation. Some people get clear answers about what they hope to get out of practicing mindfulness, and others reflect on the question, yet no answers arise. Some people find that the answers they get at the surface of the lake are the more obvious ones but, as the pebble falls deeper, their reasons to practice clarify and deepen too. If the exercise was helpful, great; if not, don't be concerned — there are other exercises to do later in this chapter.

Discovering your intention: Sentence completion

TIP

Take a piece of paper or your journal, and write as many answers as you can to the following questions in one minute, without thinking about them too much:

I want to practice mindfulness because . . .

I'm hoping mindfulness will give me . . .

If I'm more mindful I'll . . .

The real reasons I want to practice mindfulness are to . . .

Ultimately mindfulness will give me . . .

Mindfulness is . . .

These sentence-completion exercises may help to clarify your motivation and intentions for mindfulness.

Now read and reflect on your answers. Did any of your answers surprise you? Why is that? You may like to come back to these answers when you're struggling to motivate yourself to be mindful; reading your answers then can be a way of empowering yourself to practice some mindfulness.

Developing a vision

A *vision* is a long-term aspiration: something you're willing to work toward. By having a clear vision, you have an idea of where you need to get to. Think of it in terms of any journey you make, for which you need to know two things: where you are now, and where you need to get to.

Mindfulness is about being in the present moment and letting go of goals. Why think about visions and intentions? Why not just be in the here and now and for-get about aspirations? Well, the vision gives you the energy, the motivation, and the strength to practice mindfulness, especially when you really don't feel like practicing.

For example, your mind may be jam-packed with thoughts, ideas, and opinions to such an extent that you can't easily calm down. Your vision may be to be a calm and collected person, someone who never really worries about things too much, and who others come to for advice. With this in mind, you know why you're practicing mindfulness and *are committed* to sticking at it. This doesn't mean that the goal of each and every mindful meditation is calmness, and that if you're not calm you've failed; a vision is bigger than that — a long-term objective rather than a short-term goal.

TIP

If you're not too sure what your vision is, come back to this section after doing some mindfulness exercises. Doing this may give you a clearer idea of a vision to work toward. The practice of mindfulness itself helps to develop an unambiguous vision as you begin to experience some benefits.

Try the following two exercises to help clarify your vision.

Writing a letter to your future self

This is a wonderful way to develop a long-term vision of what you hope to achieve through mindfulness.

TIP

Reflect on your future self in five or ten years. This is your chance to let go and dream. How will you feel? What sort of person do you hope to be? How do you cope with challenges in your life? Write a letter to yourself about it, or if you're a visual person, draw pictures. This vision gives your brain something to work toward, and the opportunity to begin discovering a path for you to tread to get there.

Pin the letter up on the wall at home, or ask a good friend to post the letter back to you any time in the next year. Most people feel great receiving a letter from themselves dropped in the mail, and the self-reflection always seems to arrive at the right time in your life.

TIP

You can even send an email to yourself from your future self. The website www. futureme.org allows you to do this for free.

Attending your own funeral

Try to overcome any reluctance about this exercise, because it's very moving and powerful. Imagine being at your own funeral service. You're aware of family and friends around you. Consider each person and imagine everyone saying what you'd *like* them to say about you. Really hear the positive things they're saying about you and your life. What do they value about you? What sort of aspects of your personality would you like them to talk about? What have they admired about you? After the exercise, think about it. How did you feel? What did people say about you?

The exercise helps to put things into context and clarifies your values — what's really important to you. How can you use what was said to create a vision of the kind of person you want to become? How can that vision help motivate your mindfulness practice?

TIP

Ask yourself the following question every day for a couple of weeks: "If today were the last day of my life, would I want to do what I'm about to do today?" Whenever the answer is no for too many days in a row, you know that you need to change something. Even if you don't explicitly ask this question, you get a flavor of the value of considering death to help you wake up and focus on what's most important in life.

Chapter **4**

Humans Being Versus Humans Doing

Human beings love doing stuff. You go to work, have hobbies, socialize, and become an adept multi-tasker trying to fit everything into the day. But what about the *being* in human being?

Every day, in everything you do, your mind switches between *doing* mode and *being* mode. This doesn't mean that you switch between, say, typing an email and staring into space. Instead, it means *being* in the moment as you're *doing* a task. One mode of mind isn't better than the other. They're both helpful in different ways. However, using the wrong mode of mind for a particular situation can cause difficulties.

This chapter explains how spending some of your time just *being* has huge and far-reaching advantages. You also find out how to "just be it."

Delving into the Doing Mode of Mind

You know the feeling. You've got to get the kids ready, drop them off at school, pay the gas bill, pop that letter in the mail, renew the car insurance, and make sure that you call your sister to see if she's feeling better. You're exhausted just thinking about everything! But you know you have to do it all. Your mind is in *doing* mode.

Doing mode is a highly developed quality in humans. You can think and conceptualize how you want things to be, and then work methodically to achieve them. That's part of the reason why people have been able to design computers and land on the moon — the products of doing mode.

Doing mode is certainly not a bad thing. If you want to get the shopping done, you need some doing mode! However, sometimes doing mode goes too far, and you start doing more and more without taking a break. That can certainly be draining.

Here are the hallmarks of the doing mode of mind:

>> **You're aware of how things *are*, and how they *should* be.** For example, if you need to renew your home insurance, you're aware that you currently haven't renewed the insurance, and that you need to at some point soon.

>> **You set a goal to fix things.** If you're in doing mode, you're setting goals for the way things should be. This problem-solving happens all the time without you being conscious of it. In the home insurance example, your goal may be to call several insurance companies or visit several websites to find the right deal for you.

>> **You try harder and harder to achieve your goal.** In doing mode, you feel driven. You know what you want and you try hard to get it. Doing mode is all about getting to the destination rather than considering anything else. So if an insurance company puts you on hold for too long, you begin to feel tense and frustrated. In this driven state of mind, you don't come up with creative solutions such as calling a different company or just trying at a quieter time.

>> **Most of your actions happen automatically.** You're not really aware when you're in doing mode. You're completing tasks on automatic pilot. Thoughts pop into your head, emotions emerge, and you act on them largely unconsciously. If the person you're speaking to on the telephone is rude, you may automatically react, making you both feel bad, rather than considering that the phone operator may have had a really long and bad day too.

>> **You're not in the present moment.** When engaged in doing mode, you're not connected with your senses, in the now. You're thinking about how things should be in the future, or replaying events from the past. You're lost in your head rather than focused in the moment. While you're placed on hold on the telephone, your mind may wander into anxious thoughts about tomorrow's meeting rather than you just taking the chance to have a break and look at the sky or gaze at the beautiful tree through the window.

REMEMBER

Doing mode isn't just the mode you're in when you're doing stuff. Even when you're sitting on the sofa, your mind can be spinning. You're in doing mode. Trying to run away from negative emotions or toward pleasant ones is also part of doing mode's specialty.

WARNING

Doing mode is most unhelpful when applied to emotional difficulties. Trying to get rid of or suppress emotions may seem to work in the very short term, but before long the emotions rise up again. Being mode is a more helpful state of mind for understanding and finding out about emotions, particularly negative ones. See the later section "Dealing with emotions using being mode."

Embracing the Being Mode of Mind

Society values people achieving goals. You see people in the papers who have record amounts of money, or who've climbed the highest mountain. How many times has someone made the headlines for living in the moment?

People are very familiar with and almost comforted by the doing mode of mind. To stop doing so much, whether physically or mentally, isn't easy. Doing feels attractive and exciting. However, people are beginning to realize that too much doing is a problem. In fact, a whole philosophy has arisen and lots of books have been written all about how you can slow down.

On the surface, the realm of *being* appears lifeless and boring. In actual fact, this couldn't be farther from the truth. Being mode is a nourishing and uplifting state of mind that's always available to you, in the midst of busy activity. You can be trading in the stock market or teaching young children math — if you're conscious of your physical, emotional, and psychological state of mind — you're in being mode. In some ways, being mode isn't easy to cultivate, yet the rewards of accessing this inner resource far outweigh any difficulties in reaching it.

Here are some of the qualities of the being mode of mind:

>> **You connect with the present moment.** When you're in being mode, you're mindful of sight, sound, smell, taste, or touch. Or you're consciously aware of your thoughts or emotions, without being too caught up by them. You're not intentionally getting lost in regrets about the past or concerns about the future.

>> **You accept and allow things to be as they are.** You're less goal-oriented. You have less of a burning desire for situations to change. You accept how things are before moving to change anything. Being mode doesn't mean

resignation; it means active acceptance of the way things are at the moment. If you're lost but you have a map, the only way of getting anywhere is to know where you are to start with. Being mode is about acknowledging and accepting where you are.

>> **You're open to pleasant, unpleasant, and neutral emotions.** You're willing to open up to painful and unpleasant sensations or emotions without trying to run away from them. You understand that avoiding an emotion just locks you into the feeling more tightly.

The being mode of mind is what mindfulness endeavors to cultivate. Being mode is about allowing things to be as they are already. When you stop trying to change things, paradoxically they change by themselves. As Carl Jung said: "We cannot change anything until we accept it."

TIP

Don't accept an emotion just to try to make it go away. That's not acceptance. For example, say you're feeling a bit sad. If you accept it with a secret desire that the sadness will go away, you haven't fully accepted it yet. It's like offering to hug a friend but then not actually participating in the hugging. Instead, accept an emotion wholeheartedly if you can. After all, emotions are here to teach you something. Listen to your emotions and see what they have to say. This skill is certainly not easy at first, but with time and practice, you'll get better and better at accepting and making peace with your emotions.

Combining Being and Doing

Think of your mind as like the ocean. The waves rise and fall, but the still, deep waters are always there underneath.

You're tossed and turned in the waves when you're on the surface in doing mode. The waves aren't bad — they're just part of the ocean. Going farther down, the waves of doing rest on the still waters of being, as shown in Figure 4-1. Being is your sense of who you are. Being is characterized as a state of acceptance, a willingness to be with whatever is. Being is tranquil, still, and grounding.

REMEMBER

Experience itself is neither doing nor being mode. You determine the mode by how you react or respond to the experience. Doing is getting actively involved in the experience to change it in some way. Being is simply seeing it as it is. That lack of fixing can result in a sense of calmness even when things are tricky.

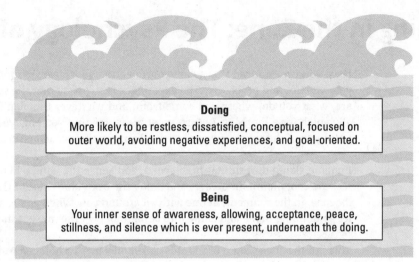

Doing
More likely to be restless, dissatisfied, conceptual, focused on outer world, avoiding negative experiences, and goal-oriented.

Being
Your inner sense of awareness, allowing, acceptance, peace, stillness, and silence which is ever present, underneath the doing.

FIGURE 4-1: The ocean of doing and being.

© *John Wiley & Sons, Inc.*

Switching from doing to being doesn't require years of mindfulness training. It can happen in a moment. Imagine walking to work and worrying about all the things that you need to get done, and planning how you'll tackle the next project with the manager away on vacation. Suddenly you notice the fiery red leaves on a tree. You're amazed at the beauty of it. That simple connection with the sense of sight is an example of being mode. The mode of mind changes by shifting the focus of attention to the present moment. You're no longer on automatic pilot with all its planning, judging, criticizing, and praising. You're in the present moment.

Even something as seemingly mundane as feeling your feet in contact with the ground as you walk is a move toward being mode, too. You can also notice the beauty of a tree, the sounds of birds chirping, or the gentle sun on the back of your neck. Changing modes may not seem easy at first, especially when you're preoccupied by thoughts, but it gets easier through practice. You don't have to rush through life.

REMEMBER

The key to a mindful way of living is to integrate both doing and being modes of mind into your life. Become aware of which mode you're operating in and make an appropriate choice about which is most helpful for the situation. You need to know where you are on the map before you can move on. Doing mode is important. You need to plan what you're going to do today, what food to buy, how to give feedback to a colleague, and how best to respond when your children start arguing. These activities make you human. However, as a human *being*, you need to integrate a being mode of mind into your doing to be fully awake to your life.

Being in the Zone: The Psychology of Flow

Have you ever noticed that when you're eating your favorite food, you forget all your worries and problems? The experience is so lovely that the sense of who you are, what you do, where you come from, and whatever the plan is for tomorrow all vanish for a moment. In fact, most pleasures that you engage in result in you letting go of the sense of "you" with all your problems and issues.

Imagine skiing downhill at high speed. You sense the wind whooshing past you, feel the cool mountain breeze, and enjoy the deep blue color of the sky. You're *in the zone*, in the moment, at one with all around you. When you're in the zone, you let go of doing mode and come into being mode — the present moment.

This "in the zone" state of mind is called *flow* by psychologist Mihaly Csíkszentmihályi. But what's flow got to do with the being mode of mind? Surely being in the zone is always about doing? Not quite. Practicing mindfulness helps to generate flow experiences directly. Everything you do, you can do in the moment, giving you a deeper sense of aliveness.

Here's what you experience when you're in a state of flow:

>> You feel at one with the world.

>> You let go of your sense of being an individual and any worries and problems.

>> You're completely focused.

>> You feel very satisfied with what you're doing.

>> You're happy, although you don't really notice it at the time because you're so engrossed in whatever you're doing.

Understanding the factors of mindful flow

Csíkszentmihályi found some key factors that accompany an experience of flow. They've been adapted here so you can generate a mindful flow experience. As long as you do a task mindfully, it's potentially going to be a flow experience.

Here are some key factors of mindful flow and how you can generate them using mindfulness:

>> **Attention:** Flow experiences need attention. Mindfulness is all about attention, and mindfulness increases your level of attention with practice. Through regular mindfulness practice, your brain becomes better at paying

attention to whatever you choose to focus on, making a flow experience far more likely. When driving, you simply pay attention to your surroundings rather than letting your mind wander off.

>> **Immediate feedback:** Flow needs immediate feedback as to how you're doing. When you're practicing mindfulness, you're getting immediate feedback because you know at any time if you're paying attention or if your mind has wandered off for the last few minutes. So, if driving, you notice when your mind has drifted into dreaming about what's for dinner tonight, and you bring your attention gently back to the here and now.

>> **Sufficiently challenging:** Mindfulness is an active process of repeatedly rebalancing to come back to the present moment while the mind — doing what minds do — wants to pull you away into other thoughts. To drive in a mindful way from work to home would be a suitable challenge for anyone, potentially creating a flow experience.

>> **Sense of control:** When you're mindful of your thoughts and feelings that are arising, you've created a choice. You don't have to react to your thoughts or do what they tell you to do. This generates a sense of control as you become aware of the choices you have. If, while you're driving, someone cuts in front of you, you've got the choice to either react and feel annoyed, or practice letting it go. Even if you do react, you can notice how you react and what effect the reaction has on your thoughts and feelings. Eventually, mindfulness goes beyond trying to control — you discover the flow experience is accessed through letting go rather than controlling your attention.

>> **Intrinsically rewarding:** As you carry out a task, you're doing it for the sake of itself. If you're driving your car to get home as fast as possible to make dinner, you're not going to be in a flow experience. If you drive to simply enjoy each moment of the journey, that's different. You can feel the warmth of the sunshine on your arms, appreciate the color of the sky while sitting in traffic, and marvel at the miracle of the human body's ability to do such a complex task effortlessly. You're in a flow experience.

WARNING

Normally, mindfulness would make you a safer driver rather than a more dangerous one. However, begin by being mindful of safer tasks such as washing dishes or going for a walk before you attempt mindfulness of driving, just so you get used to being mindful. Don't use mindfulness of driving if you find the experience distracting.

Discovering your flow experiences

Everyone's had flow experiences. By knowing when you've been in flow, you can encourage more opportunities to experience it in the future. The following are some typical activities that people often find themselves flowing in. You may even find something here to try yourself:

>> **Reading or writing:** When you're fully engaged in a good book full of fascinating insights or a challenging storyline, you're in flow. You forget about everything else and time flies by. When writing in flow, words simply pop into your head and onto your page with effortless ease. You stop criticizing what you're creating, and enjoy seeing the report or book pouring out of you. One example of mindful writing is to write whatever words arise into your awareness first, and avoid all self-judgment. Then you can go back and edit the writing later. In this way, the writing seems to flow naturally.

>> **Art or hobbies (such as drawing, painting, dancing, singing, or playing music):** Most artistic endeavors involve flow. You're directly connected with your senses, and people often describe themselves as being "at one with the music." If you're forced to do a particular hobby, it may or may not be a flow experience, because the intrinsic motivation isn't there. Picture a friend being dragged onto the dance floor before they've had a drink and you'll understand.

>> **Exercise (walking, running, cycling, swimming, and so on):** Some people love exercise so much that they get addicted to it. The rush of adrenaline, the full focus in the present moment, and the feeling of exhilaration make for a flow experience.

>> **Work:** Perhaps surprisingly, you can be in flow at work. Research has found that people are happier at work than they are in their leisure time. Work encourages you to do something with a focused attention, and often involves interaction with others. You need to give something of yourself. This can set the stage for flow. In contrast, watching television at home can drain your energy, especially if you're watching unchallenging programs.

>> **Anything done mindfully:** Remember, anything that you do with a mindful awareness is going to generate a flow state of mind, from making love to making a cup of tea. Just let go of your judgment, be fully present as best you can, and see whether you can enjoy the experience.

Encouraging a Being Mode of Mind

Generally speaking, most people spend too much time in doing mode and not enough in being mode. Doing mode results in chasing after goals that may not be what you're really interested in. Being mode offers a rest — a chance to let go of the usual, habitual patterns of the mind and drop into the awareness that's always there.

REMEMBER

You can be in being mode even though you're doing something. Being mode doesn't necessarily mean that you're doing nothing. You can be busy working hard in the garden, and yet if your attention is right in the moment, and you're connecting directly with the senses, you can be in being mode.

TIP

Here are ten ways of switching from doing mode to being mode:

» **When walking from place to place, take the opportunity to feel your feet on the floor, see the range of different colors in front of you, and listen to the variety of different sounds.** By walking in a mindful, calm, and relaxed way, you arrive at your destination feeling refreshed and energized.

» **When moving from one activity to another, take a moment to rest.** Feel one complete in-breath and out-breath.

» **Establish a regular mindfulness routine using formal mindfulness meditation practices.** Examples include mindful eating meditation, mindful breathing meditation, and mindful movement.

» **Use the three-minute mini mindfulness meditation several times a day (see Chapter 5 in Book 1).** Whenever you catch yourself becoming excessively tense or emotional, use the mini meditation to begin moving toward being mode and opening up to the challenging experience, rather than reacting to try to avoid or get rid of the experience.

» **Avoid multi-tasking whenever you can.** Doing one thing at a time with your full and undivided attention can engage being mode. Doing too many things at the same time encourages your mind to spin.

» **Find time to do a hobby or sport.** These activities tend to involve connecting with the senses, which immediately brings you into being mode. Painting, listening to music, playing an instrument, dancing, singing, walking in the park, and many more activities all offer a chance to be with the senses.

» **When taking a bath or shower, use the time to feel the warmth of the water and the contact of the water with your skin.** Allow all your senses to be involved in the experience; enjoy the sound of the water and breathe in the scent of your favorite soap or body wash.

» **When you're eating, pause before your meal to take a few conscious breaths.** Then eat the meal with your full attention.

» **Treat yourself to a half day or full day of mindfulness once in a while.** Wake up slowly, feel your breath frequently, and connect with your senses and with other significant people around you as much as you can. Chapter 6 in Book 1 sets out some suggestions for having a mindful day.

Dealing with emotions using being mode

Using doing mode in the area of thoughts and emotions is like using the wrong remote control to change the channel on your television. No matter how hard you push the buttons, the channel isn't going to change — and pushing the buttons harder just makes you more tired and breaks the remote control. You're using the wrong tool for the job.

Say you're feeling sad today. Doing mode may feel the emotion and use the problem-solving, goal-oriented mind to try to fight it, asking, "Why am I sad? How can I escape from it? What will I do now? Why does this always happen to me? Let me try watching television. Oh, I feel worse. What if this feeling never goes away? What if I feel depressed again?"

Doing mode sets thoughts spinning in your head, which just makes you feel worse. Your focus is on getting rid of the feeling instead of feeling the emotion. The more you fight the emotion, the stronger it seems to get. So, what's the solution?

Next time you have an uncomfortable feeling such as sadness, anger, frustration, or jealousy, try this exercise to get into being mode:

1. Set your intention. Let your intention be to feel the emotion and its effects as best you can with a gentle curiosity, kindness, and acceptance. You're not doing so as a clever way to get rid of it. You're just giving yourself space to learn from the emotion rather than running away.

REMEMBER

All emotions, no matter how strong, have a beginning and an end.

2. Feel the emotion. Feel the emotion with care, kindness, and acceptance, as best you can. Open up to it. Notice where the emotion manifests itself in your body. Breathe into that part of your body and stay with it. Allow the emotion to be as it is. You don't need to fight or run away. Be with the experience.

3. Step back from the emotion. Notice that you can be aware of the emotion without being the emotion itself — create a space between yourself and the feeling. This is an important aspect of mindfulness. As you observe the feeling, you're separate from it in the sense that you're free from it. You're watching it. It's like sitting on a riverbank as the water rushes by rather than being in the river itself. As you watch the water (emotion) pass by, you're not in the river itself. Every now and then, you may feel like you've been sucked into the river and washed downstream. As soon as you feel this, simply step back out of the river again. Figure 4-2 illustrates this idea.

4. Breathe. Now simply feel your breath. Be with each in-breath and each out-breath. Notice how each breath is unique, different, and vital for your health and wellbeing. Then continue with whatever you need to do in a mindful way.

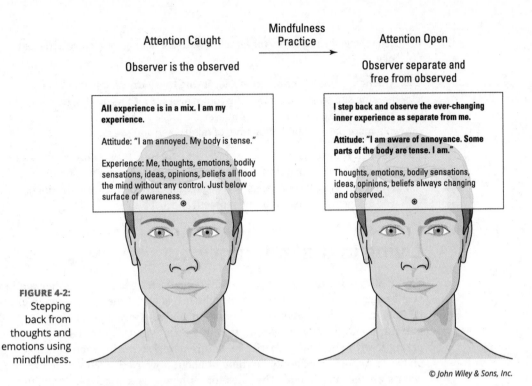

Attention Caught

Observer is the observed

Mindfulness Practice →

Attention Open

Observer separate and free from observed

All experience is in a mix. I am my experience.

Attitude: "I am annoyed. My body is tense."

Experience: Me, thoughts, emotions, bodily sensations, ideas, opinions, beliefs all flood the mind without any control. Just below surface of awareness.

I step back and observe the ever-changing inner experience as separate from me.

Attitude: "I am aware of annoyance. Some parts of the body are tense. I am."

Thoughts, emotions, bodily sensations, ideas, opinions, beliefs always changing and observed.

FIGURE 4-2: Stepping back from thoughts and emotions using mindfulness.

© *John Wiley & Sons, Inc.*

Finding time to just be

Are you a busy bee? Do you have too much to do to have time to be? One of the attractive things about mindfulness is that you don't have a fixed amount of time that you're "supposed" to practice for. Your daily practice can be a mindfulness exercise for one minute or one hour — it's up to you. The other great thing about mindfulness is that you can simply be mindful of your normal everyday routine and in that way build up your awareness and *being* mode. That takes no time at all; in fact, it can save time because you're more focused on your activities.

TIP

These mindful practices require almost no time at all:

>> **When waiting in a line, rather than killing time, engage your awareness.** Time is too precious to be killed. Notice the colors and sounds around you. Or challenge yourself to see whether you can maintain the awareness of your feet on the floor for ten full breaths. Even engaging in a friendly chat with someone can help you practice mindful listening.

>> **When you stop at a red traffic light, you have a choice.** You can let yourself get frustrated and impatient, or you can do traffic light meditation! Close your eyes and nourish yourself with three mindful breaths — very

refreshing! If you get into this practice, you'll be hoping for red lights instead of green lights.

>> **The next time the phone rings, let it ring three times.** Use that time to breathe and smile. Telemarketing companies know that you can "hear the smile" on the phone and ask employees to smile when they're on a call. You're in a more patient and happy state of mind when you speak.

>> **Change your routine.** If you normally drive to work, try walking or cycling for part of it. Speak to different friends or colleagues. Take up a new hobby. When you change your habits, you engage different pathways in the brain. You instinctively wake up to the moment and just be.

Living in the moment

You're always in the present moment. You've never been in any other moment. Don't believe me? Every time your mind worries about the past, when does it do it? Only in the present moment. Every plan you've ever made is only made in the present too. Right now, as you're thinking about what you're reading and comparing it with your past experience, you're doing so in this moment, now. Your plans for tomorrow can only be thought about now. Now is all you're ever in. So what's all the fuss about? The question is how you can connect with the here and now.

Here are some tips for living in the present moment:

>> **Value the present moment.** Spend time considering that the present moment is the *only* moment that you have. You then discover the value of focusing on the here and now. And once you experience how enjoyable present-moment living can be, you've created a powerful shift into a more mindful and happy lifestyle.

>> **Focus on whatever you're doing.** Be present in the little moments that fill your day, because the little moments aren't little; they're life. When you type, feel the contact between your fingers and the keyboard. When getting dressed, try giving it your full attention rather than allowing your mind to wander. When setting the table for dinner, feel the weight of the plates and utensils as you carry them. Appreciate how the table looks once you have set it. Enjoy doing tasks to the best of your ability. Living in the present is trickier than it sounds, but each time you try, you get a little better at it. Slowly but surely, you start really living in the moment.

>> **Reduce activities that draw you out of the moment.** You may need to reduce the time you spend on social media or surfing websites. Or it may be as simple as not lying in bed in the morning for too long, allowing yourself to

worry unnecessarily about the day. Nothing's wrong with any of these activities, but they don't encourage moment-by-moment living. They capture your attention and lead to a passive state of mind. Watching too many hours of Netflix while slumped on the sofa drains your energy much faster than an activity done with a gentle awareness.

>> **Establish a daily mindfulness practice.** Doing so strengthens your ability to stay in the present rather than being drawn into the past or pulled into the future. The strength of your daily habit extends into your everyday life, without you even trying. You hear the sound of that bird in the tree, or find yourself listening intently to your colleague in an effortless way. Now mindfulness becomes fun. See Chapter 3 of Book 1 to find out how to incorporate mindfullness into your daily life.

>> **Look deeply.** Consider and reflect on all the people and things that come together in each moment. For example, you're reading this book. The book's paper came from trees that needed sunshine and rain, soil, and nutrients. The book was edited, marketed, printed, transported, distributed, and sold by people. It also required the invention of the printing press, language, and more. You were taught English by someone to enable you to understand the words. This awareness of all that's come together and been provided for you to enjoy naturally creates gratitude and present-moment awareness. This is called *looking deeply*. You're connecting in the moment, and also seeing the bigger picture of how things have come together in an interconnected way. Looking deeply isn't thinking about your experience, but seeing your experience in a different way. You can try it in any situation — it transforms your perspective, and perspective transforms experience.

TIP

If you want to let go of your baggage from the past and future, try this mindful exercise discovered from a mindfulness teacher and monk named Ajahn Brahm. To let go of the weight of the past and future, follow these steps:

1. **Find a nice comfortable position to sit or lie in.** Be kind to yourself, and ensure you're in a relaxed posture, loosening any tight clothing, removing any glasses you're wearing, and slipping off your shoes if you wish.

2. **Take your time to take a few deep, smooth breaths.** Let each in-breath represent nourishment and energy. Let each out-breath signify letting go.

3. **Gently close your eyes. Imagine you're holding two heavy shopping bags. Imagine how heavy they feel.** Feel the strain on your fingers and how much effort it takes to hold both bags. Their weight is pulling you down. The strain makes you feel tired and tense.

4. **Let the bag in one hand represent your past.** Imagine the bag is labelled "past." The bag contains all your regrets and mistakes. All your successes and failures. Past relationships. The choices you've made and the sorrows you've felt. You may even be able to visualize all your past experiences contained within this heavy bag. Holding this bag all day is tiring.

5. **Imagine that you decide it's time to let go of the "past" bag.** You want to put the bag down and have a rest. So imagine slowly lowering the bag to the ground. Eventually the bag makes contact with the ground, and as it does so, immediately you begin to feel a release. Eventually your whole bag, representing all your past, is down on the ground. You smile as you let go completely. Imagine your hand opening and imagine yourself feeling so much better. You're liberated from carrying your past around with you.

6. **In your other hand, you're holding a heavy bag signifying your future.** Imagine the word "future" written on the bag. The bag contains all your hopes, dreams, and plans. And also all your anxieties and worries. All your concerns and fears about what may or may not happen. Holding this hefty burden is no joke. The bag slows you down. But now you know how to put this bag, which is full of your future, down.

7. **Imagine that you slowly lower the "future" bag until the bottom of the bag starts to make contact with the ground.** You begin to feel a relief. As you continue to lower the bag, all the weight is transferred to the earth. You feel an immense burden lifted. Your hand is now free, and you completely let go of your worries about the future.

8. **Imagine yourself standing with a bag representing your past on the floor on one side, and a bag representing your future on the floor on the other side.** Because you're standing between the past and future, where are you? You're in the best place to be: the present moment. Give yourself the go-ahead to feel free. The bags are perfectly safe on the ground. Rest in the joy of being in the present moment. Rejoice in the childlike innocence of the here and now — timelessness.

9. **Spend as much time as you want to in this experience of the present moment. And any time you feel you're carrying too much weight from the past or future, practice this mindful exercise and put the weights down again.**

Chapter 5

Using Mindfulness for Yourself

Y ou probably appreciate the need to look after others. But are you aware of the need to look after yourself as well? You need to eat a balanced diet and exercise regularly for your health and wellbeing. You need to have the right amount of work and rest in your life. And you need to challenge yourself intellectually, to keep your mind healthy. You need to socialize and also save some time just for yourself. Achieving all this perfectly is impossible, but how can you strive to take care of yourself in a light-hearted way, without becoming overly uptight and stressed?

A caring, accepting awareness of your thoughts, emotions, and body is the key to healthy living. Mindfulness is a wonderful way to develop greater awareness. This chapter details suggestions for looking after yourself through mindfulness.

Using a Mini Mindful Exercise

You don't need to practice mindfulness meditation for hours and hours to reap its benefits. Short and frequent meditations are an effective way of developing mindfulness in your everyday life.

Introducing the breathing space

When you've had a busy day, you probably enjoy stopping for a nice hot cup of tea or coffee, or another favorite beverage. The drink offers more than just liquid for the body. The break gives you a chance to relax and unwind a bit. The three-minute mini meditation, called the *breathing space* (illustrated in Figure 5-1 and 5-2), is a bit like a coffee break, but beyond relaxation, the breathing space enables you to check what's going on in your body, mind, and heart — not getting rid of feelings or thoughts, but looking at them from a clearer perspective.

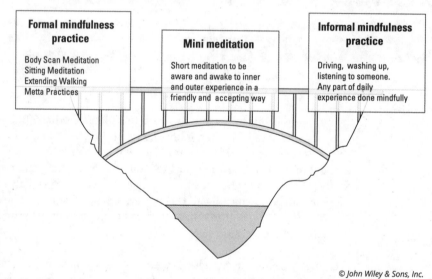

Formal mindfulness practice

Body Scan Meditation
Sitting Meditation
Extending Walking
Metta Practices

Mini meditation

Short meditation to be aware and awake to inner and outer experience in a friendly and accepting way

Informal mindfulness practice

Driving, washing up, listening to someone. Any part of daily experience done mindfully

FIGURE 5-1: How the breathing space acts as a bridge between formal and informal mindfulness practice.

© John Wiley & Sons, Inc.

REMEMBER Mindfulness is an awareness and acceptance exercise — not a relaxation exercise. Relaxation may come as a welcome side benefit. Let your intention be to become aware of your thoughts and emotions and allow them space to just be as they are, with curiosity and kindness, as best you can.

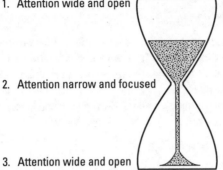

1. Attention wide and open

Step A – Open awareness of experience just as it is. What is happening in your body, thoughts, emotions?

2. Attention narrow and focused

Step B – Breathing–Gathering your attention on the feeling the breath

3. Attention wide and open

Step C – Consciously expanding awareness to whole body and breath in a spacious awareness. Getting a sense of the whole body breathing

FIGURE 5-2:
The three-minute breathing space meditation progresses like an hourglass.

© *John Wiley & Sons, Inc.*

Practicing the breathing space

TIP

You can practice the breathing space at almost any time and anywhere. The meditation is made up of three distinct stages, which are called A, B, and C to help you to remember what to practice at each stage. The exercise doesn't have to last exactly three minutes: you can make it longer or shorter depending on where you are and how much time you have. If you only have time to feel three breaths, that's okay; doing so can still have a profound effect.

1. **Sit comfortably with a sense of dignity, but don't strain your back and neck.** You can sit upright or stand; even lying down on your back or curling up is acceptable. Sitting upright is helpful, because it sends a positive message to the brain — you're doing something different.

2. **Practice step A for about a minute or so, then move on to B for a minute, ending with C also for a minute — or however long you can manage.**

    Step A: Awareness:

    Reflect on the following questions, pausing for a few seconds between each one:

    i. **What bodily sensations am I aware of at the moment?** Feel your posture, become aware of any aches or pains, or any pleasant sensations. Just accept them as they are, as far as you can.

    ii. **What emotions am I aware of at the moment?** Notice the feelings in your heart or belly area or wherever you can feel emotion.

    iii. **What thoughts am I aware of, passing through my mind at the moment?** Become aware of your thoughts, and the space between yourself and your thoughts. If you can, simply observe your thoughts rather than becoming caught up in them.

Step B: Breathing:

Focus your attention in your belly area — the lower abdomen. As best you can, feel the whole of your in-breath and the whole of each out-breath. You don't need to change the rate of your breathing — just become mindful of it in a warm, curious, and friendly way. Notice how each breath is slightly different. If your mind wanders away, gently and kindly guide your attention back to your breath. Appreciate how precious each breath is.

Step C: Consciously expanding:

Consciously expand your awareness from your belly to your whole body. Get a sense of your entire body breathing (which it is, through the skin). As your awareness heightens within your body, notice its effect. Accept yourself as perfect and complete just as you are, just in this moment, as much as you can.

TIP

Experiment with having a very gentle smile on your face as you do the breathing space, no matter how you feel. Notice whether doing so has a positive effect on your state of mind. If it does, use this approach every time. You don't even need to say "cheese"!

TIP

Imagine the breathing space as an hourglass (refer to Figure 5-2). The attention is wide and open to start with and then narrows and focuses on the breath in the second stage, before expanding again with more awareness and spaciousness.

The breathing space meditation encapsulates the core of mindfulness in a succinct and portable way. The full effects of the breathing space are as follows:

>> **You move into a restful "being" mode of mind.** Your mind can be in one of two very different states of mind: *doing* mode or *being* mode. Doing mode is energetic and all about carrying out actions and changing things. Being mode is a soothing state of mind where you acknowledge things as they are. (For lots more on being and doing mode, refer to Chapter 4 in Book 1.)

>> **Your self-awareness increases.** You become more aware of how your body feels, the thoughts going through your mind, and the emotion or need of the moment. You may notice that your shoulders are hunched or your jaw is clenched. You may have thoughts whizzing through your head that you hadn't even realized were there. Or perhaps you're feeling sad, or are thirsty or tired. If you listen to these messages, you can take appropriate action. Without self-awareness, you can't tackle them.

>> **Your self-compassion increases.** You allow yourself the space to be kinder to yourself, rather than self-critical or overly demanding. If you've had a tough day, the breathing space offers you time to let go of your concerns, forgive

your mistakes and come back into the present moment. And with greater self-compassion, you're better able to be compassionate and understanding of others too.

» **You create more opportunities to make choices.** You make choices all the time. At the moment, you've chosen to read this book and this page. Later on you may choose to go for a walk, call a friend, or cook dinner. If your partner snaps at you, your reaction is a choice to a certain extent too. By practicing the breathing space, you stand back from your experiences and see the bigger picture of the situation you're in. When a difficulty arises, you can make a decision from your whole wealth of knowledge and experience, rather than just having a fleeting reaction. The breathing space can help you make wiser decisions.

» **You switch off automatic pilot.** Have you ever eaten a whole meal and realized that you didn't actually taste it? You were most likely on automatic pilot. You're so used to eating, you can do it while thinking about other things. The breathing space helps to connect you with your senses so that you're alive to the moment.

Try this thought experiment. Without looking, remember whether your wrist watch has roman numerals or normal numbers on it. If you're not sure, or get it wrong, it's a small indication of how you're operating on automatic pilot. You've looked at your watch hundreds of times, but not really looked carefully.

» **You become an observer of your experience rather than feeling trapped by it.** In your normal everyday experience, no distance exists between you and your thoughts or emotions. They just arise and you act on them almost without noticing. One of the key outcomes of the breathing space is the creation of a space between you and your inner world. Your thoughts and emotions can be in complete turmoil, but you simply observe and are free from them, like watching a film at the cinema. This seemingly small shift in viewpoint has huge implications, which are explored in Chapter 4 of Book 1.

» **You see things from a different perspective.** Have you ever taken a comment too personally? Everyone certainly has. Perhaps someone is critical about a piece of work you've done, and you immediately react or at least feel a surge of emotion in the pit of your stomach. But you have other ways of reacting. Was the other person stressed out? Are you making a big deal about nothing? The pause offered by the breathing space can help you see things in another way.

» **You walk the bridge between formal and informal practice.** Formal practice is where you carve out a chunk of time in the day to practice meditation. Informal practice is being mindful of your normal everyday activities.

The breathing space is a very useful way of bridging the gap between these two important aspects of mindfulness. The breathing space is both a formal practice because you're making some time to carry it out, and informal because you integrate it into your day-to-day activities.

>> **You create a space for new ideas to arise.** By stopping your normal everyday activities to practice the breathing space, you create room in your mind for other things to pop in. If your mind is cluttered, you can't think clearly. The breathing space may be just what the doctor ordered to allow an intelligent insight or creative idea to pop into your mind.

Using the breathing space between activities

Aim to practice the breathing space three times a day. Here are some suggested times for practicing the breathing space:

>> **Before or after meal times:** Some people pray with their family before eating a meal to be together with gratitude and give thanks for the food. Doing a breathing space before or after a meal gives you a set time to practice and reminds you to appreciate your meal too. If you can't manage three minutes, just feel three breaths before diving in.

>> **Between activities:** Resting between your daily activities, even for just a few moments, is very nourishing. Feeling your breath and renewing yourself is very pleasant. Research has found that just three mindful breaths can change your body's physiology, lowering blood pressure and reducing muscle tension.

>> **On waking up or before going to bed:** A short meditation before you jump out of bed can be a wholesome experience. You can stay lying in bed and enjoy your breathing. Or you can sit up and do the breathing space. Meditating in this way helps to put you in a good frame of mind and sets you up for meeting life afresh. Practicing the breathing space before going to bed can calm your mind and encourage a deeper and more restful sleep.

>> **When a difficult thought or emotion arises:** The breathing space meditation is particularly helpful when you're experiencing challenging thoughts or emotions. By becoming aware of the nature of your thoughts, and listening to them with a sense of kindness and curiosity, you change your relationship to them. A mindful relationship to thoughts and emotions results in a totally different experience.

Using Mindfulness to Look After Yourself

Have you ever heard the safety announcements on a plane? In the event of an emergency, cabin crew advise you to put your own oxygen mask on first, before you help put one on anyone else, even your own child. The reason is obvious. If you can't breathe yourself, how can you possibly help anyone else? Looking after yourself isn't just necessary in emergencies. In normal everyday life, you need to look after your own needs. If you don't, not only do you suffer, but so do all the people who interact or depend on you. Taking care of yourself isn't selfish: It's the best way to be of optimal service to others. Eating, sleeping, exercising, and meditating regularly are all ways of looking after yourself and hence others.

Exercising mindfully

You can practice mindfulness and do physical exercise at the same time. In fact, Jon Kabat-Zinn, one of the key founders of mindfulness in the West, trained the USA men's Olympic rowing team in 1984. A couple of the men won gold — not bad for a bunch of meditators! And in more recent Olympics, several athletes claimed that mindfulness helped them to reach peak performance and achieve their gold medals.

TIP

Regular exercise is beneficial for both body and mind, as confirmed by thousands of research studies. If you already exercise on a regular basis, you know the advantages. If not, and your doctor is happy with you exercising, you can begin by simply walking. Walking is an aerobic exercise and a great way to practice mindfulness. Then, if you want to, you can build up to whatever type of more strenuous exercise you fancy. Approach each new exercise with a mindful attitude: be curious of what will happen, stay with uncomfortable sensations for a while, explore the edge between comfort and discomfort, and look around you.

TIP

Whatever exercise you choose, allow yourself to enjoy the experience. Find simple physical activities that make you smile rather than frown, and you're much more likely to stick with the discipline. And if you find the word "exercise" a turn off, call it "physical activity" or simply "moving your body" every day. Use words that are appealing to you.

To start you off, here are a few typical physical exercises and ideas for how to suffuse them with mindfulness.

Mindful running

Leave your music and phone at home. Try running outside rather than at the gym — your senses have more to connect with outside. Begin by taking ten mindful breaths as you walk along. Become aware of your body as a whole. Build up from normal walking to walking fast to running. Notice how quickly your breathing rate changes, and focus on your breathing whenever your mind wanders away from the present moment. Feel your heart beating and the rhythm of your feet bouncing on the ground. Notice whether you're tensing up any parts of your body unnecessarily. Enjoy the wind against your face and the warmth of your body.

Observe what sort of thoughts pop up when you're running, without being judgmental of them. If running begins to be painful, explore whether you need to keep going or slow down. If you're a regular runner, you may want to stay on the edge a little bit longer; if you're new to it, slow down and build up more gradually. At the end of your run, notice how you feel. Try doing a mini meditation (described in the first section of this chapter) and notice its effect. Keep observing the effects of your run over the next few hours.

Mindful swimming

The experience of mindful swimming can be very meditative. Begin with some mindful breathing as you approach the pool. Notice the effect of the water on your body as you enter. What sort of thoughts arise? As you begin to swim, feel the contact between your arms and legs and the water. What does the water feel like? Be grateful that you can swim and have access to the water. Allow yourself to get into the rhythm of swimming. Become aware of your heartbeat, breath rate, and the muscles in your body. At times, you may even feel at one with the water — enjoy that experience. When you've finished, observe how your body and mind feel.

Mindful cycling

Begin with some mindful breathing as you sit on your bike. Feel the weight of your body, the contact between your hands and the handlebars, and your foot on the pedal. As you begin cycling, listen to the sound of the wind. Notice how your leg muscles work together rapidly as you move. Switch between focusing on a specific part of your body like the hands or face to a wide and spacious awareness of your body as a whole. Let go of wherever you're heading and come back to the here and now. As you get off your bike, perceive the sensations in your body. Scan through your body and detect how you feel after that exercise.

Preparing for sleep with mindfulness

Sleep, essential to your wellbeing, is one of the first things to improve when people do a course in mindfulness. People sleep better, and their sleep is deeper. Studies found similar results from people who suffered from insomnia who did an eight-week course in MBSR (mindfulness-based stress reduction).

Sleep is about completely letting go of the world. Falling asleep isn't something you *do* — it's about *non-doing*. In that sense sleep is similar to mindfulness. If you're *trying* to sleep, you're putting in a certain effort, which is the opposite of letting go.

TIP

Here are some tips for preparing to sleep using mindfulness:

>> **Stick to a regular time to go to bed and to wake up.** Waking up very early one day and very late the next confuses your body clock and may cause difficulties in sleeping.

>> **Avoid over-stimulating yourself by watching television or being on the computer or your phone before bed.** The light from the screen tricks your brain into believing it's still daytime, and then it takes longer for you to fall asleep.

>> **Try doing some formal mindfulness practice such as a sitting meditation or the body scan before going to bed.**

>> **Try doing some yoga or gentle stretching before going to bed.** Cats naturally stretch before curling up on the sofa for a snooze. Stretching may help you to relax and your muscles unwind. Try purring while you're stretching, too — maybe that's the secret to their relaxed way of life!

>> **Do some mindful walking indoors before bed.** Take five or ten minutes to walk a few steps and feel all the sensations in your body as you do so. The slower, the better.

>> **When you lie in bed, feel your in-breath and out-breath.** Rather than trying to sleep, just be with your breathing. Count your out-breaths from one to ten. Each time you breathe out, say the number to yourself. Every time your mind wanders off, begin again at one.

>> **If you're lying in bed worrying, perhaps even about getting to sleep, accept your worries.** Challenging or fighting thoughts just makes them more powerful. Note them, and gently come back to the feeling of the breath.

REMEMBER

If you seem to be sleeping less than usual, try not to worry about it too much. In fact, worrying about how little sleep you're getting becomes a vicious circle. Many people sleep far less than eight hours a day, and most people have bad nights once in a while. Not being able to sleep doesn't mean something is wrong with you. A regular mindfulness practice will probably help you in the long run.

Looking at a mindful work–life balance

Work–life balance means balancing work and career ambitions on the one side, and home, family, leisure, and spiritual pursuits on the other. Working too much can have a negative impact on other important areas. By keeping things in balance, you're able to get your work done quicker and your relationship quality tends to improve.

With the advent of mobile technology, or a demanding career, work may be taking over your free time. And sometimes you may struggle to see how you can re-dress this imbalance. The following mindful reflection may help.

TIP

Try this little reflection to help reflect on and improve your work–life balance:

1. Sit in a comfortable upright posture, with a sense of dignity and stability.

2. Become aware of your body as a whole, with all its various changing sensations.

3. Guide your attention to the ebb and flow of your breath. Allow your mind to settle on the feeling of the breath.

4. Observe the balance of the breath. Notice how your in-breath naturally stops when it needs to, as does the out-breath. You don't need to do anything — it just happens. Enjoy the flow of the breath.

5. When you're ready, reflect on this question for a few minutes:

    What can I do to find a wiser and healthier balance in my life?

6. Go back to the sensations of the breathing. See what ideas arise. No need to force any ideas. Just reflect on the question gently, and see what happens. You may get a new thought, image, or perhaps a feeling.

7. When you're ready, bring the meditation to a close and jot down any ideas that may have arisen.

TIP

Refer to *Work/Life Balance For Dummies* by Katherine Lockett and Jeni Mumford (Wiley) or *Mindfulness at Work For Dummies* by Shamash Alidina and Juliet Adams (Wiley) for more on this topic.

Building a better relationship with yourself

Trees need to withstand powerful storms, and the only way they can do that is by having deep roots for stability. With shallow roots, the tree can't really stand upright. The deeper and stronger the roots, the bigger and more plentiful are the branches that the tree can produce. In the same way, you need to nourish your relationship with yourself to effectively branch out to relate to others in a meaningful and fulfilling way.

TIP

Here are some tips to help you begin building a better relationship with yourself by using a mindful attitude:

>> **Set the intention.** Begin with a clear intention to begin to love and care for yourself. You're not being selfish by looking after yourself; you're watering your own roots, so you can help others when the time is right. You're opening the door to a brighter future that you truly deserve as a human being.

>> **Understand that no one's perfect.** You may have high expectations of yourself. Try to let them go, just a tiny bit. Try to accept at least one aspect of yourself that you don't like, if you can. The smallest of steps make a huge difference. Just as a snowball starts small and gradually grows as you roll it through the snow, so a little bit of kindness and acceptance of the way things are can start off a positive chain reaction to improve things for you.

>> **Step back from self-criticism.** As you practice mindfulness, you become more aware of your thoughts. You may be surprised to hear a harsh, self-critical inner voice berating you. Take a step back from that voice if you can, and know that *you're not your thoughts*. When you begin to see this, the thoughts lose their sting and power.

>> **Be kind to yourself.** Take note of your positive qualities, no matter how small and insignificant they seem, and acknowledge them. Maybe you're polite, or perhaps you're generous or a good listener. Whatever your positive qualities are, notice them rather than looking for the negative aspects of yourself or what you can't do. Being kind to yourself isn't easy, but through mindfulness and by taking a step-by-step approach, it's definitely possible.

>> **Forgive yourself.** Remember that you're not perfect. You make mistakes; so does everyone. Making mistakes makes us human. By understanding that you can't be perfect in what you do, and can't get everything right, you're more able to forgive yourself and move on. Ultimately, you can learn only through making mistakes: If you did everything correctly, you'd have little to discover about yourself. Give yourself permission to forgive yourself.

>> **Be grateful.** Develop an attitude of gratitude. Try being grateful for all that you do have, and all that you can do. Can you see, hear, smell, taste, and touch? Can you think, feel, walk, and run? Do you have access to food, shelter, and clothing? Use mindfulness to become more aware of what you have. Every evening before going to bed, write down three things that you're grateful for, even if they're really small and insignificant. Writing gratitude statements each evening has been proven to be beneficial for many people. Try this for a month, and continue if you find the exercise helps you in any way.

» **Practice metta/lovingkindness meditation.** *Metta* is a Buddhist term meaning lovingkindness or friendliness. Metta meditation is designed to generate a sense of compassion both for yourself and toward others. All mindfulness meditations make use of an affectionate awareness, but metta meditations are specifically designed to deepen this skill and direct it in specific ways. When you practice a metta meditation, certain phrases may arise from your heart for what you most deeply desire for yourself in a long-lasting way, and ultimately for all beings. Phrases may include these: *May I be well. May I be happy. May I be healthy. May I be free from suffering.* This is probably the most effective and powerful way of developing a deeper, kinder, and more fulfilling relationship with yourself.

REMEMBER

Practicing any one of the preceding activities regularly, even for just a minute or two per day, can help to raise your own wellbeing and help increase the quality of your relationships with others too. The secret is in regular practice rather than the length of the practice.

Chapter **6**

Using Mindfulness in Your Daily Life

Mindfulness is portable: You can be mindful anywhere and everywhere, not only on the meditation cushion or yoga mat. You can engage in a mindful state of mind while giving a presentation, feeding the cat, or hugging a friend. By cultivating a mindful awareness, you deepen your day-to-day experiences and break free from habitual mental and emotional patterns. You notice that beautiful flower on the side of the road, you become aware and release your tense shoulders when thinking about work, and you give space for your creative solutions to life's challenges. All the small changes you make add up. Your stress levels go down, your depression or anxiety becomes a bit more manageable, and you begin to be more focused. You need to put in some effort to achieve this, but a totally different effort to the kind you're probably used to; you're then bound to change in a positive way. This chapter offers some of the infinite ways of engaging this ancient art and modern science of mindfulness in your daily life.

Using Mindfulness at Work

Work. A four-letter word with lots of negative connotations. Many people dislike work because of the high levels of stress they need to tolerate. A high level of stress isn't a pleasant or healthy experience, so you should welcome any way of managing that stress with open arms.

So how can mindfulness help with work?

>> Most importantly, mindfulness gives you the space to relate to your stress in a more healthy way.

>> Mindfulness has been found to lower levels of stress, anxiety, and depression.

>> Mindfulness leads to a greater ability to focus, even when under pressure, which then results in higher productivity and efficiency and more creativity.

>> Mindfulness improves the quality of relationships, including those at work.

REMEMBER

Mindfulness isn't simply a tool or technique to lower stress levels. Mindfulness is a way of being. Stress reduction is the tip of the iceberg. One business organization aptly said: "Mindfulness goes to the heart of what good business is about — deepening relationships, communicating responsibly, and making mindful decisions based on the present facts, not the limits of the past." When employees understand that giving mindful attention to their work actually improves the power of their brain to focus, their work becomes more meaningful and inspiring.

Beginning the day mindfully

Watching the 100-meter race in the Olympics, you see the athletes jump up and down for a few minutes before the start, but when they prepare themselves in the blocks, they become totally still. They focus their whole being completely, listening for the gunfire to signify the start. They begin in stillness. Be inspired by the athletes: Begin your day with an inner stillness, so you can perform at your very best.

TIP

Start the day with a mindfulness exercise. You can do a full formal meditation such as a body scan or a sitting meditation, or perhaps some yoga or stretching in a slow and mindful way. Alternatively, simply sit up and feel the gentle ebb and flow of your own breath, or listen to the sounds of the birds as they wake up and chirp in the morning. Other alternatives include waking up early and eating your breakfast mindfully, or perhaps tuning in to your sense of smell, sight, and touch fully as you have your morning bath or shower; see what effect that has. That's better than just worrying about your day.

Dropping in with mini meditations

When you arrive at work, you can easily be swept away by it all and forget to be mindful of what you're doing. The telephone rings, you get email after email, and you're called into endless meetings. Whatever your work involves, your attention is sure to be sucked up.

This habitual loss of attention and going from activity to activity without really thinking about what you're doing is called *automatic pilot mode.* You simply need to change to mindful awareness mode. The most effective way of doing this is by one- to three-minute mini meditations, by feeling the sensation of your own breath as it enters and leaves your body. (Head to Chapter 4 in Book 1 for more about changing from automatic pilot.)

REMEMBER

The breathing space meditation (a type of mini meditation) consists of three stages. In the first stage you become aware of your thoughts, emotions, and bodily sensations. In the second stage you become aware of your own breathing. And in the third and final stage you expand your awareness to the breath and the body as a whole. For lots more on how to do the breathing space meditation, check out Chapter 5 in Book 1.

TIP

When you're at work, give a mini meditation a go:

>> **When?** You can do a mini meditation at set times or between activities. So when you've finished a certain task or job, you take time to practice a mini meditation before heading to the next task. In this way you increase the likelihood of being calm and centered, rather than flustered, by the time you get to the end of the day or working week. If you don't like the rigidity of planning your mini meditations ahead of time, just practice them whenever the thought crosses your mind and you feel you need to go into mindfulness mode.

Additionally, you can use the meditation to cope with a difficult situation, such as your boss irritating you. One way of coping with the wash of emotion that arises in such situations is to do a three-minute coping (breathing space) meditation (described in full in Chapter 5 of Book 1).

>> **How?** Use any posture you like, but sit up if you wish to energize yourself through the practice. The simplest form of mini meditation is to feel your breathing. If you find your mind wanders a lot when feeling your breath, you can say to yourself "in" as you breathe in, and "out" as you breathe out. Alternatively, count each out-breath to yourself, going from one to ten. As always, when your mind drifts off, simply guide the attention gently and kindly back, even congratulating yourself for noticing that your mind had wandered

off the breath. Remember to accept and embrace mind wandering as part of the mindfulness process.

>> **Where?** You can do a mini meditation anywhere you feel comfortable. Usually, meditating is easier with your eyes closed, but that's not so easy at work! You can keep your eyes open and softly gaze at something while you focus your attention inwards. One practitioner goes to a special room at work for prayer and uses the space to meditate at lunchtime. If you work outside, try going for a slow walk for a few minutes, feeling your breathing and noticing the sensations of your feet as they gently make contact with the earth. Or if the weather is nice, perhaps you can lie down in the sunshine while lying on some grass as you practice some mindfulness.

TIP

You may dearly want to try out the mini meditation at work, but you simply keep forgetting. Well, why not make an appointment with yourself? Perhaps set a reminder to pop up on your computer, or a screen saver with a subtle reminder for yourself. One practitioner popped a card on her desk with a picture of a beautiful flower. Each time she saw the picture, she took three conscious breaths. This helped to calm her and had a transformative effect on the day. Or, try a sticky note or a gentle alarm on your mobile phone. Be creative in thinking of ways to remind yourself to be mindful.

Going from reacting to responding

A *reaction* is your almost automatic thought, reply, and behavior following some sort of stimulus, such as your boss criticizing you. A *response* to a situation is a more considered, balanced choice, often creative in reply to the criticism, and leads to solving your problems rather than compounding them.

You don't have to react when someone interrupts you in a meeting, takes away your project, or sends a rude email. Instead, having a balanced, considered response is most helpful for both you and your relationship with colleagues.

For example, say you hand in a piece of work to your manager, and she doesn't even say thank you. Later on you ask what she thinks of your work, and she says it's okay, but you can tell she doesn't seem impressed. You spent lots of time and effort to do a superb report, and you feel hurt and annoyed. You *react* by either automatically thinking negative thoughts about your manager and avoiding eye contact with her for the rest of the week, or you lash out with an outburst of accusations and feel extremely tense and frustrated for hours afterwards. Here's how you can turn this into a mindful response.

TIP

Begin to feel the sensations of your breath. Notice whether you're breathing in a shallow or rapid way because of your frustration, but try not to judge yourself. Say to yourself, "in . . . out" as you breathe in and out. Expand your awareness to a sense of your body as a whole. Become mindful of the processes taking place inside you. Feel the burning anger rising from the pit of your stomach up through your chest and throat, or your racing heart and dry mouth when you're nervous. Honor the feeling instead of criticizing or blocking the emotion. Notice what happens if you don't react as you normally do or feel like doing. Imagine your breath soothing the feeling. Bring kindness and curiosity to your emotions. This isn't an easy time for you — acknowledging that is an act of self-compassion.

You may discover that the very act of being aware of your reaction changes the flavor of the sensation altogether. Your relationship to the reaction changes an outburst, for example, to a more considered response. Your tone of voice may subtly change from aggressive and demanding to being slightly calmer and more inquisitive. The point is not to try to change anything, but just to sit back and watch what's going on for a few moments.

TIP

To help you to bring a sense of curiosity when you're about to react to a situation at work, try asking yourself the following questions slowly, one at a time, and giving yourself time for reflection:

>> What feeling am I experiencing at the moment, here at work? How familiar is this feeling? Where do I feel the feeling in my body?

>> What thoughts are passing through my mind at the moment? How judgmental are my thoughts? How understanding are my thoughts? How are my thoughts affecting my actions at work?

>> How does my body feel at the moment? How tired do I feel at work? What effect has the recent level of work had on my body? How much discomfort can I feel at the moment in my body, and where is the source of it?

>> Can I acknowledge my experiences here at work, just as they are? Am I able to respect my own rights as well as responsibilities in the actions I choose? What would be a wise way of responding right now, instead of my usual reaction? If I do react, can I acknowledge that I'm not perfect and make my next decision a more mindful response?

Perhaps you'll go back to your manager and calmly explain why you feel frustrated. You may become angry too, if you feel this is necessary, but without feeling out of control. Perhaps you'll choose not to say anything today, but wait for things to settle before discussing the next step. The idea is for you to be more creative in your *response* to this frustration rather than *reacting* in your usual way, if your usual way is unhelpful and leads to further problems.

The benefits of a considered, balanced response as opposed to an automatic reaction include

>> Lower blood pressure. (High blood pressure is a cause of heart disease.)

>> Lower levels of stress hormones in your blood stream, leading to a healthier immune system.

>> Improved relationships, because you're less likely to break down communication between colleagues if you're in a calmer state of mind.

>> A greater feeling of being in control, because you're able to choose how you respond to others rather than automatically reacting involuntarily.

REMEMBER

You don't sweep your frustration or anger under the carpet. Mindfulness isn't about blocking emotions. You do the opposite: You allow yourself to mindfully feel and soothe the emotions with as much friendliness and kindness as you can muster. Even forcing a smile can help. Mindfulness is a great way to effectively overcome destructive emotions. Expressing out-of-control anger leads to more anger: You just get better at it. Suppressing anger leads to outbursts at some other time. Mindfulness is the path to easing your frustration through being genuinely curious and respectful of your own emotional experiences.

Solving problems creatively

Your ideas need room. You need space for new perceptions and novel ways of meeting challenges, in the same way that plants need space to grow, or they begin to wither. For your ideas, the space can be in the form of a walk outside, a three-minute mini meditation, or a cup of tea. Working harder is often not the best solution: working smarter is.

If your job involves dealing with issues and problems, whether that involves people or not, you can train yourself to see the problems differently. By seeing the problems as challenges, you're already changing how you meet this issue. A *challenge* is something you rise to — something energizing and fulfilling. A *problem* is something that has to be dealt with — something draining, an irritation. Studies have found people who learn to see problems as positive challenges have a more enjoyable experience of navigating a solution.

TIP

To meet your challenges in a creative way, find some space and time for yourself. Write down *exactly* what the challenge is; when you're sure what your challenge is, you find it much easier to solve. Try to see the challenge from a different person's perspective. Talk to other people and ask how they'd deal with the issue. Become mindful of your immediate reactive way of dealing with this challenge, and question the validity of it.

Practicing mindful working

Mindful working is simply being mindful of whatever you do when you work. Here are some examples of ways of being mindful at work:

» **Start the day with a clear intention.** What do you need to get done today? What attitude do you wish to bring to your day? Perhaps kindness or focus, for example. How will you ensure you're best able to achieve what you intend to do? What barriers could prevent you achieving your intention and how can you best remove or manage them? For example, if your intention is to be focused and you're likely to get distracted in the office, can you work from home or in another part of the office?

» **Be mindful of your everyday activities.** For example, when typing, notice the sense of touch between your fingers and the keyboard. Notice how quickly your mind converts a thought into an action on keys. Are you striking the keys too hard? Are your shoulders tense; is your face screwing up unnecessarily? How's your posture? Are you taking breaks regularly to walk and stretch?

» **Before writing or checking an email, take a breath.** Is this really important to do right now? Reflect for a few moments on the key message you need to get across, and remember it's a human being receiving this message — not just a computer. After sending the message, take time to feel your breath and, if you can, enjoy it. Notice how easy it is to be swept away for hours by the screen.

» **When the telephone rings, let the sound of the ring be a reminder for you to be mindful.** Let the telephone ring a few times before answering. Use this time to notice your breath and posture. When you pick it up, speak and listen with mindfulness. Notice both the tone of your own voice and the other person's. If you want to, experiment by gently smiling as you speak and listen, and become aware of the effect that has.

» **When you get a text message or other ping sound from your smart-phone, just pause for a moment.** Do you need to check your phone right now or are you in the middle of something? If it's not an ideal time to check, is now a good time to switch off your phone so that you can focus and finish the work you're doing? These small moments of choice can make a difference to your whole day.

» **No matter what your work involves, do it with awareness.** Awareness helps your actions become clear and efficient. Connect your senses with whatever you're doing. Whenever you notice your mind drifting out of the present moment, just gently bring it back.

>> **Make use of the mini meditations to keep you aware and awake at work.** The meditations are like lampposts, lighting wherever you go and making things clear.

USING MINDFUL LEADERSHIP

If you're a leader in an organization, responsibility goes with the job. Good leaders need to make effective decisions, manage emotions successfully, and keep their attention on the big picture. In their book *Resonant Leadership* (Harvard Business School Press), Richard Boyatzis and Annie McKee highlight the need for mindfulness for leadership to be most effective. They found that the ability to manage your own emotions and the emotions of others, called *emotional intelligence,* is vitally important for an effective leader, and to achieve this, you need to find a way to renew yourself.

Renewal is a way of optimizing your state of mind so you're able to work most effectively. The stress generated through leadership puts your body and mind on high alert and weakens your capacity for focus and creativity. Renewal is a necessary antidote for leadership stress, and one key way science has found to achieve this is through mindfulness.

Neuroscience has shown that optimistic, hopeful people are naturally in an *approach* mode of mind. They *approach* difficulties as challenges and see things in a positive light. Other people have more *avoidant* modes of mind, characterized by *avoiding* difficult situations and denying problems rather than facing up to them. Mindfulness practiced for just eight weeks has been shown to move people from unhelpful, *avoidant* modes to more helpful, creative, emotionally intelligent, *approach* modes of mind, leading to a greater sense of meaning and purpose, healthy relationships, and an ability to work and lead effectively.

For example, a CEO of a medium-sized corporation felt isolated and highly stressed. Through practicing tailor-made mindfulness techniques, he began to renew himself, see the business more holistically, take greater time to make critical decisions, and communicate more effectively with his team about the way forwards. He now practices mindfulness on a daily basis for 10 minutes, as well as using other strategies during the day, to create renewal.

Trying single-tasking

Everyone does it nowadays: texting as we walk, or checking emails as we speak on the phone. People multi-task to be efficient, but most of the time it actually makes you *less* efficient. And from a mindfulness perspective, your attention becomes hazy rather than centered.

Many studies by top universities show that multi-tasking leads to inefficiency and unnecessary stress. Some reasons to avoid multi-tasking and to mindfully focus on just one task at a time instead are that doing so will help you to

>> **Live in the moment:** In one hilarious study, researchers asked people who walked across a park whether they noticed a clown on a unicycle. People who were glued to their phones didn't notice it! Others did.

>> **Be efficient:** By switching between two tasks, you take longer. It's quicker to finish one task and then the other. Switching attention takes up time and energy and reduces your capacity to focus. Some experts found a 40 percent reduction in productivity due to multi-tasking.

>> **Improve relationships:** A study at the University of Essex found that just by having a phone nearby while having a person-to-person conversation had a negative impact. Give your partner your full attention as much as possible. Most people don't realize how much of a positive effect simply giving your partner your mindful awareness has.

>> **De-stress:** A study by the University of California found that when office workers were constantly checking email as they were working, their heart rates were elevated compared with those of people focusing on just one task.

>> **Get creative:** By multi-tasking, you over-challenge your memory resources. There's no space for creativity. A study in Chicago found that multi-taskers struggled to find creative solutions to problems they were given.

Finishing by letting go

You may find letting go of your work at the end of the day very difficult. Perhaps you come home and all you can think about is work. You may spend the evening talking angrily about colleagues and bosses, or actually doing more work to try to catch up with what you should've finished during the day. This impacts the quality and quantity of your sleep, lowering your energy levels for the next day. This unfortunate negative cycle can spin out of control.

REMEMBER

You need to draw a line between work and home, especially if your stress levels feel unmanageable. Meditating as soon as you get home, or on your way home (see the following section), provides an empowering way of achieving this. You're saying "enough." You're taking a stand against the tidal wave of demands on your limited time and energy. You're doing something uplifting for your health and wellbeing, and ultimately for all those around you too. And you're letting go.

To let go at the end of the day most powerfully, choose a mindful practice that you feel works best for you (like one in Chapter 5 of Book 1). Or take up a sport or hobby in which you're absorbed by gentle, focused attention — an activity that enables the energy of your body and mind to settle, and the mindfulness to indirectly calm you.

Using Mindfulness on the Move

Some people from abroad on the Underground transport system in London look at the trains with awe and take plenty of photos. Other commuters look up, almost in disgust, before burying their heads back in a book or newspaper or checking their phones. When people are on vacation, they live in the moment, and the present moment is always exciting. The new environment is a change from their routine. Traveling is another opportunity to bring mindfulness to the moment.

Walking mindfully

Take a moment to consider this question: What do you find miraculous? Perhaps you find the vastness of space amazing; perhaps you find your favorite book or band a wonder. What about walking? Walking is a miracle too. Scientists have managed to design computers powerful enough to make the Internet work and for man to land on the moon, but no robot in the world can walk anywhere nearly as smoothly as a human being. If you're able to walk, you're lucky indeed. To contemplate the miracle called walking is the beginning of walking meditation.

Normally, in a formal walking meditation, you aren't trying to get anywhere. You simply walk back and forth slowly, being mindful of each step you take, with gratitude. However, when walking to work or wherever you're going, you have a goal. You're trying to get somewhere. This creates a challenge, because your mind becomes drawn into thinking about when you're going to arrive, what you're going to do when you get there, and whether you're on time. In other words, you're not in the moment. The focus on the goal puts you out of the present moment.

TIP

Practice letting the destination go. Be in the moment as you walk. Feel the breeze and enjoy your steps if you can. If you can't enjoy the walk, just feel the sensations in your feet — that's mindfulness. Focus more on the process and less on the out-come. Keep bringing your mind back into the moment, again and again, and, hey presto, you're being mindful as you walk.

Driving mindfully

If everyone did mindful driving, the world would be a safer and happier place. Don't worry: It doesn't involve closing your eyes or going into a trance! Try this mindful driving exercise, and feel free to be creative and adapt it as you like. Remember, don't read this book while you're driving: that would be dangerous.

1. **Set your intention by deciding to drive mindfully.** Commit to driving with care and attention. Set your attitude to be patient and kind to others on the road. Leave in plenty of time to get to where you're going, so you can let go of overly focusing on your destination.

2. **Sit in the driver's seat and practice a minute or so of mindful breathing.** Feel your natural breath as it is, and come into the present moment.

3. **Start your car.** Get a sense of the weight and size of the car — a machine with tremendous power, whatever its size, and with the potential to do much damage if you drive irresponsibly, or to be tremendously helpful if you drive with mindful awareness and intelligence. Begin making your way to your destination.

4. **Be alert.** Don't switch on the music or news. Instead, let your awareness be wide and perceptive. Be aware of what other vehicles and people are doing all around you. Let your awareness be gentle, rather than forcing and straining it.

5. **See how smoothly you can drive.** Brake gradually and accelerate without excessive revving. This type of driving is less stressful and more fuel efficient.

6. **Every now and then, briefly check in with your body.** Notice any tension and let it go if you can, or become aware and accept it if you can't. You don't need to struggle or fight with the tension.

7. **Show a healthy courtesy to your fellow drivers.** Driving is all about trusting and co-operating with others. Use any opportunities you can to be kind to your fellow drivers.

8. **Stay within the speed limit.** If you can, drive more slowly than you normally do. You'll soon grow to enjoy that pace, and may be safer.

9. **Take advantage of red traffic lights and traffic jams.** If the lights are about to change to red, stop rather than speed through. Smile when you meet traffic. Getting annoyed will not get you to your destination any faster. This is a great opportunity to do traffic meditation! This is a time to breathe. Look out of the window and notice the sky, the trees, and other people. Let this be a time of rest for you, rather than a time to become anxious and frustrated. Note that stress isn't caused by the situation but by the attitude you bring to the circumstance. Bring a mindful attitude, just as an experiment, and see what happens. You may discover a different way of living altogether.

Traveling mindfully on public transport

If you travel on a bus, train, or plane, you're not in active control of the transport itself, and so you can sit back and be mindful. Most people plug themselves into headphones or read, but mindfulness is another option. Why not exercise your mind while traveling? If commuting is part of your daily routine, you can listen to a guided mindfulness exercise or just practice by yourself. If you think you'll go deeply into meditation, ensure that you don't miss your stop by setting the alarm on your watch or phone.

The disadvantage of practicing mindfulness in this way is the distractions. You may find yourself being distracted by sudden braking or the person who keeps snoring right next to you. Consider practicing your core mindfulness meditation in a relatively quiet and relaxed environment, such as your bedroom, and using a mindfulness exercise while traveling as a secondary meditation. Ultimately there are no distractions in mindfulness: Whatever you experience can be the object of your mindful attention.

TIP

Here are some specific mindfulness experiments to try while on the move:

>> **See whether you can be mindful of your breath from one station to the next, just for fun.** Whether you manage isn't the issue: This is just an experiment to see what happens. Do you become more mindful or less? What happens if you put more or less effort into trying to be mindful?

>> **Hear the various announcements and other distractions as sounds to be mindful of.** Let the distractions be part of your mindful experience. Listen to the pitch, tone, and volume of the sound, rather than thinking about the sound. Listen as you'd listen to a piece of music.

>> **See whether you can tolerate and even welcome unpleasant events.** For example, if two people are talking loudly to each other, or someone is listening to noisy music, notice your reaction. What particular thought is stirring up emotion in you? Where can you feel the emotion? What happens when you imagine your breath going into and out of that part of your body?

>> **Allow your mindful awareness to spill into your walk to wherever you're going.** As you walk, feel your feet making contact with the ground. Notice how the rate of your breathing changes as you walk. Allow your body to get into the rhythm of the walk, and enjoy the contact of the surrounding air with your skin as you move.

Using Mindfulness in the Home

Not only is doing mindfulness meditation and exercise at home convenient, but it also helps you to enjoy your everyday activities as well. Then, rather than seeing chores as a burden, you may begin to see them as opportunities to enjoy the present moment as it is.

Waking up mindfully

When you wake up, breathe three mindful breaths. Feel the whole of each in-breath and the whole of each out-breath. Try adding a smile to the equation if you like. Think of three things you're grateful for — a loved one, your home, your body, your next meal — anything. Then slowly get up. Enjoy a good stretch. Cats are masters of stretching — imagine you're a cat and feel your muscles elongate having been confined to the warmth of your bed all night. If you want to, do some mindful yoga or tai chi.

Then, if you can, do some formal mindful meditation. You can do five minutes of mindful breathing, a 20-minute sitting meditation, or a body scan meditation — choose what feels right for you.

Doing everyday tasks with awareness

The word *chore* makes routine housework unpleasant before you've even started. Give your chores a different name to help spice them up, such as dirt-bursting, vacuum-dancing, mopping 'n' bopping, or home sparkling!

The great thing about everyday jobs, including eating, is that they're slow, repetitive physical tasks, which makes them ideal for mindfulness. You're more easily able to be mindful of the task as you do it. Here are a few examples to get you started.

Washing dishes

Recently, one practitioner who works from home found mindful dishwashing a transformative experience. She realized that she used to wash dishes to have a break from work, but when washing up she was still thinking about the work. By connecting with the process of dishwashing, she felt calmer and relaxed, renewed and ready to do a bit more creative work.

Have a go:

1. **Be aware of the situation.** Take a moment to look at the dishes. How dirty are they? Notice the stains. See how the dishes are placed. What color are they? Now move into your body. How does your physical body feel at the moment? Become aware of any emotions you feel — are you annoyed or irritated? Consider what sort of thoughts are running through your mind; perhaps, "When I finish this, then I can relax," or "This is stupid."

2. **Begin cleaning, slowly to begin with.** Feel the warmth of the water. Notice the bubbles forming and the rainbow reflections in the light. Put slightly less effort into the scrubbing than you may normally, and let the soap do the work of cleaning. When the dish looks completely clean, wash the bubbles off and see how clean the plate looks. Allow yourself to see how you've transformed a grimy, mucky plate into a spotless, sparkling one. Now let it go. Place the dish on the side to dry. Be childlike in your sense of wonder as you wash.

3. **Try to wash each dish as if for the first time.** Keep letting go of the idea of finishing the job or of the other things you could be doing.

4. **When you've finished, look at what you've done.** Look at the dishes and how they've been transformed through your mindful awareness and gentle activity. Congratulate yourself on having taken the time to wash the dishes in a mindful way, thereby training your mind at the same time.

REMEMBER

All meditation is like mindfully washing dishes. In mindfulness you're gently cleaning your mind. Each time your attention wanders into other thoughts and ideas, you become aware of the fact and gently step back. Each step you take back from your unruly thoughts is a cleansing process.

Vacuuming

Using the vacuum cleaner, another common activity in many people's lives, is usually done while your mind is thinking about other things — which isn't actually experiencing the process of vacuuming. Try these steps to experience mindfulness while vacuuming:

1. **Begin by noticing the area you want to clean.** What does it look like and how dirty is the floor? Notice any objects that may obstruct your vacuuming. Become mindful of your own physical body, your emotions, and thoughts running through your mind.

2. **Tidy up the area so you can use the vacuum cleaner in one go, without stopping, if you can.** This ensures you have time to get into the rhythm of the activity without stopping and starting, helping you to focus.

3. **Switch the vacuum cleaner on.** Notice the quality of the sound and feel the vibrations in your arm. Begin moving the vacuum cleaner, getting into a calm rhythm if possible, and continue to focus your mindful attention on your senses. Stay in the moment if you can, and when your mind takes your attention away, acknowledge that and come back into the here and now.

4. **When you've finished, switch off and observe how you feel.** How was the process different to how you normally vacuum the floor? Look at what you've done and be proud of your achievement.

Eating mindfully

Regular, daily mindfulness practice is a key aspect of mindful eating. This acts as a foundation from which you can build a mindful–eating lifestyle. The discipline of mindfulness makes you aware of your emotions and thoughts. You begin to notice the kinds of situations, thoughts, and emotions that lead you to eating particular foods.

Here's how to eat a meal mindfully:

1. **Remove distractions.** Turn off the television, radio, and all other electronics. Put aside any newspapers, magazines, and books. All you need is you and your meal.

2. **Carry out three minutes of mindful breathing.** Sit with your back upright but not stiff, and feel the sensations of your breathing. Alternatively, try the three-minute breathing space detailed in Chapter 5 of Book 1.

3. **Become aware of your food.** Notice the range of colors on the plate. Inhale the smell. Remember how fortunate you are to have a meal today and be grateful for what you have.

4. **Observe your body.** Are you salivating? Do you feel hungry? Are you aware of any other emotions? What thoughts are going through your head right now? Can you see them as just thoughts rather than facts?

5. **Now slowly place a morsel of food into your mouth.** Be mindful of the taste, smell, and texture of the food as you chew. Put your cutlery down as you chew. Don't eat the next mouthful until you've fully chewed this one. At what point do you swallow? Have you chewed the food fully?

6. **When you're ready, take the next mouthful in the same way.** As you continue to eat mindfully, be aware of your stomach and the feeling of being full. As soon as you feel you've had enough to eat, stop. Because you've been eating slowly, you may find that you feel full sooner than usual.

7. **If you feel full but still have the desire to eat more, try doing another three minutes of mindful breathing.** Remember that the thought "I need to eat" is just a thought. You don't have to obey the thought and eat if that's not the best thing for you.

Try eating in this way once a day for a week or two, and become mindful of the effect it has.

Second hunger: Overcoming problem eating

When you eat, you need to

>> Eat the right amount of food, neither too much nor too little, to maintain a healthy weight.

>> Eat the right types of food for you to meet your daily nutritional needs. (See Book 5 for details on eating clean.)

However, you may not eat just to meet those needs. In reality you may eat to

>> Avoid feeling bored.

>> Cope with a sense of anger.

>> Fill a feeling of emptiness within you.

>> Satisfy a desire for some taste in particular (such as sweet or fatty food).

>> Help you cope with high levels of stress.

This "comfort eating," or emotional eating as it's sometimes called, tends to operate on an unconscious level, driving your cravings for food.

Emotional eating is like a second hunger, to satisfy the need for psychological wellbeing. Your emotions are eating rather than your stomach. You're using the food to calm your mind. This can lead to an unhealthy eating cycle. You experience a negative emotion, so you eat food to cope with the emotion, which leads to a temporary feeling of satisfaction, but before long, the negative emotion returns.

Mindful eating offers a way of becoming more aware of the inner thoughts and emotions driving your tendency to eat. Through a mindful awareness you begin naturally to untangle this web and begin to discover how to eat in a healthy and conscious way, making the right choices for you.

TIP

Additionally, you may like to try these strategies:

>> **Do a hunger reality check.** Before eating, notice whether your hunger is physical or emotional. If you've eaten recently and your tummy isn't rumbling, perhaps you can wait a little longer and see whether the sensation passes.

>> **Keep a food diary.** Simply writing down everything you eat for a few weeks is often an eye-opener. You may begin to see patterns emerging.

>> **Manage boredom.** Rather than using boredom as a reason to eat, try doing an activity such as mindful walking, or call a friend and be really aware of your conversation.

>> **Avoid extreme dieting.** By depriving yourself of certain foods, you may end up fueling your desire for that food. Instead, treat yourself occasionally and eat the food mindfully. Actually tasting the treat makes it even tastier!

2

Treating Yourself with Compassion

Contents at a Glance

CHAPTER 1: Exploring Self-Compassion 93

Befriending Yourself: A Splendid New Relationship. 94

Understanding Self-Compassion. 95

Looking at the Yin and Yang of Self-Compassion 100

Asking the Fundamental Question of Self-Compassion 102

Activating Your Secret Weapon for Safety, Warmth, and
Connection 103

Introducing the Mindful
Self-Compassion Program 105

CHAPTER 2: The Self-Compassion Road Ahead 109

Why Self-Compassion Isn't Always Easy. 110

Getting the Most Out of a Self-Compassion Practice. 112

The Four Noble Truths: A Buddhist Perspective on
Being Human 118

Finding What You Need to Feel Safe and Courageous. 120

**CHAPTER 3: Common Humanity: Connection and
Belonging** 129

The Inescapable Truth: We Need Each Other 130

Acknowledging Our Universal Human Need. 133

Two Tasks to Embrace Common Humanity 142

Practice: Just Like Me 145

CHAPTER 4: Cultivating Your Innate Kindness 149

We All Just Want to Be Happy 150

Investing in Your Capacity to Be Kind. 152

Practice: Lovingkindness for a Loved One. 153

**CHAPTER 5: Discovering Core Values: Your Inner
Compass** 159

Core Values Guide Us and "Re-Mind" Us 160

Dark Nights and Dark Clouds: Wisdom Gleaned from
Life's Challenges 168

Chapter 1

Exploring Self-Compassion

Welcome to the next step on a journey to greater self-compassion in your life. Take a moment to appreciate the road you have traveled thus far and how you came to be holding this book. It is probably safe to say that, if you are reading these words, you do not consider yourself skilled at being kind to yourself or treating yourself compassionately when you have a hard time. After all, *those* people don't buy books like this. Maybe you're "self-compassion-curious," and you are here because you have become increasingly aware that being hard on yourself, perfectionistic, and prone to bouts of shame and maybe even self-loathing is not serving you. In fact, this way of being with yourself has caused you a great deal of emotional pain and impacted your ability to do what you want to do in life and to have the things you most desire, such as joy, happiness, and satisfaction. Maybe you've observed a repeating pattern of destructive relationships, unfulfilling jobs, or unhealthy habits that you engage in to mute the pain you feel.

It may be pain or struggle or stress that brought you through the door, so to speak, but before you move on, consider looking just a little bit below the surface of those painful challenges. Specifically, the reason you took action and are seeking to find out about self-compassion is actually *not* because of the discomfort or pain that you feel. Instead, it is another part of you, that deeply understands that you deserve better, that motivated and moved you. At your very core is a deep desire to be happy and free from suffering. It is this quiet but persistent voice and inclination of the heart that moves you to seek something better for yourself.

The practice of self-compassion is really about accessing that small voice and giving it space to grow and expand. Becoming more self-compassionate is like pulling weeds around a tender seedling full of potential and beauty and bounty so that it can reach its full potential. In this metaphor, you are both the seedling and the gardener, so with a fair amount of patience, persistence, and kind intention toward yourself, you can tend this garden and harvest the fruits of your labor. You actually have everything you need inside of you to do this kindhearted, important work.

Befriending Yourself: A Splendid New Relationship

If you're like most people, you are a really good friend. When your pals have a hard time, when they miss out on a promotion or go through a divorce, you know how to respond in just the right way. You can comfort and soothe if needed, you may inspire self-confidence or cheer them on at other times, and you're generally their "rock" when times are tough. It's what you do. You're a mensch as they say in Yiddish, a good person, a stand-up guy. Not always, not perfectly, but you do your best, and friends appreciate your kind intention.

But maybe something different happens when the one who struggles is *you*. Take a moment to pause and consider this brief, guided reflection drawn from the Mindful Self-Compassion program:

1. **Pause for a moment to allow your mind to settle and to become aware of your body as it sits just where it is.**

   Create a brief pause between reading and reflecting.

2. **Call to mind a situation when a close friend was having a hard time.**

   Perhaps they failed a test in school, or they interviewed for a desirable job and they didn't get it, or they accidentally said something that made someone angry at them.

3. **See if you can recall how you responded to your friend in this situation.**

   Maybe recall how you found out about the situation and what you did upon hearing of it. What were the kinds of things you said to your friend? See if you can remember the tone of voice you used or your body posture at the time.

4. **Now take a moment to consider another scenario. Think of a time when *you* faced a misfortune.**

   Maybe you made a proposal at work that was rejected by management, or you said something that upset a romantic partner and they ended the relationship.

5. **Call to mind what went on inside your mind and heart at the time.**

   Again, how did you react? See if you can recall the words you used with yourself in the aftermath of the event. And even if you can't recall the exact words, you may recall the tone of your inner voice. You may even recall how your body felt to hear this or what emotions came up.

6. **Compare these two situations. Is there a difference in how you respond to a friend versus how you respond to yourself under similar circumstances?**

If what you discovered in the previous reflection was that you are harder on yourself than you are on your friends when things go wrong, you are in very good company. Researchers have found that the vast majority (78 percent) of the general population (at least in the United States) shares your bias toward cutting more slack to your friends. Sixteen percent report that they are more balanced in their treatment of themselves and others. And finally, 6 percent say that they are more compassionate to themselves than others (those folks are unlikely to buy this book!).

But the point of this reflection is not to highlight yet another way that you are not perfect or to imply that there is something wrong with you for being so hard on yourself. Instead, you can actually take heart! Consider the fact that you already know how to cultivate compassion and kindness, because you admitted you can do it for your dear friends.

TIP

All you have to do is orchestrate a U-turn on that compassion for others and, bingo, you've befriended yourself and you are on the road to more self-compassion. Simple. But of course, not so easy. Whenever you may struggle to offer yourself compassion in a difficult moment, consider starting by asking yourself, "How would I treat a good friend if they were going through what I'm going through? What would I say? What tone of voice would I use? What might I do to let them know that I'm here for them?" Asking yourself this question can "jump-start" your practice when your self-compassion "battery" has run down.

Understanding Self-Compassion

It's important to begin by being completely clear on what, exactly, self-compassion *is*, so that you can then proceed to cultivate it in your life. By necessity, this discussion must begin with Dr. Kristin Neff, an author and social psychologist who is the world's leading researcher and authority on self-compassion. Kristin's work, in collaboration with clinical psychologist Dr. Chris Germer, who is a pioneer in exploring the integration of psychology and contemplative practice, has resulted in the empirically supported Mindful Self-Compassion (MSC) program (described later in this chapter). But beyond the development of MSC, Neff and Germer (through their writing, speaking, and research) have raised the profile of self-compassion in the popular consciousness and contributed to a new appreciation in clinical and contemplative circles for the role of self-compassion in resilience, wellbeing, and the relief of human suffering.

Kristin Neff's research on the topic of self-compassion arose out of her own experience of discovering just how hard she was on herself as a graduate student. She thought it might be possible to cultivate a more harmonious relationship with herself through cultivating self-compassion. This direct personal experience led her to want to study the concept and understand it in a way that had not yet been researched. In turn, this led to a remarkable body of research that is cited widely around the globe, pointing to the benefits of self-compassion. Kristin developed the empirically supported Self-Compassion Scale, which enabled her and her colleagues to more directly study self-compassion and begin to understand how it is related to various other things such as mood, wellbeing, motivation, behavior change, and so on. (You can test your self-compassion at self-compassion.org/self-compassion-test/.)

If you're particularly interested in the research aspect of this topic, see Kristin's website (self-compassion.org) for a huge bibliography of published research studies on self-compassion.

Compassion at the core

First and foremost, it's important to be completely clear that compassion is the foundation for everything that you discover and practice in Book 2. Whether you direct that compassion at others or yourself, the definition of compassion remains the same. A number of different authorities, from the Merriam-Webster Dictionary to the Dalai Lama, essentially define compassion in similar terms: the awareness of distress and the desire to alleviate that distress. (Some use the term "suffering" instead of "distress," but again, it's easiest to think of these as equivalent: distress, suffering, stress, pain.)

This two-part definition (awareness of distress and the desire to alleviate it) helps to also clarify the difference between empathy and compassion, which is another question that people often have. In simple terms, empathy is the first part of the definition of compassion, without the second part. Empathy is the human capacity to relate to and sense another person's pain. Period. You can say that "empathy is a one-way street" in this regard, and it lacks the action component of compassion. One can have empathy for another person's struggle without having compassion.

Most people tend to think of compassion as it relates to compassion for other people, which is probably why self-compassion gets lost in the shuffle and so many of us are in need of a "booster" when it comes to directing this warmth toward ourselves! Self-compassion is simply the capacity to include ourselves within the circle of our compassion, a kind of "compassionate U-turn." This may sound simple on the one hand, but if you've tried, you know that it can be challenging. To appreciate the elements involved in self-compassion, it may help to start with unpacking the experience of compassion for others. By doing so, you begin to see the connection between this and self-compassion.

Take a moment to imagine a scenario where you are walking down the street and encounter a homeless woman sitting on the curb, rumpled, dirty, holding a paper cup for donations, and clearly suffering. As you consider this situation, what do you think would have to be present in you for compassion for this woman to arise? When this exercise is presented in talks about self-compassion, invariably, the responses are very similar, group after group. You can easily group the responses into three general areas that, remarkably enough, align with what Kristin Neff's research has uncovered regarding self-compassion:

» **"You have to even notice that the person is there."** This is a way of saying that one has to first be mindful to actually notice that a person in front of you is suffering. Without awareness, there is no possibility of compassion, and this awareness is referred to as mindfulness. The simple capacity to notice what is present in the moment, without judgment, is not so easy sometimes, but each of us possesses the ability.

» **"I realize that there but for the grace of God go I."** The recognition that this person is a fellow human being, who just like you, wants to be happy and free from suffering, is a powerful acknowledgement of what Kristin Neff calls common humanity. This ability to remember that all of us are human, all of us are imperfect, and that we need each other to survive is often forgotten when you are feeling isolated and different from others. But when you connect with it, it provides a solid support.

» **"I feel the desire to do something to help them out."** Simply being aware, or even noticing the common humanity, does not automatically mean that compassion has arisen, unless it includes that action component of wanting to relieve the suffering or the difficulty. You can't always actively change the circumstances, but even in this scenario, noting the desire to relieve her suffering or offering the simple gift of eye contact or a smile may be an act of kindness that is possible in the moment.

Mindfulness, common humanity, and kindness. These are the three components of self-compassion that have emerged from Kristin Neff's research, and they point the way forward for developing self-compassion if they are directed inwardly in the same way that most of us easily direct them outwardly. One way to capture this self-compassionate stance is by boiling it down to what therapist Michelle Becker coined as a "loving, connected presence."

REMEMBER

When you can be a loving (self-kindness), connected (common humanity) presence (mindfulness) for yourself, you are practicing self-compassion. Much, much easier said than done, but a nice way to keep a simple vision of your intention going forward.

Mindfulness

Book 1 explores the topic of mindfulness in greater depth, but for now it's helpful to get a basic grasp of how mindfulness plays a role in self-compassion and to contrast it with other ways of being that are less helpful or counterproductive to becoming more self-compassionate. With each of the three components — mindfulness, common humanity, and self-compassion — you may find it helpful to think of it as falling in the center of a continuum. In the case of mindfulness, it is the middle point between over-identification and being completely avoidant and checking out.

For example, consider the situation where your partner is facing a difficult medical procedure and you are concerned, worried, or afraid about the outcome of the procedure. From the standpoint of awareness, you would be most supported by finding a space between the two possible extremes:

» Constantly ruminating over potential outcomes and becoming paralyzed with anxiety constitutes over-identification

» Being totally checked out and in denial that something significant is happening to your beloved partner

Instead, you would want to stay connected, in tune with your reasonable fears but not overwhelmed by them, so that you can be present and supportive of your partner in the process. This attentional middle ground is mindfulness.

Common humanity

Chapter 3 in Book 2 covers the important role of common humanity in more detail, but getting a general sense of it here can help ground you in the foundation of self-compassion. Returning to the metaphor of balance when looking at common humanity, you can probably relate to all points on that continuum. The extremes look like this:

>> On one end of the scale is a deep and painful sense of isolation, loneliness, and feeling different from others, especially when you fail or fall short. When something goes wrong, you are convinced it is because *you* are somehow wrong or flawed or uniquely imperfect.

>> On the other end of the spectrum are those times when you become so swallowed up in another's troubles that you lose yourself in the process and become overwhelmed.

Calmly in the middle between these two extremes is a balanced sense of connection and commonality with your fellow human beings, a deep awareness that at times we all suffer, fall short, and fail. When you are resting in a sense of common humanity after having flubbed an important job interview, you recognize that your imperfections are not actually *yours* in the sense that all humans (and the other candidates for the job) are imperfect. Rather than feeling uniquely flawed and fatally doomed to a life of mediocrity and solitude, you see this as one episode in a larger life. You can learn from your errors and perhaps seek the comfort of friends and colleagues who can relate with having had unfortunate experiences in key important situations. This is the healing power of common humanity.

Self-kindness

Our innate inclination toward kindness and happiness is further explored in Chapter 4 of Book 2, and as the third component of self-compassion, it is the warm ribbon that ties all three together into a package of goodwill in the face of difficulty. As nice as you may feel when you can muster up some kindness for yourself in challenging times, it may feel incredibly elusive at other times. Opposite ends of the self-compassion spectrum look like this:

>> Many people are more acutely aware of self-criticism, self-deprecation, and self-recrimination. You may be someone who lives with the voice of a harsh and judgmental inner critic: a constant badgering, undermining, and demeaning voice that pokes you unmercifully and may have been with you for as long as you can remember.

>> The other end of the spectrum is slightly more seductive and seems quite nice at first glance, but self-indulgence, just doing what feels good in the moment regardless of whether it is exactly what you need or even in your best interests, is another extreme that does not support self-compassion.

Self-kindness is that middle space that you might think of as the good parenting that you may or may not have had growing up. As an adult, you understand how to keep the big picture in mind when your son stays out past curfew because he was with friends having fun and lost track of the time. You know that berating him for being irresponsible and lazy is not a helpful way to react (however afraid you were that something had happened to him when he wasn't home at the appointed time). On the other hand, simply shrugging it off and saying, "That's okay, I'm just glad you're fine" may not be appropriate either if you want him to develop responsibility and maturity. The reasonable, compassionate response is somewhere in between, where you make clear your expectations and how he violated them, provide appropriate consequences, and emphasize your love and respect for him. This is the balanced essence of kindness that is not indulgent but not overly critical either.

Looking at the Yin and Yang of Self-Compassion

Self-compassion suffers from what people in the public relations business call "an image problem." Think about what comes to mind when you first see the phrase "self-compassion," or what a stranger might think when they see the title of this book. Perhaps something comforting or soothing or cuddly springs to mind. Maybe the term conjures the image of a rustic hot tub on a chilly autumn evening or a warm cup of cocoa by the fire in the ski lodge. You might think of this practice as soothing, comforting, and nurturing — something to do when you hit a bumpy stretch that helps you settle down and meet yourself with patience and kindness, the way you would counsel a good friend to handle such a situation. And you would not be wrong about that. But there is a whole other side of the practice that balances this softer side of self-compassion and is equally important.

You may have a tendency to see self-compassion as nurturing and soothing because your mental model of what compassion looks like usually comes from the example of how a mother may nurture or comfort her child when the child is upset or suffering. As a result, you are likely to link compassion more broadly to a more traditional feminine gender role, and therein lies the flaw in your appreciation of what compassion really includes.

The goal here is to help illuminate your understanding of self-compassion so that you can appreciate its full expression, which will likely dispel some myths or misunderstandings you may have about the practice and allow you to open to it more easily.

Compassion can best be thought of as a complete whole that has a complementary side to this soft side as well. The other side of compassion (including self-compassion) is more stereotypically masculine and linked to action-oriented gender roles.

Consider the job of a brave Coast Guardsman (the official title for a uniformed member of the U.S. Coast Guard, irrespective of gender). These individuals risk their lives, dangling out of helicopters to pluck hapless boaters from the icy waves and pulling shivering fishermen from the hulls of capsized boats. It's hard to imagine a more compassionate act than putting aside one's own safety for the good of another. There's nothing warm and fuzzy about that!

Or, in another scenario, imagine facing someone making an unwanted and uninvited romantic advance, and needing to firmly say "no!" to protect yourself. This is also an act of self-compassion that is more about strength and speaking your truth than soothing or comforting yourself.

Taken together, you can appreciate that self-compassion has both tender (stereotypically feminine) and fierce (stereotypically masculine) sides. They complement each other in a beautiful dance between "being with" ourselves in a compassionate way and "acting in the world" to get things done. In Chinese philosophy this combination is represented by yin and yang, and indicates that all seemingly opposite attributes, such as masculine-feminine, light-dark, and active-passive, are complementary and interdependent. This idea is represented by the familiar symbol shown in Figure 1-1.

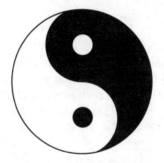

FIGURE 1-1: The yin-yang symbol.

© John Wiley & Sons, Inc.

The *yin* side is most associated with the tender aspect of comforting, soothing, and validating ourselves in times of great difficulty. On the flip side, the *yang* aspect of self-compassion is linked to fiercely protecting ourselves, providing for our needs, and motivating ourselves to take action. All of these are self-compassion, and all are ultimately in our own best interests, but in quite different and complementary forms.

REMEMBER

It is notable that each side of the symbol contains a dot of the other side within it, showing that neither side loses touch with the other. For example, imagine finding out that you failed an important test because your professor accidentally told you to read the wrong chapter in the textbook. You are fuming over the unfairness of it and considering writing a nasty email to the professor that vents a semester's worth of frustration in a couple of paragraphs. You pause for a moment and simply acknowledge the situation by saying to yourself, "This is really unfair, and it hurts to feel this anger right now." In this moment you are both validating your anger in a yin way by naming it and acknowledging that it is hard, but it also requires a "dot" of yang strength and resolve to be willing to turn toward your anger first, when you really want to discharge it with a nasty email that will certainly make things worse.

Taken together, the yin and the yang energy of self-compassion support you in making wiser, more effective choices that are ultimately in your best interests.

Asking the Fundamental Question of Self-Compassion

In the end, for all the components and facets and considerations about self-compassion, it boils down to developing the capacity to ask and respond to a very simple question:

What do I need?

That's it. It's no more complex than simply stopping in a moment (or a whole stream of moments) and checking to respond to what is present for you and to see what you need. The act of stopping itself is an act of kindness, and it creates a space for you to step out of the stream (or raging river!) of life and to see with clarity and kindness what you may need.

Okay, although it is simple, it's not easy; otherwise, Kristin Neff and Chris Germer would not have dedicated their entire professional careers to understanding, exploring, and sharing the practice. But at its core, it comes down to this simple question and how you answer it. As noted earlier, this is generally easy enough for you to do for your friends and loved ones when *they* struggle, face failure, or have a hard time, but so often you look past your own struggles and pain, ignore them, deny them, or push them aside for whatever reason.

REMEMBER

But there is profound truth in the statement (sometimes attributed to the Buddha): "You, yourself, as much as anybody in the entire universe, deserve your love and affection." Why not? Who are you *not* to deserve your own kindness, patience, and care?

Activating Your Secret Weapon for Safety, Warmth, and Connection

We all possess the necessary neural and biochemical circuitry to access our innate instincts to foster safety, warmth, and connection. You can think of it as your "mammalian secret weapon" that's always at the ready and always available to you in all situations, not just to connect with others but to feel safe and secure in your own skin too.

You may be wondering about how to access your secret weapon, and there, the science is quite clear. The mammalian caregiving system is triggered by two primary means that are both relatively easy for you to engage: soothing touch and gentle vocalization. Think about how you may soothe a screaming child, and it becomes quite obvious how you can meet yourself in the same way. You reach to caress or reassure the child with your kind and gentle touch, and you may coo or whisper or hum a lullaby in the child's ear with the sweetest of tones. Together, these simple things release the cuddle hormone and the body's built-in opiates to foster a tiny little cocoon of safety and security around you. The same things happen to your adult self when you meet yourself with your own touch and compassionate self-talk.

REMEMBER

By offering yourself soothing touch and warm, gentle vocalizations (the Mammalian Secret Weapon), you activate your innate mammalian caregiving system, counteract the fight-or-flight you may be experiencing, and ultimately reclaim your place as a mindful, compassionate, evolved being. For now.

Discovering which form of touch works for you

TIP

To develop a practice of offering yourself compassion when you struggle and suffer to engage the mammalian caregiving system, you can begin by experimenting with what sort of soothing touch *you* can offer yourself. It can be your go-to recipe for self-kindness in a difficult moment. Here are some tips:

>> You may want to stand up for this little experiment or at least take a short stretch break so you can fully tune in to how your body feels. Allow your eyes to close if you like to focus more specifically on the senses you feel during this exercise.

>> Begin by gently pressing your palms against one another and just notice whatever sensations you feel. Continue to do this with each subsequent instruction, pausing for a few seconds between each.

>> Try cupping one hand in the other or grasping one hand with the other so that you are effectively holding your own hand.

>> Gently place the open palm of one hand over your heart and then place the other open palm over the first.

>> Try forming a fist with one hand over your heart and placing an open palm over the fist.

>> Try placing just one palm over the heart.

>> Place one hand over the heart and the other over the belly.

>> Try placing both hands over the belly.

>> Experiment with placing one hand on one cheek.

>> Try placing one hand on each cheek, cradling your face in your hands.

>> Try crossing your arms across your torso and giving yourself a gentle hug. (Think of this as the surreptitious self-hug).

>> Gently stroke one arm with the hand of the other arm.

Take some time to go back and linger among these various forms of soothing and supportive touch to find which one "clicks" for you and perhaps unlock a little cuddle hormone in *your* body when you offer it to yourself. Some of these gestures are likely to be more pleasant than others, and some may actually be unpleasant. Remember that there is no one right way or one right form of touch. What works for you?

Knowing that sometimes it's all in the tone

Most of us have had the experience (especially when we were teenagers) of having had someone (usually a parent) say, "Don't use that tone with me!" Whether you were the parent or the teen (or both) in that scenario, you know the bottom line: Tone matters.

So it's not surprising that the way in which you speak to yourself in your own head also matters. In this context, you don't have to think about words just yet, but just gentle, soothing vocalizations like what you might offer the upset child. And these sounds just ooze compassion and kindness.

TIP

Pause for a moment and take a deep breath or two. Then, at the end of a nice deep in-breath, let yourself vocalize the natural sound of a nice, long, delicious out-breath as you release it. The sound is "Ahhhhhhhhh." Let it extend as long as it feels comfortable. Notice how you feel in your body in the aftermath of this soothing sound of letting go and becoming present. In other words, this is the sound (and the feel) of mindfulness.

Now, when you're ready, take another deep breath and maybe imagine you just saw the cutest baby photo of a beloved friend or a basset puppy trip over his long ears. Let your exhale be one of warmth and tenderness, sounding something like "Awwwwwww" and extending again as long as you like. Let this feeling of affection and compassion linger and notice how it feels as the oxytocin floods your system.

Introducing the Mindful Self-Compassion Program

In 2009, Chris Germer published *The Mindful Path to Self-Compassion,* which was the culmination of many years of contemplative practice, clinical experience, and training. Chris's personal journey (much like Kristin's, which was detailed in her own book, *Self-Compassion*) had led him to his life's work of teaching and speaking about integrating self-compassion practice into daily life and into psychotherapy to support people in feeling happier, more fulfilled, and able to overcome challenging histories. In 2008 Chris and Kristin (at the time, mere distant colleagues) were invited to participate in an important meeting of the Mind and Life Institute in upstate New York and Chris offered to give Kristin a ride to that conference. On the auspicious journey back to the airport after the conference, the Mindful Self-Compassion (MSC) program was born.

Kristin was the social psychologist who had done significant research on self-compassion but never considered herself someone who could teach the practice to others. Chris was a well-respected clinical psychologist with years of experience, study, and teaching of the practical application of self-compassion with a relatively modest research background. Chris and Kristin each started suggesting the other was the perfect person to create a self-compassion training program and ultimately decided that they were better together than apart.

Working together and drawing on their respective experience and study, Chris and Kristin developed the program that they first offered at a workshop in 2010 at the fabled Esalen Institute on the central California coast. Despite the later success, it was an inauspicious beginning, as 12 people had signed up for the course and three dropped out within a day or so. (These days, their programs draw huge crowds.) Kristin and Chris later conducted a randomized controlled trial of the MSC program with very promising results, pointing to increased self-compassion as a result of the training (an important first point to establish — that one can actually learn to be more self-compassionate), as well as improved mood and greater quality of life, among other findings.

The MSC program has since grown and improved year by year, with the help and support of the nonprofit Center for Mindful Self-Compassion, and over 2,700 people are now trained to teach the program worldwide. Research on MSC continues, and it is estimated that over 100,000 people worldwide have experienced the program in one form or another. The teachers continue to report remarkable impact on the participants in their courses.

Book 2 and the vast majority of meditations, exercises, and topics in it are largely inspired by and drawn from the MSC program. It is a powerful and empirically supported way of systematically developing greater self-compassion. MSC is highly recommended for those who find the material in Book 2 to be helpful. The opportunity to discover and practice self-compassion in the context of a group (whether in-person or online) is tremendously valuable because of the greater sense of common humanity, among many other reasons.

Practice: The Self-Compassion Break

This is the quintessential practice taken directly from the Mindful Self-Compassion program and is perfectly suited to support you in deploying the three components of self-compassion in a moment of difficulty. It's presented here like a formal meditation, but this is only to help you become familiar with the practice. The real value is in practicing it when you face a difficult moment or a time when you are feeling distressed or upset in some way. But for now, give yourself this opportunity to become familiar with the practice. Follow these steps:

1. **Begin by taking some time to relax.**

   Allow your gaze to soften and your face to relax. Notice your body sitting here. Perhaps take note of your breath moving in and out, over and over, as it does whether you are attending to it or not.

2. **Call to mind a situation in your life that is difficult right now and causing you stress.**

   It may be a health issue, a challenging relationship, a work problem, or perhaps stress related to one of your identities, such as your gender, race, ethnicity, age, or ability. Do your best to choose a problem in the mild to moderate range, not a big problem. Remember, this time through you are just learning this skill of self-compassion, perhaps for the first time.

3. **Give yourself time to really bring the situation to mind, to see, hear, and feel your way into the problem, perhaps enough so that you notice some uneasiness or discomfort in your body associated with it.**

   Where do you happen to feel it the most just now? See if you can have a sense of where it is in the body and simply open to noticing it as it is.

4. **As you sense the discomfort in your awareness, note to yourself, slowly and clearly, "This is a moment of suffering."**

This is *mindfulness*, simply opening awareness to what is present. Other words you might use are "Ouch!" or "This hurts," or "This is painful." Take your time and acknowledge what is here for you.

5. **Say to yourself, slowly and clearly, "Suffering is a part of living."**

This is *common humanity* as you note that all humans have moments like this. You may say instead, "I'm not alone," or "Me too," or "Others in my community would feel a lot like me in a situation like this." Remember that suffering is a universal experience, even though it is not equal across individuals or groups. Maybe you can have a sense of at least one person similar to yourself who may feel this like you do.

6. **Place your open palms over your heart or wherever it may feel support-ive to you, feeling the warmth and tenderness of your touch.**

You might say to yourself, "May I be kind to myself," or "May I give myself what I need." This is the self-kindness that you often long for but may not receive from yourself.

You can even explore just what kind of self-compassion you need just now, whether it is yin compassion or yang compassion. Yin might be "May I accept myself as I am" or "May I bring tenderness to myself just now." If you feel that yang is more appropriate, you might say, "No. I will not allow this to continue," or perhaps "May I have the courage and strength to make a change when I can."

TIP

If you find it hard to locate just the right words for yourself at any point in this Self-Compassion Break, you might consider imagining what would flow from your heart and mouth if a dear friend were facing a similar situation. What would you say to them, heart to heart, if they were feeling this discomfort? Once you've identified some words, can you offer those same words to yourself as well?

7. **Whenever you are ready and you feel you've given yourself what you need, allow your gaze to raise and your eyes to take in your surroundings.**

Take some time to settle, reflect, and perhaps take notes.

Inquiring: What arose for you when you took a Self-Compassion Break?

Notice that the Self-Compassion Break incorporates the three components of self-compassion (mindfulness, common humanity, and self-kindness) as well as the two sides of self-compassion (yin and yang), all wrapped up in a fairly straightforward practice. As noted in the preceding section, this practice is intended for you to deploy at a moment's notice when you become aware of struggle, pain, or stress in a moment. It can be as simple and brief as stepping through the three components in a cascade for a few seconds or creating some time and space to linger with each element of the break, whatever is needed and possible in a moment.

Reflect on the break afterward by considering the following questions:

>> When you called to mind the difficult situation, how was that for you? What was most noticeable when you imagined the difficult situation?

>> What was your experience in each of the three steps of the Self-Compassion Break? What was it like to acknowledge mindfulness, common humanity, and self-kindness?

>> Do you think you could use this practice in the future, the next time you face a challenge or difficulty?

Give it a try and see if you can do a Self-Compassion Break a time or two in the next day or so and see what happens and what you notice. Let go of needing anything to change just yet, and be patient with yourself as you slowly develop this capacity to respond differently in challenging situations. This will all take time, and you are only just beginning!

By the way, it is possible that you found placing your hands over your heart not particularly supportive or pleasant. A certain percentage of people find this to be the case. For now, be willing to experiment and see if there are other places on the body that may be better for you. You can explore other options for this soothing and supportive touch earlier in this chapter.

One last note: This practice run includes calling to mind a difficult situation so that you have a problem to work with as you begin to practice the process. As you continue to practice self-compassion, you don't need to pause to call to mind a challenging situation. Life will do quite a good job of handing you all the difficulties you need to master the practice; there's no need for you to open yourself to additional, unnecessary suffering. Just be patient and begin to notice when it happens. And it will.

IN THIS CHAPTER

» Facing the challenges of self-compassion

» Getting the most out of self-compassion practice

» Understanding the four noble truths

» Practicing from a place of courage and safety

Chapter **2**

The Self-Compassion Road Ahead

Simply having enough information, science, or even inspiration won't necessarily turn you into a more self-compassionate human being. You can read a hundred books on swimming, watch dozens of YouTube videos of Olympic swimming competitions, and talk to all your friends who swim, but you're not a swimmer until you get into the water and do it. And the same is true of self-compassion.

Fortunately, with self-compassion, you don't have to just plunge into the deep end of the pool, so to speak, and flounder around until you either swim or drown. But you do need the willingness to change some old habits and patterns, to do some things that may not feel completely familiar or comfortable or even easy, and to have an open mind and patience about the whole process as you dip your toe in the waters of self-compassion practice. This chapter shows you some ways to take care of yourself so that you can get the most out of this challenging practice.

REMEMBER

Don't lose hope if you are thinking right now that your particular feelings are just too painful, too overwhelming, or too pervasive to be helped by self-compassion. This is simply not the case. You have come to the right place, and the secret is all in how you pace yourself and take care of yourself while making this important change.

This chapter prepares you well for the challenges ahead. You belong here, and if you remember that, even when the going gets tough, you will be glad you stayed.

Note: For ease of communication here, this book uses the umbrella term "suffering." Many of us equate the word "suffering" to the kind of intense unfortunate suffering that people experience in abuse, neglect, war, and other violence. This level of suffering is what you may refer to as "Capital 'S' Suffering." This book uses "suffering" to encompass any form of discomfort, stress, uneasiness, pain, or distress — it may be helpful to think of it as "lowercase 's' suffering." This is the kind of suffering that we all experience as humans in our everyday lives. Some call it "struggle" or "stress" instead.

Why Self-Compassion Isn't Always Easy

Perhaps the most difficult part of self-compassion is the fact that you need to encounter and work with pain and suffering to practice it. The joke among Mindful Self-Compassion teachers is that the program is really more like the "Opening to Pain and Suffering Program," but if they actually called it that, nobody would sign up! Who wants to experience challenging emotions or difficult thoughts? Did you buy this book because you wanted to experience discomfort? Probably not. As a matter of fact, it may have been your suffering or discomfort that drove you to explore this practice in the first place. In other words, you came here to *get rid* of suffering and find more ease, and now you're finding out that in order to find ease, you may have to feel the things you least want to feel.

At this point, you may be feeling betrayed and disillusioned, and you may be entertaining a few thoughts of quitting now and trying something else to control, avoid, or reduce the suffering in your life. But before you do this, take a little journey down memory lane to review your path to this particular moment. (This exercise is drawn from the innovative *Acceptance and Commitment Therapy* developed by Stephen Hayes and colleagues.) Carefully consider your answers to the following prompts:

>> Have there been times in your life when you found yourself suffering and wanting to somehow control these feelings through avoiding, suppressing, or ignoring them?

>> What, specifically, did you do in response to those feelings to try to control them? (For example: Did you distract yourself; deny the feelings; do relaxation exercises or meditate; drink alcohol, eat, or take drugs; go to a therapist or doctor?)

>> Whatever coping strategy you chose (and you may have chosen several over the years), how did each one work at first? Did you feel better or get some relief?

>> What happened over time if you persisted with each of those same coping strategies? Did you continue to feel better or were there "diminishing returns" on your efforts? In other words, was the strategy less and less effective over time? And were there additional consequences to your coping strategy that may have made things worse? For example: Maybe you started drinking too much, over-relied upon anxiety medication, or got into trouble because you resisted or denied the feelings and actually worsened them by doing so.

>> If you think about what motivated you to try these various things to control, avoid, or eliminate your difficult emotions, is it possible that the same motivation led you to pick up this book and explore self-compassion?

If you are like most people (and frankly, aren't we all?), then the previous reflection led you to discover that you have been on a long (perhaps lifelong) quest to get rid of your suffering through various means of controlling, avoiding, or suppressing it. In the words of a certain famous TV psychologist: "How's that been working out for you so far?" It probably hasn't gone well in the long run.

So before deciding to make self-compassion your next thing in a long line of attempts to control these feelings, what would it be like to consider that perhaps the *real* problem here is not that you *have* suffering but actually the attempt to *control* these feelings in the first place? The common thread in your various attempts to contend with your suffering so far (without sustained effect) is that you have, in fact, been trying to control it. To put it another way, control is the problem.

If you instead consider self-compassion as a means of *encountering* these feelings, not to control them but to *change your relationship* with them, then there is some possibility of real, substantial change to happen. As Chapter 1 of Book 2 notes, one of the three components of self-compassion is common humanity, and it is reflected in the simple phrase from the Self-Compassion Break: "Suffering is a part of life." If you admit that these feelings are a part of the human experience, like gravity, imperfection, and death, you begin to slowly loosen the grip that they have on you because you recognize that they are experiences to be accommodated rather than problems to be solved.

Using gravity as one example, we all acknowledge that gravity exerts an influence on our lives (in practical terms, "gravity sucks," especially when we regard ourselves in the mirror periodically and see how things aren't quite where they used to be . . . thanks for that, gravity). However, despite the reality of gravity, nobody wakes up in the morning and gets out of bed, only to exclaim "Damn! I'm still stuck to the earth!" This is because we have come to terms with the reality of gravity and we work with it, rather than rail against it. The question is whether you can do the same with your very human emotions and suffering.

The pages ahead map some ways you can begin to alter your relationship with suffering, but for now just pause and consider what it takes to do this. It means that when you feel pain or discomfort, you need to let go of trying to control it, push it away, or avoid it, and instead, to some extent, be willing to lean into it and see if there is something to be gained from doing so. The idea of leaning into pain that you would rather avoid may sound awful or even terrifying (like the idea of jumping into the pool when you can't swim), but even this can be done gradually, in line with what you can manage and nothing more.

This process takes no small measure of courage now and then, but the potential payoff can be tremendous. Take some time in the following pages to consider how to chart a course for relief of your suffering that is likely to take you on some bumpy roads and take some twists and turns. And know that, like life itself, this is where the really fruitful discoveries usually happen and where we truly grow as humans.

REMEMBER

While this section speaks about difficult emotions in a somewhat lighthearted, breezy way, you may struggle mightily with incredibly painful, intense, pervasive, and debilitating emotions that are crippling at times and may seem just too overwhelming and powerful to work with in any meaningful way. This is true of large numbers of people who come to self-compassion and mindfulness courses. If this is true of you, you are not alone. Know that the guidance provided here still applies to you, but it is of paramount importance that you read this chapter carefully and follow the guidance to go slowly, allow yourself to ease into this approach, and know that balancing curiosity and self-care, safety and courage, will support you.

Getting the Most Out of a Self-Compassion Practice

Have you considered what your relationship is to this practice of self-compassion? Probably not; it's not something that most of us do on a regular basis. But if you pause and consider it, you probably do actually have a relationship to this material and practice. Perhaps you are feeling intrigued or enthralled at what you have read so far, excited even. Or perhaps your relationship to all of this is a bit more cautious and skeptical. Maybe your attitude could be summed up in the body language of sitting back with arms crossed and saying (with your eyes and your posture): "Show me what you've got." Or maybe you're feeling relieved, as if this is the thing that will finally solve the problems you face in your life. Take a moment and check in with yourself to see what your relationship is just now with the idea of being kinder to yourself when you struggle.

There is room here for all attitudes. Your attitude makes a difference in how you experience something. Think about the last time you had your favorite food. What was your attitude about that food? If you were ravenous and super-excited to be having your favorite pizza, you may have had a great deal of excitement, eaten quickly, and exclaimed loudly about how awesome it was. Or perhaps you had been anticipating it for many days and fantasizing about what it would be like, and when the day finally came, maybe you savored each bite, letting your eyes roll up in your head in delight (like they do on the TV commercials) as if the whole experience were one of pure ecstasy. Or perhaps the last time you had that favorite pizza you were engrossed in a Netflix binge-watching frenzy, and frankly, you don't really remember what the pizza tasted like. Attitudes are like that. They lead to different experiences.

And so, you're invited to have what experienced meditators call "beginner's mind" about self-compassion practice. This means letting go of your expectations and preconceived notions about self-compassion and seeing it with an open mind, like a beginner. Think of the first time you learned to do something that you now do relatively well. Everything is a discovery; there is curiosity, patience, maybe some confusion, a few missteps, but all in the service of opening to a new experience, having a new adventure. This is your invitation to approach self-compassion practice with a sense of adventure and an open mind.

Having the spirit of an adventurer

Thus far this book has spoken of your foray into self-compassion as a kind of personal journey. Notice how that notion feels in your body: You are on a journey. If you feel anything noteworthy, it may be a kind of heaviness or even fatigue in your body, as you contemplate putting one foot in front of the other for many, many steps. A journey is a task, a thing to be accomplished, a kind of solemn and noble obligation to get from here to there.

Now consider a different possibility: What if instead of a journey, you are on an adventure? Let that sink in and check in to see how that feels to you. Try it on and wear it around a little bit. It feels a bit different, right? There may be a spark of excitement, maybe a flareup of curiosity, a twinge of apprehension or even fear. When you contemplate going on an adventure, perhaps it gets your juices flowing and you have a sense of heightened awareness. Perhaps your sympathetic nervous system just dumps a few drops of adrenaline into your system.

So consider the idea that this journey is actually an adventure for you. See if you can approach it with the spirit of an adventurer, not only with a sense of beginner's mind, but also with a bit of anticipation of . . . something, though you don't yet know what. An adventure takes you into uncharted territory where you may very well encounter surprises, unanticipated obstacles, and glorious discoveries.

The obstacles in self-compassion practice may include strong emotions, hidden memories, or frustrating old patterns that try to keep you stuck in old, unworkable ways of being. Discovering these twists and turns on the adventure — the raging stream of pent-up, painful emotions; the deep ravine of untended shame; the perilous paths of persistent anxiety — is all part of the adventure of self-compassion.

Consider adopting the attitude of ancient explorers when all the maps of the earth still extended out to the distances that people had traveled, and then there were labels for the uncharted territories where it said "beyond there be dragons" to discourage future explorers from going into the unknown. Think about adventuring into these regions of the unknown, acknowledging that there is not only some fear or apprehension, but also the promise of new discoveries. You can achieve a greater sense of mastery of the inner terrain and confidence in yourself for having gone there. Be curious, patient, and willing to stretch yourself on an inner adventure.

Being a self-compassion scientist

While this book provides a guide and a map for your adventure, and accompanies you on this journey, it is up to you to explore the terrain and decide for yourself how it may suit you and what you may gain from becoming more self-compassionate. Consider adopting the attitude of a researcher: Think of what this book describes to you as your working hypothesis, use your own inner experience as your "laboratory," and observe your own "data" to come to your own conclusions.

The qualities of a good scientist include being open-minded about what you may discover (beginner's mind) and cultivating curiosity about whatever you witness. Recognizing that you are human, and as such, have various ideas (*theories*) about how things are or should be, can be a challenge to maintaining an open, curious mind. Our brains try to be efficient and like to create scripts for how things work (called *schemas*) and to summarize complex processes into simple labels (such as "successful" or "easy" or "deserving"). But as a rigorous, objective scientist, you want to look a bit closer at these assumptions and test them by studying them more closely.

For example, if you practice a meditation and find yourself characterizing it as "hard," don't settle for that label, but ask yourself, "What led me to call that meditation 'hard'? What was the *data* that led me to that conclusion?" Many times, things are not what your brain tells you they are, but you only know if you adopt the conservative approach of the researcher.

TIP

One last note about letting this process of self-compassion become a grand personal experiment: See if you can put aside the question of "why" and instead focus upon the "what" and the "how" instead. Ask yourself

>> *"What* am I aware of right now?"

>> *"What* did I notice when I was kind to myself?"

>> *"How* did I respond to a moment of struggle?"

These are the fruitful questions that researchers ask in order to gather good data.

You may wonder what's wrong with asking yourself "why" and that's a reasonable question to ask. In fact, even asking that question is actually a form of "why" question in itself ("Why can't I ask why?")! *Why* is a beautiful, deep, and thoughtful kind of question, and one that humans are uniquely able to ask and even answer sometimes. *Why* can bring some order and meaning to your experience, but when it comes to the complex world inside our hearts and minds, *why* becomes a bit of a rabbit hole down which you can easily disappear if you aren't careful. Wondering *why* you are having an emotion may lead you down a path of trying to eliminate or avoid the emotion, which is a nearly impossible thing to do. And even if you do know *why* you are feeling something, the question becomes what you can do about it if the *why* is in the past.

Sometimes the *why* question can also lead to trying to assign blame for a feeling or experience. While blame may be important in some circumstances, when speaking about your own internal experiences, it is not at all helpful. If someone else did something to lead to the feeling you have, you are still having to contend with that feeling, regardless of blame. Blame leaves you stuck and powerless when you most need to access your own compassion to support and encourage yourself.

REMEMBER

When you notice that you have an emotion, say shame, your natural human tendency is to wonder why you feel that shame and to try to ascribe a cause or a condition that led you to this feeling. But in your best scientific approach (picture yourself in the white coat of a lab researcher, looking through the microscope), your job is to simply observe what can be seen and described so that you can put this data with other data, to begin to understand your experience in a larger context. Give yourself permission to be free from the entanglement of *why* and explore the rich and fruitful world of *what* and *how* instead.

Being willing to be a slow learner and your own best teacher

In the pages ahead you will discover quite a number of different tips, tricks, meditations, exercises, and informal practices to help you develop your capacity to become more self-compassionate. As a package, it could seem impossibly hard to digest and integrate all these different elements, but luckily, you don't have to (and most people don't). What this book lays out ahead is a variety of options, a veritable self-compassion buffet, and your heart and mind (like your plate at a buffet) is only so big. Each of us has a different plate, so to speak, but the key is to not overload your plate and know that you can always come back for more, if you want. The self-compassion buffet is an all-you-can-eat affair, and fresh plates are always available. If you find a practice or way of thinking that suits you, come back for seconds and thirds. Feel free to skip other things that just don't inspire or move you. Of course, consider trying everything at least once, but don't feel obligated to embrace everything you find.

If you think of your introduction to self-compassion here as only the beginning of your adventure, then you can give yourself permission to go slowly and take it in at your own pace. In the Mindful Self-Compassion program, you can be a *slow learner* and move, as the motivational speaker Stephen Covey likes to say, at the speed of trust. Specifically, the speed of trust is the speed that is *right for you*. Don't force yourself to move faster than you are able to assimilate the material. Just because you *can* move faster doesn't mean you *should*. You can easily defeat the whole purpose of self-compassion by flogging yourself to do more, to do better, and to do faster.

REMEMBER

Learning from your own experience, relying on your inner wisdom, and moving at the speed of trust are all powerful ways of letting you be your own teacher, if you are willing to do so. You may not be confident that you have anything to offer yourself, but you do. Take some time and listen, be curious, and be patient. Only take from the buffet the things that nourish and support you, and, voilà, you've just been both student and teacher!

If it's a struggle, it's not self-compassion

As you review the challenges of practicing self-compassion, you may be wondering just exactly what you've gotten yourself into. There's some good news in all of this that you ought to know. While this work can be occasionally challenging, the ultimate goal is to find a way to practice that is actually easy and pleasant. Moments of self-compassion are actually moments of ease, comfort, and encouragement, not striving, forcing, or berating. Your aim in this practice is to reduce stress and let go of your striving for something else and working so hard to find ease. More work is not the path to ease, just as more self-criticism does not lead to self-acceptance. The ironic pirate saying is that "the beatings will continue until morale improves." Struggling to practice self-compassion is likely to be just as fruitless.

TIP

In fact, as you make your way through this practice, if you find yourself struggling, pushing yourself, or in some other way trying to make something happen, this is not actually self-compassion at all, and it's time to pause and take stock of the situation. You may wonder how to recognize and work with those moments of struggle. Here are a few tips:

1. **Notice your body.**

   If you find that your jaw is clenched, your brow is furrowed, your butt cheeks are clenched, or your shoulders are somewhere in the vicinity of your ears, you may just be trying a bit too hard. See what you can possibly let go of in the way of tension, clenching, or bracing, and see what unfolds.

2. **Listen for the sounds of resistance and forcing.**

   A moment of resistance or trying too hard can sound a bit like the sounds those Olympic weightlifters make when they thrust a barbell that weighs more than your sofa (with you on it) into the air. If the sound is something like "grrrrrr" or "aaarrrrrgggghhhh," then you are struggling and not practicing self-compassion.

3. **Take a moment to practice the sound of mindfulness.**

   The pause and letting go of needing things to be different can elicit a delicious exhale that sounds like "ahhhhhhhhh." Try it now: "ahhhhhhhhh." Notice how this feels in your body.

4. **Try a little tenderness.**

   If you're having a hard time, see if you can tap into your mammalian caregiving system for a little warmth and soothing vocalization (see Chapter 1 in Book 2). Offer yourself the quintessential sound of tender self-compassion: "awwwww-www." Try it now: "awwwwwwwww." Notice how that feels in your body. You can almost feel the endorphins flooding your bloodstream.

5. **Listen past your inner critic.**

   If you find the inner critic nattering on inside your head about what's wrong with you, see if you can simply listen *past* the critic for a few moments and listen to the other voice inside you that's been a bit quieter and wants the best for you. Maybe you can hear the whispers of self-compassion that can help you through the tough spots if you only listen.

The Four Noble Truths: A Buddhist Perspective on Being Human

While compassion and mindfulness are universal aspects of being human, various spiritual traditions have examined these qualities of mind and heart and spoken about them in quite eloquent and helpful ways. Buddhism has perhaps explored these phenomena more than most, and while self-compassion is not a Buddhist practice per se, it may help you to shift your relationship with life's suffering by looking at how they speak of suffering.

Buddhism abounds with lists of things (for example, The Three Refuges, The Eightfold Path, The Four Foundations of Mindfulness, The Seven Dwarfs — okay, maybe not the last one. . .). This book does not delve into most of these, as interesting and practical as they may be upon closer inspection, but there is one list that helps you see your own struggles in a larger context that can loosen the grip of suffering on your life and make room for a more self-compassionate stance toward life.

The Four Noble Truths comprise the essence of the Buddha's teaching and lay out, in very concrete and concise terms, what he observed about life and suffering from being a keen observer of people and experience. Therefore, these are scientific observations made in the same spirit that you're encouraged to be a scientific observer of your own experience so that you can draw your own conclusions. The Buddha came to the conclusion that if you are aware of these truths and accept or embrace them, you can find a way to liberate yourself from suffering.

TECHNICAL STUFF

A brief note on the label "The Four Noble Truths": The word "noble," in this case, refers to the discoveries made by people on the "noble path" or those who routinely embody admirable personal qualities such as honesty, generosity, and courage. And the word "truth" refers to the predictability with which these things arise in daily life. So, The Four Noble Truths arise from direct observation of *the way things are for people* in the mental/emotional world, just as we know the truth of the laws of physics and thermodynamics by observing them in the physical world. These are not platitudes handed down from an ethereal or mythical being, but instead scientific observations made by wise and intentional humans who have sought to make sense of their experience.

First noble truth: Suffering exists

REMEMBER

It seems simple enough, but this first truth is worth taking note of because it acknowledges that suffering is not something that intrudes into our lives or impedes our lives as humans, but is actually an integral *part of our lives*. When you can fully acknowledge that life *always* includes some suffering (in both obvious and subtle forms), it can begin to help you loosen your grip on trying to make it disappear. Like gravity mentioned earlier, when you acknowledge the reality of it, you can then find a way to live alongside it.

It's also worth noting that even when things seem good to you, you still feel some undercurrent of anxiety, dissatisfaction, or uncertainty. This is a part of being human. It is one aspect of our common humanity, and it binds us to each other because we all experience it.

Second noble truth: The cause of suffering

Seeing our suffering as having an explainable cause, rather than being random, chaotic, or inflicted by a source outside ourselves, is particularly helpful. The second truth says that the source of our suffering is desire (or craving) and the opposite of desire, which we could call aversion. Aversion is actually just craving in reverse, meaning that you are grasping for something other than what you already have. For example, "I ordered the fish, but I wish I'd ordered the chicken instead." Yes, you have to admit that, although you may often blame things outside of yourself for your suffering, such as circumstances, luck, or other people, the cause is actually you, or more accurately, your attitude toward the realities you face. This is not to say that you are to blame for the circumstances you find yourself in, but it is in *wanting it to be different than it is* where your suffering arises.

In a rather benign case that you are sitting in a boring lecture, wishing you were someplace else and feeling as if the boredom is unbearable and even painful, the suffering in this equation does not come from the lecture itself. The lecture is just the lecture. The degree to which you suffer during this lecture is the degree to which you are craving *the experience of not being there because of your boredom.* Suffering can actually be summed up as "the struggle with *what is.*"

Third noble truth: The end of suffering

"Finally!" you are saying to yourself. "Enough with all the suffering and stress and pain, I want to know if it can end." The Buddha says that there is indeed an end of suffering because these ideas of deeply craving things and pushing things away that you are not willing to accept are just thoughts or ideas and not fixed realities. A thought that "this pain is unbearable" or "I don't deserve this kindness" is really only a brain secretion, a semi-random electrical firing of a few thousand neurons in your brain that is here one moment and gone the next. They have no palpable or persisting reality and are instead like clouds floating on the horizon or leaves on a stream. They come and they go, and they only influence you to the degree that you get caught up in them. Therefore, you can find a way out of your suffering by becoming aware of this, awakening to the actual reality of the workings of your mind, so that you are not enslaved by it.

"Don't believe everything you think," says a popular bumper sticker. The comedian Emo Philips famously said: "I used to think that the brain was the most wonderful organ in the body. Then I realized which organ was telling me this." Not falling for the tricky antics of your clever human brain is the essence of hope for the relief of your suffering.

Fourth noble truth: The path to relief of suffering

The Buddha didn't own a prescription pad to write it for you, but thankfully he spelled out the path for all of us in his many talks to his followers over the years. Those steps have been laid out very clearly in something called The Eightfold Path (yes, another list). The important point for your purposes here is that he prescribed a simple path of living ethically, practicing mindfulness and compassion, and developing wisdom through doing exactly what is proposed in these pages. In other words, not avoiding or denying the reality of suffering, but instead being willing to directly meet and get to know the suffering with clear eyes, steady concentration, a warm heart, and patient but persistent effort.

If you've been wondering as you read this whether we will *ever* dispense with all the preparations and get on to the *actual* practice of self-compassion in this book, perhaps now you can see why we've spent so much time on the preliminaries. The goal is to help you cultivate a certain attitude that will allow you to fully realize the potential of these Four Noble Truths and find a truly sustainable and effective way of alleviating your suffering. Thank you for being patient. It will be worth the wait.

Finding What You Need to Feel Safe and Courageous

Now is your big chance to try your hand (or maybe it's your heart?) at self-compassion. Yes, *finally* you get to unleash the power of your own kindness, albeit in the service of sorting out just what you need to proceed to the next chapters.

If you were planning on growing a beautiful garden, this would be the stage where you would be tilling the soil, fertilizing, and choosing exactly what seeds you will sow in your garden. It's not nearly as showy and fun as harvesting big juicy tomatoes or cauliflower as big as your head, but it's no less important (and perhaps even more so).

The process, not surprisingly, begins with that fundamental question of self-compassion: "What do I need?" If you're on board with the idea that this process will likely require you to be courageous and potentially lean into and encounter some of your more challenging emotions, then you should be well-prepared to do this to the extent that it feels right to you. In other words, you get to choose just exactly how much challenge you take on to explore the possibility of change while maintaining a sense of safety and internal support.

If you walk into the gym and head to the heaviest barbells, you won't be doing yourself any favors (unless, of course, you're one of those muscley gym rats who wears sweatshirts with the sleeves torn off because your biceps don't fit in regular sleeves). The same is true with self-compassion. Ambition is useful in some areas, but unbridled, unrealistic ambition simply doesn't work here because it just opens you to too much emotional "weight" to manage as you ease into the practice. You won't be able to gain as much as you could if you took a more measured approach.

REMEMBER

Here is the opportunity to *customize* your experience and exploration of self-compassion. By asking yourself "What do I need?" you are able to assess your readiness and capacity for this work and find just the right dosage for you. Make no mistake: Adjusting the dosage (either up or down) has absolutely nothing to do with the value of the practice. In other words, if you decide you need a lighter "dose" because you are feeling a bit depleted or overwhelmed or tentative, making that adjustment will actually make the practice *more* valuable because it will be matched to exactly what you need. In fact, even choosing to adjust your dosage is an act of self-compassion all by itself! And, sadly for you if you are the competitive type, upping the dosage of self-compassion beyond your capacity (like lifting the heaviest weights) earns you no extra credit in the self-compassion game and can have a downside. Find your own sweet spot by using some of the approaches that follow, and you'll be set up for success in this self-compassion adventure.

Opening and closing to adjust your "dosage"

We are all well aware of how our amazing human body tends to its needs through the process of self-regulation. The eyes dilate and constrict, our blood vessels do the same, our heart valves open and close, our lungs expand and contract; the examples are endless. This capacity to open and close in various ways is the key to maintaining the body at its optimal capacity. If you give it some thought, you will see that our hearts and minds do the same.

You are not "always on" just as you are not always "shut down," but you do have a sense of when you are "on" and when you are "off" — when you are receptive and when you can't take on any more challenge. You have a natural internal regulatory process for giving yourself just the right amount of whatever you need, even if you don't always heed the inner signals about this process. It may be helpful to consider how you can tell when you are opening or closing so that you can use these signs as cues and listen and respond to them when it comes to self-compassion practice.

Here are four indications that you may be opening:

>> **Your body feels relaxed but alert.** Your body has a way of letting go of tension so that you can focus and become receptive to new things. When you are open, you feel just the right amount of arousal in your body, like when you listen carefully to a new song or someone says something provocative and you tilt your head in interest.

>> **Thinking is vivid and clear.** The brain is able to engage and process information in efficient ways when you are opening, and you become more creative and inquisitive. When you are opening, there is a playful quality to your attention that facilitates savoring an experience, exploring an idea, or testing a hypothesis.

>> **Laughter happens.** When you are open, it means you have let go of tunnel vision. You can see the big picture and are willing to be surprised and delighted by the experience. Surprise is the essence of humor, so when you are open and willing to be surprised, you often find a smile on your lips and in your eyes.

>> **Tears may flow.** This one may surprise you, but crying is really the body's way of letting go of stress. In a moment of fear, for example, you are hyper-focused on the task at hand, such as finding the lost child at the amusement park, and nothing can deter you in your efforts. But when the child is finally found safe, it is then that the tears can flow (for both parent and child!) because you are letting go of the fear and stress.

So when your heart is open to your feelings (including the sad ones) your tears can naturally flow. A Buddhist teacher, Lama Yeshe, says, "The way to practice compassion is with wet eyes." And never fear — if you are not so much of a "leaky person," that's okay too. We are all different in our tendency toward tears, and it's not a problem if your eyes are dry.

Following are four indications that you may be closing:

» **Huh? Distraction.** Our brains have an amazing capacity to "titrate" their dosage and to disengage from challenging tasks when they have had enough. The mind begins to wander in these moments and suddenly the tiniest thing seemingly becomes the most fascinating thing in the world. The stray dog hair on your pant leg or the amazing resemblance between the speaker and your Uncle Isaac suddenly swells up to fill your awareness, and you lose track of whatever you started attending to.

» **Anger and irritation arise.** You know the drill. You've had an especially hard day at work, and you come home to your loving partner only to have them greet you at the door with a request to take out the trash and "speak to *your* son about his room." You're a responsible spouse and parent, but today this is more than you can manage. You feel the irritation rise up and you may give vent to the hurtful comments that your mind offers. You are closed (or closing), and this is your mind's way of fending off one more demand that it can't adequately process at this time.

» **The inner critic chimes in.** When you have some awareness that you should be open (say to listening to an important talk by your supervisor) and you're simply struggling to focus and process what is being said, you may find yourself further compounding the situation by criticizing yourself for not being able to concentrate. "You're just not smart enough for this job," your ever-present, ever-nasty inner critic whispers in your ear. "You have no business even being here if you can't grasp what she's saying to you." Your inner critic likes to take a natural process (like closing when you reach capacity) and turn it into a character flaw or weakness that needs fixing.

» **Boredom and sleepiness arise.** Sleepiness is your body's last-ditch effort to get you to close, by essentially beginning to shut down the attentional processes and force you to close. A close cousin to sleepiness is boredom, of course, and they often co-exist. While you can't always do something about a feeling of boredom or sleepiness (indulging in a nap by placing your head down on the conference table during a meeting is generally frowned upon in modern corporate culture), you can see it as a sign that you are naturally closing.

Once you recognize that your body and mind naturally give you cues when it is opening and closing, you can then take a more proactive role in both responding to these cues and managing the process to your best advantage. If you are naturally closing, then perhaps the self-compassionate thing to do would be to allow yourself to close. In the context of this book, if you have been voraciously consuming page after page of this material and trying all the practices, and now you are feeling "full," then maybe it would be kind to pause and put the book aside to give yourself time to digest what you've taken in. Or maybe you will want to honor when you are opening and set aside some time to delve back into the material or the practice with a renewed sense of adventure. There is no reward for "pushing through" the opening or closing process and forcing yourself to open or close.

REMEMBER

It may be helpful to think of this process of opening and closing as a continuous range and not a binary choice. In other words, instead of thinking of opening and closing like flipping a light switch on the wall, think of it as turning on the faucet, or better yet, adjusting the temperature of the water to just the right balance of hot and cold to suit the situation. You can adjust your degree of openness to match your needs in any given moment (and it changes constantly). Sometimes the circumstances call for a deep and steamy soak in the tub, sometimes you want an icy drink of water, and still other times a warm flow is just the right thing for washing the mutt after a romp in the mud. Customize your degree of openness and you will be able to explore the practice of self-compassion in a meaningful and sustainable way.

Finding your sweet spot of tolerance

When Goldilocks of fairy-tale fame tried the different beds belonging to the three bears, one was found to be "too hard," one was "too soft," and the final one was "just right." When you ask yourself what you need in the practice of self-compassion, you need to feel your way into the "just right" zone, the "sweet spot" that best suits you. You can adjust the degree of opening and closing as you've just explored, but how do you end up knowing just what is the right temperature for healing and growth? If it's bathwater, you dip your toes in the water, and frankly, the same is true of self-compassion. But there are some rough parameters for what is likely to work best.

REMEMBER

Specifically, there is an optimal place, a sweet spot of learning and growth that comes somewhere between total safety and maximum risk. Scientists refer to this phenomenon as the Yerkes-Dodson Law, which states that there is a relationship between pressure and performance, such that performance increases with physiological or mental arousal, but only up to a point. When arousal becomes too high, performance then decreases. Think of the athlete who needs a certain amount of stimulation to approach peak performance, but at a certain point if they bear down too much or try too hard, their performance actually decreases. When it comes to self-compassion, we need to challenge ourselves but not overwhelm ourselves.

If you think in terms of Figure 2-1, you can begin to feel your way into your particular sweet spot.

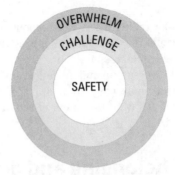

FIGURE 2-1:
Zones of
Emotional
Tolerance.

© John Wiley & Sons, Inc.

The middle circle is the Safety Zone and reflects the place where you can stay all day without any danger of feeling pushed or pulled in any direction. A participant in a self-compassion course several years ago said, "Oh, I know that place. I call it a 'duvet day' when I don't even want to get out of bed and do anything; I just want to curl up under the duvet and be safe and comfy." It's a sweet place to be, under that duvet, but one doesn't grow or change or move in valued directions from that safe space.

When you begin to edge out of that safe space and put yourself into the tug of war of life as it is, where there are unexpected things and delightful things and opportunities to make choices and pursue goals, you begin to find yourself in the fruitful sweet spot of life that is the Challenge Zone. Extending the tug-of-war analogy, the Safety Zone is where the rope is coiled at your feet, limp and unthreatening. In the Challenge Zone you are feeling a tug but holding your own, engaged in the struggle and finding your strengths but not outmatched.

If the force on the other end of the rope begins to tug you farther than you are willing to go and the imbalance is too strong, then you are in the Overwhelm Zone, and nothing fruitful can happen here. If you are the ambitious sort, you may think that you can multiply the impact of your practice by recklessly putting yourself into overwhelm. You will quickly realize that Dr. Yerkes and Dr. Dodson were onto something with their law, and your performance will suffer tremendously.

REMEMBER

Inevitably, because self-compassion is an ongoing and varied human process, like all human processes, you will find yourself constantly treading and retreading this same journey out from Safe, into Challenge for a while, accidentally falling into Overwhelm, and then catching yourself and wending your way back to the platform of Safety so you can catch your breath, find your feet, and explore Challenge again. And what allows you to move back and forth between these zones? You guessed it, opening and closing! The two processes work hand in glove to help you find your optimal dosage, your sweet spot.

TIP

You may find it helpful to consider taking a few notes about how to recognize when you are in each zone, especially the Overwhelm Zone, so that when it happens (and it will) you catch yourself sooner, spare yourself a lot of difficulty, and get yourself back to safety so you can regroup and move forward. Maybe you will find yourself unable to focus, or feel emotionally numb or disconnected, or possibly feel a rising sense of panic as if you want to run out of the room. Make a note for yourself. You'll be glad you did.

The experience of belonging and deserving

Thus far this chapter has talked about safety as a kind of simple state of feeling sheltered and secure, but there are many dimensions of safety in the context of self-compassion. For those who are seeking to become more self-compassionate, it is especially important to look a bit closer at the feeling of safety to explore two related qualities: a sense of belonging and a sense of deserving.

For you to feel safe to practice self-compassion, you must feel as if you have come to the right place to do so. What that means in this context is that you may need to feel that we share something in common as humans, such that you feel welcomed and embraced, as if you, specifically, were invited. This may sound quite obvious to you, especially if you are a member of the dominant culture and hold identities that are largely privileged, embraced by society, and in the majority, but that is not the case for so many who have identities or histories that have caused them to be (or feel) marginalized, excluded, discriminated against, or mistreated.

REMEMBER

If you have any concerns about belonging here, know that from the point of view of self-compassion practice, everybody who wants to become more self-compassionate belongs here. Everyone has a voice; everyone is valued and appreciated. We are all humans, but we are all different, and yet we all are much more alike than different when you look past the superficial differences between us. We all just want to be happy and free from suffering, and at our very foundations, we all simply want to be loved.

There are those among us who have been the victim of terrible treatment in various forms and who emerged from those experiences with a deep sense of inadequacy, self-doubt, shame, and self-hatred. If you, in your life, faced anything like this, we're overjoyed that you are here and so excited for you in making this difficult journey to healing and growth. But for now, you may be plagued by feelings of not deserving. This may be a sense of not deserving to have access to this practice, or not deserving of being free from your suffering, or simply not deserving of anything good. Our hearts ache for you if you feel that you don't deserve ease and peace and joy in your life.

But in the meantime, you need to contend with this nagging fear that you do not deserve this practice. As noted before, arguing with this insidious inner voice is fruitless and may actually take away from your potential to grow and change. However, you're urged to consider that your inner critic only gets one voice in your own inner poll of what is right for you. Consider what your heart whispers about what you *really* deserve. Think about the child version of you and what it wishes for you. What do the people who love and care about you most believe about what you deserve? Those are all votes that sway the results of your poll in favor of you belonging here and being deserving of your own good wishes and kind intentions.

REMEMBER

If you struggle, you deserve to be free of struggle sometimes. If you hurt, you deserve to be free of hurt sometimes. If you have unease, you are worthy of peace. If you have sadness, you deserve joy. If you are imperfect, you deserve to feel perfectly imperfect. You deserve your own kindness, even if there is a voice to the contrary. See what you can do to acknowledge that nagging, irritating voice that has been with you for years, and simply let it natter on while you tend to the task at hand.

Chapter **3**

Common Humanity: Connection and Belonging

"I'm only human."

How often have you heard this statement (or said it) and not given it much thought? Usually, we say this when people or circumstances are demanding that we be much more than human. In other words, when we are being asked to *do* more than we reasonably can, to *be* more than is within our grasp, or to simply be perfect. We offer the statement as a kind of apology or excuse for being what we are: human. Perhaps the origin is from the days when many humans believed in a pantheon of gods and amidst those exalted beings we were "mere mortals."

But as Marianne Williamson has said, "Your playing small does not serve the world." Not only that, but your playing small doesn't even serve you! We humans spend a remarkable amount of emotional and cognitive energy denying and avoiding the miracle of our existence as human beings. But "only" human? Are you kidding? With all that our human minds and hearts can accomplish; all that we have built, created, discovered, harnessed, and celebrated through our collective efforts as social and creative beings, how can we disown that heritage through apology for not being better or more or perfect? Just the simple fact that we have the capacity to think ahead and plan and execute that plan (like making breakfast) is a uniquely human capability that can be celebrated.

REMEMBER

You don't need to excel or achieve great things to be a part of the human race. Sometimes simply surviving life's challenges is an incredible accomplishment. For now, just let that sink in.

If you ever feel particularly isolated or different from other people, then you have yet another reminder of our common humanity, and you've come to the right place. As another component of self-compassion, this awareness is a powerful force for healing and growth because it dispels the illusion of isolation from each other and from our common human existence, and instead reminds us of our shared experience so that we feel less alone and more connected to each other.

In fact, the road to joy and understanding is paved with recognizing and embracing our common humanity and finding the common ground upon which we all stand. The pages ahead allow you to explore and experience our common humanity as an important element of a more self-compassionate you.

The Inescapable Truth: We Need Each Other

The image of the rugged individualist is embedded in our Western culture and is often a point of pride for those who have achieved greatness in various ways. Certainly, nothing is wrong with being bold, charting your own path, or overcoming peer pressure to strike out in a new direction. Self-reliance and independence are admirable traits and much of what we aim to instill in our offspring as dutiful parents (so that our children aren't still asking us to make them peanut butter and jelly sandwiches at the age of 30).

But the truth is that, however independent and self-reliant we may be or become, we are social beings who need each other for our very survival. As mammals, we are born helpless and dependent upon our parents or other caregivers to make sure that we have food, clothing, and shelter. And this reliance on others is only the beginning, as we continue to exist in community and connection. We collaborate to accomplish many of the great things that mankind has created (from the banking system to bridges to sliced bread). As John Donne famously said:

> "No man is an island entire of itself; every man is a piece of the continent, a part of the main; if a clod be washed away by the sea, Europe is the less, as well as if a promontory were, as well as any manner of thy friends or of thine own were; any man's death diminishes me, because I am involved in mankind. And therefore never send to know for whom the bell tolls; it tolls for thee."

We are all "involved in mankind," which is to say that we are actually all engaged together in this business of being members of the human race, and we are interconnected in this way. Hesitation arises when people start saying "We are all connected," because it sounds a bit New Agey to some. But this reality of interconnection is nothing weird or metaphysical or theoretical. It is observable, irrefutable fact that we are *inter*dependent beings who can't survive or thrive without each other. But we like to tell ourselves that we can. We can say "I am independent because I make my own cheese." But if someone else milked the cow, another person transported the milk, and someone else sold you the milk, then the illusion of your independence begins to fade. And this doesn't even take into account how the cow got there in the first place, where its food came from, and who made the container that you carried home to "independently" make your own cheese.

When we see ourselves as wholly independent beings not reliant on others or subject to the same conditions as all other human beings, it gives us a sense of self-efficacy and self-determination that can motivate us to persist against the odds or in difficult circumstances, and potentially triumph in whatever we aim to accomplish. This is quite powerful if all our ideas are flawless, all our efforts succeed, and we never make mistakes. But here in the real world, human activities don't go like that. The smartest scientists form hypotheses and test them, with a humble willingness to refine those ideas if the data doesn't support the original hypothesis. These same scientists know that they stand on the shoulders of those scientists who came before them, and most scientists do not resemble the movie characterizations of them as crazed and passionate loners in the attics of castles with burbling test tubes. (Even the fictional Dr. Frankenstein had his faithful assistant, Igor.) Imperfection and interconnection are accounted for in every successful human endeavor, even something as seemingly tangible and concrete as science.

The point is that we are fooling ourselves if we think that we are truly independent of our larger human condition. Even more relevant to the practice of self-compassion, we are setting ourselves up to amplify our suffering when we perpetuate this fantasy that we are not a part of a larger "tribe" or collective.

If the previously mentioned scientist discovers that their hypothesis was flawed or their experiment was based on a miscalculation, she has two options. If she is enlightened and recognizes that one of her human inheritances is fallibility (in other words, she knows she is human and therefore subject to making mistakes), she will correct the error, inform her team, learn from it, and move on. If the same scientist is a perfectionist (overlooking the human impossibility of perfection), a similar error could lead to a spiral of self-critical thoughts (such as "I'm a terrible scientist," "My colleagues will now find out that I'm not as smart as they thought," or "I should just quit my job and get work flipping burgers instead") that descend into shame and a lifetime of suffering.

Awareness of our common humanity, as you can see in these examples, allows for us to see past our "small selves" and into the larger perspective of ourselves as fallible but talented human beings with incredible strengths and capacities along with inevitable weaknesses and shortcomings, all just seeking to be happy and free from suffering. But to change our perspective on the fact of being human, it may be helpful to explore our tendency to overlook the fact that we do, in fact, need each other.

Albert Einstein described humankind's tendency toward separateness in this way: "He experiences himself, his thoughts and feelings, as something separate from the rest — a kind of optical delusion of consciousness."

When you shake that optical delusion and see yourself as fully connected to all your human counterparts, you can begin to be able to tolerate and even embrace the reality of your life, including the moments of imperfection, failure, and falling short.

In other words, you become more able to have compassion for yourself in these moments because of the reality that they happen to *all* humans, rather than seeing them as evidence of something fatally flawed about just you.

HOW YOU DENY YOUR HUMANITY

What are some ways that you deny your humanity? How do you routinely overlook the fact that you share your human nature with every other human who has ever lived or will ever live? Here are a few ways that you may recognize:

- You observe the fact that human beings come in separate envelopes of flesh (also known as "bodies") and mistake this for a kind of separate existence that causes you to believe that you don't need anyone else to survive. And then, when you feel the need to connect with other people (and to be seen and heard), you see it as some sort of unique weakness in your character rather than a feature of your birthright as a human.

- You (gasp!) make a mistake and immediately enter a downward spiral of self-recrimination and self-criticism. You convince yourself that you are uniquely flawed and imperfect and "less than" everyone else, whom you are convinced would *never* make such a mistake.

- You find out you weren't invited to a party to which several of your friends were invited. Although you act outwardly as if you are cool with that, inside it feels like your world is collapsing into a deep, dark hole, and you feel your heart pounding in panic over the slight.

- You find yourself having dark, shameful feelings toward your boss over a work conflict. You find yourself so mired in hurt, anger, and resentment toward them that you can't even empathically acknowledge that, just like you, they are going through life with a desire to be happy and free from suffering. Your boss is actually a fellow traveler on the human highway, but you want nothing to do with this acknowledgement. It feels better to see them as motivated by some sort of evil or destructive force that is foreign to you and needs to be defeated. As a result you harbor resentment and fear, and feel stuck and powerless in this conflict.

Acknowledging Our Universal Human Need

Why do we invest so much time and energy keeping up that optical delusion of separateness? Einstein went on to call this state "a kind of prison for us, restricting us to our personal desires and to affection for a few persons nearest to us." So the question becomes, why have we checked ourselves into this very human prison and just exactly how long is our sentence? The answer, not surprisingly, is that we get sprung from this particular joint whenever we are able to embrace our common humanity and see ourselves as part of something bigger than ourselves.

Some would call this spirituality, but you can use whatever word works for you. You may think of it as taking the wide view and seeing the whole picture of our existence.

But that still begs the question of how we have come to be imprisoned to begin with. It may have to do with the fact that we do literally need each other to survive. Starting with infancy, as mentioned earlier, we are completely reliant on the kindness and care of others. Our offspring come out with certain survival needs and few rudimentary tools at their disposal to get those needs met. Mainly those tools are confined to crying . . . and crying louder, but over time babies expand their repertoire to facial expressions and more nuanced verbalizations. Our children are not like those sea turtle babies you see hatching on nature shows, where they burst out of their little eggs in the sand, waddle on down to the water, and swim off into the sunset. Our little "hatchlings" are far more helpless, and as a result, nature (in its infinite wisdom) has endowed humans with a deep and instinctive drive to connect, to seek out sources of vitality and safety, and also, to be on alert to any threats to that short but vital food chain of survival.

It is this last bit, the fear of being cut off from others and therefore vulnerable and at risk of not surviving, that is underneath most of our illusion of separateness. Think of astronauts in the early days of the space program. These brave souls donned big shiny spacesuits with bulbous helmets and an all-important, ever-present lifeline to explore space outside the ship. The lifeline is essentially a hose that attaches them to the spacecraft and provides the oxygen (and other vital elements) they need to survive in the vacuum of space. Now imagine that you were one of these astronauts and how extremely vulnerable you would feel, how careful and alert you would be to anything threatening that lifeline, and how *mindful* you would be to make sure that the lifeline was intact and functioning.

As an astronaut, you would have learned about the importance of your lifeline, but as a human being, you are already innately hardwired to treat your own "lifeline," your connection to your caregiver, as the key to your very survival. The infant cries not because he is inconvenienced or uncomfortable; he cries because his survival literally depends upon someone providing sustenance. And this system, however crude it may seem, has worked for our entire existence on this planet.

As we grow older, we begin to engage other means to be attuned to others, including some fascinating structures in the brain referred to as *mirror neurons* that allow us to feel the feelings of others.

Survival equals love

But it's a bit more complex than this, because the baby isn't like the hungry plant Audrey in *A Little Shop of Horrors* insisting "Feed me, Seymour. Feed me!" The infant is charged with causing a broader bond to be created, a lifeline to be installed, that assures his continued existence by getting all his complex needs met (food, clothing, and shelter being only the beginning). This bond is the deeper, broader bond of love itself.

When the infant can manage to be loved by an adult, all of their needs can be met, and they can not only survive but grow and thrive. At the very foundation of our human bond, at an instinctive level, the thing that binds us together is love. Love equals survival for us, and so anything that may put that love in jeopardy is to be avoided at all costs. We want nobody to stand on our lifeline, our universal human need for love.

The poet Hafiz (loosely translated by Daniel Ladinsky) once wrote about this "great pull in us to connect" in a poem called *With that Moon Language*: "Everyone you see, you say to them, 'Love me.'" Let that sink in for a minute. Can you feel the truth of this down deep in a metaphorical sense? As Chris Germer says, "We wake up every morning with the wish to be loved and go through the entire day with the wish, although we may never realize or admit it." (What is even more intriguing is the fact that, when we can recognize and acknowledge this wish, we can more easily see the same wish in others, and suddenly we can feel less alone and afraid. More on this is in the later section "Practice: Just Like Me.")

So as human beings, we need love. It's just that simple, but it's not so easy sometimes. Usually, we think of being loved as a kind of privilege or happy circumstance that may or may not happen to us and may be fleeting. But we rarely think of love as a survival need.

REMEMBER

Perhaps it would be helpful to think more broadly about love as encompassing all the different forms of love that the ancient Greeks studied and articulated. They identified eight different forms of love: *philia*, or affectionate love; *philautia*, or self-love; *pragma*, or enduring love; *eros*, or romantic love; *ludus*, or playful love; *storge*, or familiar love; *agape*, or selfless love; and *mania*, or obsessive love. Love obviously comes in many forms and from many sources, but the point here is that we need it (in its varied forms) for our physical as well as our emotional survival. We are happiest when we feel loved and saddest when we do not. If we feel isolated or tragically different or separate from others, then we have a deep-seated feeling that our lifeline has a fatal kink in it and that we are unloved. The feeling that arises in us is akin to having your oxygen supply threatened in the vastness of the vacuum of space.

What arises if we feel unloved . . . or unlovable?

With our very survival feeling as if it is riding on feeling loved, or at least lov*able*, one can see that the stakes are high when these possibilities are threatened. In fact, the primal nature of this fear is actually the source of the most troubling of human emotional experiences: shame. Here you can explore how shame is bound up with your sense of common humanity in so many ways.

To appreciate this relationship, you need only look at one definition of shame, by W.K. Hahn (italics added): "a complex combination of emotions, physiological responses, and imagery associated with the *real or imagined rupture of relational ties*." That sounds a lot like "Excuse me, but your foot is on my lifeline." This "real or imagined rupture of relational ties" can, as you have seen, be much more than just an inconvenience because they tear at the very fabric of our existence and survival as humans.

But look beyond humans for a moment and consider the antelope. These beautiful creatures of the plains live in community and travel as a herd from place to place to eat and procreate (and to play with the deer if the old song "Home on the Range" is accurate). They don't just travel in herds because they enjoy each other's company, but because there is safety in numbers. Being in a herd protects them, to some degree, from predators such as wolves, cougars, bears, and even eagles.

It is a dangerous thing to be a lone antelope with those treacherous creatures lurking all around, so you stick to your herd and try to blend in. And when your herd is spooked by something that you don't notice and they scurry off to escape the perceived threat while you are obliviously munching on green grass, you are suddenly exposed and in potential danger. This unfortunate situation is a major rupture in your relational tie to the herd, and you may not survive it if a wolf is prowling nearby.

Take a moment to imagine how this would feel and consider that the feeling is not that different from how you might feel if you were shunned or disowned by your family when you were young, or how you might feel if you were fired from your job. In our own way, we humans are no different from herd animals like the antelope in our need to feel connected to feel safe. But antelope are concerned only with physical survival, whereas our human sympathetic nervous system does not differentiate between real and imagined threats. So these hazards can potentially come from being physically attacked, from imagining a potential injury, or even from receiving a nasty and hurtful email or phone message.

This interdependence goes two ways, of course, but mainly we've been exploring why you need everyone else. However, it's worth exploring the other direction too, because it also has some important pitfalls that are worth appreciating.

REMEMBER

Your human herd or tribe needs *you*, as it needs all its members, and this can put you in an awkward position if you don't feel as if you belong or you don't feel worthy of being a part of the collective.

In moments when we fail, fall short, or make a mistake, we can tend to attribute these unfortunate events to our flaws as individuals. We feel as if we alone have these feelings, that somehow, we are uniquely bad or stupid or ill-equipped, and that these are enduring features of ourselves and not fleeting experiences that all humans have at times. When we lack the sense of common humanity, every unfortunate experience becomes another brick in the wall of our isolation from others because we feel, at some deep, cellular level, that this flaw makes us uniquely unlovable and therefore separate from everyone.

Our relentlessly comparing minds then see us as *less than* others in a fundamental way, not measuring up and simply not worthy of the crucial love of our human clan. This is the painful experience of shame, where you feel as if you carry around a shameful and malignant truth about yourself which, if discovered by the people you need (and who need you), would cause them to reject and abandon you. The feeling of shame is that you will be left on your own in dangerous territory, vulnerable to your predators, whatever they may be.

In this case, you can feel like you alone could potentially be the cause of this rupture in your relational ties to others (you are standing on your *own* lifeline, so to speak), so you do everything in your power to hide this terrible, fatal flaw as if your life depends on it. Literally. And of course, if you fear being "found out" for the shameful "fact" of your imperfection, you hunker down to hide that flaw or run away from others. This, of course, leads you to feeling even more isolated from them and even farther from a sense of common humanity.

This scenario paints a rather dark picture of the cost of not appreciating our common humanity, but it also begins to map a course toward a way out of the clutches of Einstein's "optical delusion" and into the light of embracing our humanity as a great gift of safety, security, and strength for finding happiness and freedom from suffering. Self-compassion invites us back to humanity.

Three common blocks to embracing your common humanity

Seeing ourselves in the larger context of our human condition perhaps sounds admirable and worth exploring, but when people actually explore this possibility, many encounter some challenges. Here are three of the most common obstacles that can arise, along with some guidance to support you in overcoming them and finding your way toward feeling your deep connection to other humans as a means of becoming more self-compassionate.

THE FEAR OF BEING FOUND TO BE A FRAUD

Have you ever had a moment of relative success or paused to reflect on how fortunate you are to be doing something that you had always hoped to do? Perhaps you have been invited to give an important commencement speech at your alma mater or you've been promoted within your company to a coveted new role. You feel some gratification, you bask in the compliment that has been extended to you, and then you start to feel doubt and uncertainty taps you on the shoulder. You start to worry that you aren't up to the task, that someone (or multiple someones) has vastly overestimated your skill or talent or ability, and that when you begin to fulfil your new role, this terrible oversight will become visible. People will find out that you really don't know what you are doing and have just been a successful faker and fraud so far. And then the proverbial stuff will hit the proverbial fan.

That is a flavor of shame that many of us have experienced, and it is referred to as "impostor syndrome." At its root, it still goes back to the fear of being unloved or unlovable. "What if people find out who I *really* am?" you say to yourself, and you think, "If they knew, they would reject me. I would not be loved. I would be unlovable if people really knew me." So again, the survival instinct powers the illusion of unlovability, and we quake in our boots.

The fact that there is a name for this phenomenon should be some indication that it may be more widespread than you may have thought. In other words, most of us have some sort of self-doubt (which can be healthy to make sure we do our best), but that self-doubt can easily tip over into feeling separate, alone, and isolated from others if we lack self-compassion. So, take heart! You are among fellow imposters (also known as humans) and it's a part of our simple desire to be accepted, appreciated, acknowledged . . . and loved. When we wake up to this, we are like the two wolves dressed in sheep's clothing in a Gary Larson *Far Side* cartoon. They are standing up and have taken off their fake sheep's heads, standing amidst a whole flock of what look like "sheep" in similar makeshift costumes, with no actual sheep in sight. One is saying to the other, "Wait a minute! Isn't anyone here a real sheep?" The humor is that we are all "real sheep," which is to say that part of our reality is that we just want to be loved and accepted, and fear being found to be unworthy of love for some reason. Could you be just a little bit kind to yourself for having that fear, the way you would comfort a dear friend who was feeling unlovable?

You will see that the thread running through all three of these blocks is the strong tendency of our mind to compare and contrast everything. We find that we often learn about things by contrasting them with others. We might say "it tastes like chicken," or ask, "Is it as funny as *Caddyshack*?" (Just to be clear, nothing is as funny as *Caddyshack*.)

REMEMBER

Our human brains are efficient at this process and serve us well in many ways, but when we slip over into comparing the *facts* of things into comparing the *value* of things, we begin to get into trouble. When we decide that our own suffering is better or worse than anyone else's, or that someone else is more worthy of an experience than we are, we deny the reality of our own humanity. The goal with embracing common humanity is to stick to the *fact* of it and to let go of comparing one person's particular experience to another's.

The following sections describe those obstacles you're most likely to encounter.

Feeling unimportant

"It makes me feel like my problems are trivial compared to others'."

When we remind ourselves that other people have similar problems, we can feel as if we are dismissing our own problems as inconsequential. At a meeting once, an important authority listened to the complaints of a colleague, paused, and then responded, "and other people have other problems," and moved on. This was an unfortunate way of discounting this person's concerns by somehow suggesting that they weren't worthy of attention. When we are already inclined to feel unworthy (due to a lack of self-compassion), we are easily triggered to feel this way about our own struggles.

The key to overcoming this obstacle is to bring our practice of mindfulness to the experience and realize that acknowledging the *presence* of our problems is the point. We need to notice how the mind habitually wants to compare our experience to others, and to coax it back each time that it wanders off to comparing. We are just *making room* for our own suffering alongside that of our human brethren, acknowledging that we experience pain just as all humans do, and that this experience (regardless of the specifics) is a human one that binds us together rather than separating us.

A recent meme making the rounds in response to the COVID-19 pandemic has been, "We are not all in the same boat. But we are in the same storm, and with the support and understanding of our fellow humans, we can all come through the other side a little kinder, a little gentler, a little more human." Common humanity simply acknowledges and validates our suffering as a shared human experience, even if it manifests differently in each of us.

Feeling overwhelmed

"Even thinking about my suffering just becomes too much when I think about the enormity of it."

Often what keeps us in denial is that we build up our fear of the thing we're avoiding such that it becomes much bigger in our minds than it actually is (this is the opposite of denial). Consider this story: A man was playing golf and chasing an errant ball into the woods. As he picked up his ball to head back to the fairway, he heard rustling in the bushes. With each step he took, faster and faster, the sound continued in his direction and his fear and anxiety mounted. He imagined mountain lions, bears, and alligators chasing after him. When he finally got to "safety," breathless and sweaty, he had enough presence of mind to turn and look . . . and to see the cutest little bunny rabbit come hopping out of the shrubbery. There was indeed something alive behind him, but the rest was a construction in his imagination.

REMEMBER

Not all our pain is the equivalent of a bunny rabbit, but when we see it for what it is and not what our brain tells us it is, that is often the first powerful step to coming to terms with it. When we can let go of resistance to a feeling and simply recognize it as part of our human experience, we are taking an important step toward coming to terms with our life (including our suffering) as it actually is, rather than what we fear it may be. This is not necessarily an easy thing and takes some courage to do, but you can do this with small steps. Be willing to simply begin by touching the suffering that you carry, be patient, and always respond to what you need to embark on this exploration with attention to what you are ready to encounter. You do not have to embrace anything, but simply, slowly, kindly open up to it as you can.

Understanding that everyone suffers

"Realizing that everyone is as much of a hot mess as I am kind of freaks me out."

Far from being comforting, this awareness that everybody suffers can at first be a painful reality check, but perhaps a necessary one. At the beginning of a recent Mindful Self-Compassion course, after everyone had arrived and taken their seats in a circle, quietly whisper-chatting with people nearby, not making eye contact across the circle and generally feeling a bit self-conscious, the course began. People introduced themselves briefly one by one and made reference to what kinds of challenges and issues had brought them to the class.

The last woman to speak had the most memorable observation of all. She lit up as she said, "When I came into the room tonight I looked around and everyone looked so *normal!*" There were a few self-conscious giggles in the room, and she realized that what she'd said could have been misunderstood as unkind. "I don't mean it that way. I just felt so different from everyone else because I have always had this dark feeling inside like there's something terribly wrong with me as a person. But when you all shared some of your stories, I realized that we *all* have these feelings and we're actually more alike *because of this* and not *in spite of it.* I was doubting whether I belonged here, and now I know I do."

REMEMBER

This is the essence of common humanity and, by extension, self-compassion. As the meditation teacher Rob Nairn has said: "The goal of practice is to become a compassionate mess. This means fully human — often struggling, uncertain, confused — with great compassion."

Starting small with common humanity

Each of us has a variety of different identities that help to determine our sense of self. These identities include race, ethnicity, gender, sexual orientation, religious preference, physical ability, and any one of literally millions of other dimensions upon which we align with certain people more than with other people. We may think of these as simply features of who we are that we happen to share with other *homo sapiens.*

This concept of the things we share with all humans is actually pretty huge when you delve into it. Genetically speaking, we are more than 99.9 percent the same, which is what the Black poet Maya Angelou was referring to when she said, "We are more alike, my friends, than we are unalike." One of the more subtle stumbling blocks that people encounter when acknowledging common humanity is that, based upon their experience of particular identities that they hold, and the degree to which holding those identities has led to disenfranchisement, discrimination, marginalization, or mistreatment, people do not feel that connected to the entire human race.

If you recognize this experience, you may feel that your views, beliefs, practices, or features are not held by the larger society and as such, you may feel isolated from the rest of humanity to some degree. If that's the case, it's a pretty tall order to consider embracing all the commonality that you share with every human being who ever lived or ever will live.

People of some diverse backgrounds (especially those who identify as BIPOC: Black, Indigenous, and People of Color) struggle with the concept of common humanity because they feel as if society has constructed their particular identity as *un*common and separate from the dominant culture, and therefore somehow lower on some imagined hierarchy of humanity. So, people with these identities feel as if the talk of common humanity discounts their lived experience of society's injustice.

This is obviously a huge topic, but for our purposes here, if these ideas resonate with your lived experience, then we admire your willingness to dig in and explore this more deeply. Perhaps despite these cultural constrictions, you may begin to build and grow some common ground at the more basic level of the mere fact that each of us is human, imperfect, and subject to suffering. (And if you are someone who holds identities that have been traditionally more privileged or valued by society, it may be an opportunity to see where your own privilege may have led you to feel more separated or different from those who have not had that opportunity.)

TIP

Consistent with grasping self-compassion in the first place, you can give yourself the gift of being a brave, patient, and steady learner regarding common humanity. Think of yourself as being at the center of various concentric circles of identity and see if you can slowly find common ground and comfort in the common humanity of that circle. For example, if you are a Latinx, heterosexual, Catholic, cisgender female (to choose just a few identities) and are struggling with feelings of isolation and having difficulty fully appreciating common humanity, what if you choose to focus on one of those identities (say being Latinx) and see if you can sense whether even one other Latinx person may understand how you feel (it may or may not be a specific person you know). If you can make that connection, then you might widen the circle to include other people, for example, people who share your identities of being Latinx and Catholic. Be willing to experiment, to go slow, and to feel your way.

Common humanity does not have to be an all-or-nothing proposition. The overarching principle, the guiding intention, is to see ourselves as a part of all humanity, but we can begin with one little piece of territory that we feel we can reclaim and go from there. "Walk slowly, go farther" as someone once said.

Two Tasks to Embrace Common Humanity

In the words of Mary Oliver's poem "Wild Geese," the practical question for you becomes "How do I answer the call and claim my place in the family of things?" You may face some challenging obstacles to embracing the reality of our shared common humanity, but perhaps you are now more open to considering it. You may need to undertake a couple of important tasks to fully open yourself to your humanity and thus lead you to a more self-compassionate way of being. There is one thing you need to embrace and one thing that you need to release, and both require you to be patient with yourself and be willing to be a slow learner once again. But if you begin to travel down the road of embracing your human inheritance and releasing any tendency toward perfectionism, you will find that you can easily find "your place in the family of things."

Claiming your human birthrights

At times the term "common humanity" has been misunderstood by people as implying that everyone's experience is the same or that everyone's suffering is equal in some way. By now hopefully you see that we are not speaking in terms of the quality of suffering or the intensity of it, but just the mere fact that we all experience it. No matter who we are, we can always identify someone else who has suffered more, or more acutely, just as we can identify others who have suffered less. The common thread between us is that suffering itself is part of our makeup as humans, and it is part of our legacy.

But being human is more than just suffering; it comes with an inheritance of intrinsic value and worthiness. You are here because you belong. You are worthy, loved, needed, and have value. These are not just lofty platitudes but real truths of our existence that are easily overlooked, especially by those who have inner critical voices that speak to the contrary and may have spoken in those terms for a lifetime. We don't expect you to simply accept these things about yourself because we said them, but it is worth considering the possibility of beginning the process of exploring what it means to belong to the human race.

The suggestion here is that you look at your own good qualities and abilities as a human (and there are many) and consider making a little room for them in your heart. Take the time to actually appreciate and acknowledge the things that you bring to the table as a person, not because you are better than anyone else or the best at something, but just because you recognize that you have certain unique or admirable capabilities and talents. Start small. The fact that you are reading this book (even the fact that you *are able* to read this book) is a reflection of your deep and abiding desire to be kinder to yourself, that you seek to be happy and free from suffering, just like every human being on the planet. This is enough, but you don't have to stop there.

TIP

Make a list of ten things that you appreciate about yourself, however seemingly small and insignificant, and don't stop until you have at least ten. A hundred would be better, but you don't have to put a lot of pressure on yourself. You won't have to share this list with anyone, so you can be totally honest. If it helps, you can even take a moment to reflect on whether someone was instrumental in developing or nurturing a particular quality. A mentor, a parent, a coach or teacher, even a spiritual figure or author may have helped you unlock a natural tendency or talent that you may not have known you had. By adding that quality to your list, you are honoring that person and their contribution to your life.

This can often be a challenging exercise for people, so it's okay to go slow. Strangely enough, some people find that accepting their own flaws and inadequacies is doable, yet they find it incredibly hard to acknowledge their own strengths and accomplishments. If this is you, then this is a practice you may want to cultivate intentionally on a regular basis.

Avoiding the perils of perfection

This chapter has spent a great deal of time focusing on how much we actually depend upon each other for our survival, safety, and wellbeing. We have explored how we fear being shunned from our "herd" or "pack" and how that can cause us to feel unloved or unlovable. This chapter has painted a rather bleak picture of our deep-seated insecurity as human beings who simply seek to be loved and accepted, but constantly fear being rejected and isolated from others. This is a challenge of being human, but not an insurmountable challenge, and most of us do not give up in the face of it. We simply plod along as best we can, wishing we felt more connected than we do and wondering what is wrong with us that we don't.

Cassius proclaims in Shakespeare's *Julius Caesar:* "The fault, dear Brutus, is not in our stars, but in ourselves, that we are underlings." What Cassius is pointing to is what Marianne Williamson was also suggesting when she said, "Your playing small does not serve the world." We do not do ourselves any favors by placing ourselves one down from everyone else and seeing ourselves as underlings. It is not fate that we see ourselves as less valuable or deserving than any other human being, but simply the result of our own belief that we are not. When we see that this belief is simply an idea — another brain secretion or random neuron firing — and not a fact or immutable truth, then we can begin to loosen its hold on us.

One way that you may find yourself putting yourself down compared to others is by making the observation that you are actually not perfect. You make an error, you fall short at something you attempt, or you fail at something and immediately you are shame-stricken because you are reminded that you have imperfections. The resulting shame-spiral may even be familiar to you. The feeling of being isolated, separate, and different from everyone else begins to envelop you as you sink deeper in the mire and muck of imperfection. You may go so far as to feel as if you are uniquely flawed, tragically doomed to a life of failure, and completely unworthy of anyone's love or affection.

REMEMBER

This downward spiral unfolds because you were imperfect. All because you exhibited a trait that is true of every human being who has ever lived and ever will live on the face of the planet. In other words, in that moment of wallowing in your "unique" imperfection, you are experiencing the pain that every human feels when they make a mistake, fall short, or fail. Every single human. Ever.

In the Native American Navajo tradition (and in many other ethnic and cultural customs), rug weavers leave little imperfections in their beautiful creations to reinforce the understanding that only God is perfect and that humans should not pretend to be perfect as well. These little imperfections, called "spirit lines," are subtle reminders of the common humanity of imperfection. Taken together, this deliberate imperfection is a nod to acknowledging and embracing our shared imperfection as humans.

TIP

If you simply *must* feel perfect, then the invitation here to you is to see if you can turn this around 180 degrees and consider your own imperfections as a human being to be absolutely perfect. Could you be perfectly imperfect as you are?

Practice: Just Like Me

The invitation here is to put aside all of these ideas and concepts about common humanity, perfection, shame, survival, and the rest, and to simply see if you can begin to develop a felt sense of common humanity through a simple practice that this section guides you through. What you are tapping into here is the awareness that all of us wish for happiness and freedom from suffering, that this too is a part of our common humanity.

Just Like Me meditation

This meditation is inspired by the writing and teaching of Thupten Jinpa in his book *A Fearless Heart: How the Courage to Be Compassionate Can Transform Our Lives.*

Take some time to settle into your body for a few minutes, allowing your attention to drop inside. Take note of whatever is present in the way of sensation inside your body. You may notice the touch of clothing, the pressure of the supporting surface on certain parts of your body, or just sensations of coolness or warmth, relaxation or tension, ease or discomfort. Just take note of where and how you are in this moment. You may notice the movement of breath into and out of the body as well, recognizing that the breath has continued to breathe itself since you last attended to it.

Imagine someone whom you hold dear, someone who brings a smile to your face when you think of them, someone with whom you have a relatively easy and uncomplicated relationship. This may be a family member like a child, a grandparent, or even a pet. Try to go beyond the *idea* of this being and see if you can actually feel what it feels like to be in their presence.

Notice any pleasant feelings that may arise as you hold this beloved being in your awareness and see how easy it is to acknowledge that this one too has the same aspiration for genuine happiness that you have.

Now call to mind someone else, someone that you recognize but don't have much meaningful interaction with and don't feel any particular closeness to. This may be a person whom you see quite often, in the hallway at work, behind the counter at your favorite coffee shop, or driving the bus you take regularly. Notice what feelings arise for you as you picture this person and how these feelings may be different from what you felt in regard to the loved one you imagined first.

Usually, we don't give much thought to the happiness of people in neutral roles in our lives like this. But see if this time you can imagine what it might be like to be this person. Imagine their life, their hopes and fears, which are every bit as real, complex, and challenging as yours. You may even recognize a certain similarity between yourself and this other person at the level of your common humanity: "Just like me, she wishes to be happy and to avoid even the slightest suffering."

Next, bring to mind a person with whom you may have some difficulty, someone who irritates or annoys you, someone who may have done you harm, or someone you think might even take satisfaction in your misfortune. If you can, picture this person in front of you. If uncomfortable or painful feelings arise as you do this, maybe place a hand somewhere on your body that is comforting, soothing, or reassuring to simply acknowledge that this is difficult. See if you can acknowledge the difficult feelings, even if you find yourself recalling painful interactions with them in the past. Don't suppress the feelings, but also don't reinforce them by trying too hard to accurately recall those exchanges.

Now see if you can put yourself in this person's shoes for a moment, recognizing that he is an object of deep concern to someone, a parent or a spouse, a child or a dear friend of someone. Begin to acknowledge that even this person with whom you have challenges has the same fundamental aspiration for happiness that you have. Allow your attention to stay with this awareness for some period of time (say 20 to 30 seconds). Allow thoughts and feelings to come and go as they will, as you remain present to whatever arises, with no other agenda but to observe and be kind to yourself in that presence.

Finally, see if you can bring together these three people in one mental picture in front of you. Take some time to reflect on the fact that they all share a basic yearning to be happy and free from suffering. At this dimension, there is no difference between these three people. In this fundamental aspect, they are exactly the same. Just take the time to relate to these three beings from that perspective, from the point of view that they share the aspiration for happiness and a kind of perfect imperfection.

And be sure now to include yourself in this circle of awareness, reminding yourself that

>> These people have feelings, thoughts, and emotions, just like me.

>> These people, during their lives, have experienced physical and emotional pain and suffering, just like me.

>> These people have been sad, disappointed, angry or worried, just like me.

>> These people have felt unworthy or inadequate at times, just like me.

>> These people have longed for connection, purpose, and belonging, just like me.

>> These people want to be happy and free from pain and suffering, just like me.

>> These people want to be loved, just like me.

With this deep recognition that the desires to be happy and to overcome suffering are common to all, silently repeat this phrase: "Just like me, all others aspire to happiness and want to overcome suffering."

Take some time to sit with whatever wishes or feelings arise from this practice, allowing them to arise and fall away. Your only agenda is to notice and take note of their arising.

Inquiring: What was it like to see how others are just like you?

Take some time to settle in and reflect on your experience of the preceding meditation. See if you can adopt an open, nonjudgmental stance toward whatever comes up for you in the way of thoughts, emotions, or anything else. This is not always an easy practice, and the key to success is to be open and curious to the process and let go of specific expectations.

Consider the following questions as guides to your exploration of your own experience of the Just Like Me meditation:

>> How was it to imagine a beloved being and to acknowledge their desire to simply be happy and free from suffering?

>> When you turned your attention to a relatively neutral person, could you call them to mind? Were you able to get some sense of what it is like to be in their shoes and to live their lives? Did you sense any similarity between you and that person?

>> What came up for you when you called to mind the difficult person? Were you able to stay present and compassionate even with that person in mind and your history with that person?

>> What was it like to call this difficult person to mind and stay present with them?

>> Were you able to sense any way in which you and the difficult person have in common the simple desire to be happy and free from suffering?

>> What was your experience of holding all three people in awareness and considering how they were more alike than different?

>> How was it to contemplate the various "just like me" observations?

>> What is your relationship at this moment to the truth of common humanity?

TIP

If you found this practice fruitful in any way, consider practicing it throughout your day, especially when you encounter people from whom you feel different or separate in some way. See if, by pausing and warming up the conversation with compassion, you can see some ways in which this person shares some common humanity with you. You'll be glad you did.

Chapter **4**

Cultivating Your Innate Kindness

The journey of self-compassion begins where such journeys need to begin, with awareness, which we define as mindfulness. This basic human ability to be aware of each moment as it arises in all its fullness is an incredibly powerful capacity. It supports you in disengaging from a discursive, resistant, and wandering mind that prefers to go into the past and future rather than stay present. Mindfulness — the first component of self-compassion — is your anchor and lifeline to the present moment, which is the only place where anything can actually be accomplished.

The second component of self-compassion is common humanity. This deep awareness of our shared humanity and all that it entails is the broad and supportive base for self-compassion practice because it reminds us that we are not alone and have a shared inheritance with the entire human family. Fully embracing our common humanity allows us to see our missteps, foibles, and errors as stemming from the common imperfection of humanity.

It may seem now like you have everything you need to become more self-compassionate, and indeed you do have it within you, but this chapter helps you connect more fully and directly with the third and final component of self-compassion identified by Kristin Neff: self-kindness. Speaking more generally, lovingkindness or "boundless friendliness" is what we explore here.

This natural human tendency toward happiness and satisfaction tends to be either overlooked as just a given or overemphasized as if it is all that is required for self-compassion: to simply be nice to yourself. However, in the larger context, trying to practice self-compassion without the warmth of kindness (just relying on mindfulness and common humanity) leads to a kind of stark view of the human condition where we are acutely aware of each moment and how difficult it is for all of us, without any sense of comfort or soothing for that difficulty.

On the other hand, confusing self-kindness for the larger practice of self-compassion leaves out the grounding of mindfulness or the reality check of common humanity. What you are left with if you try to meet your suffering with just self-kindness is a kind of warm, moist, sickly sweet sentimentality that is ineffective because it is clueless (un-mindful) and ungrounded (disconnected with the human reality of suffering and imperfection).

Therefore, it's important that you tap into all three components of self-compassion to really unlock its true potential, and that includes tapping into your own natural tendency toward kindness, joy, and wellbeing.

We All Just Want to Be Happy

Following on from the Just Like Me meditation in Chapter 3 of Book 2, it is incredibly valuable to operate from a place of awareness that, regardless of how people behave or what we think of what other people think, say, or do, they are just like us in that they simply want to be happy and free from suffering. Other people may very well go about trying to be happy in ways that are sadly unfortunate, sometimes hurtful, and occasionally hard to fathom, but when we see it all in the light of this universal human desire to have joy and satisfaction, we begin to see ourselves (and others) in a new light. That new light is the light of lovingkindness, or our innate inclination of the heart toward joy and satisfaction.

REMEMBER

It's important to note that this motivation doesn't get people off the hook for truly hurtful or dangerous behavior, just because they are seeking happiness in doing it. This book only speaks to their motivation for doing it and doesn't excuse the behavior itself. And please keep in mind that the choices that people make are in the service of *seeking* happiness — it doesn't mean that they find it in these behaviors or activities. "Seek and ye shall find" does not apply when it comes to happiness, and sometimes poor choices lead to the opposite of happiness. Remember that the U.S. Declaration of Independence only grants the right to "the pursuit of happiness" and not happiness itself.

When you look at another person and scratch your head over their choices — of significant others, hobbies, or hairstyles — these choices take on a new dimension when you see them as expressions of that person's inclination toward happiness. You may see a tragic pattern in your sister's choice of partners because they tend to be charming guys who are incredibly insecure and narcissistic, and ultimately end up treating her badly. But when you see that this is just her unmindful seeking of happiness that leads her to make these choices because of how these men make her feel when she first encounters them, it changes how you view your sister. You begin to see that she is not masochistically choosing men that she knows are bad for her or seeking men who she knows you won't approve of, just because she has a problem with you. She is just charting her own idiosyncratic course toward happiness, as she knows it, with the best of intentions, but perhaps a little too much naiveté or lack of awareness that could be more protective of her tender heart.

Take a moment to call to mind someone whose behavior, attitudes, or choices are hard for you to fathom. Maybe it's the woman on Facebook who posts nothing but videos of cats in costumes, or the guy behind the meat counter with the incredibly detailed face tattoos, or maybe it's someone who supports a different political candidate than you. You may find any of these to be offensive, disturbing, or confusing and something you would never choose, but is it possible for you to not take any of these things personally?

In other words, the butcher did not choose that image of a snake wrapping around his neck to offend you personally, but because he liked how it made him look. It made him happy in some way, even if you happen to cringe inside every time you see it. This is a benign example, but even in the most challenging of cases, seeing the underlying motives of another as being essentially guided by goodness and the pursuit of happiness, and nothing intentionally hurtful to you or anyone, can change your experience.

REMEMBER

The key to being able to have this attitude is not just having the belief that all people simply want to be happy and free from suffering, but cultivating the open heart and kind intention to accept the presence of whatever is here (mindfulness) and the awareness that we share these deep motivations (if not the penchant for serpentine tattoos). This practice asks us to watch our reactivity and initial impressions and be willing to go a little deeper to tap into our *own* natural capacity for kindness and our *own* desire to be happy so that we can cultivate an inner landscape of goodwill. The more that we tend that inner garden of goodwill, the more our heart opens, and the more our heart opens, the more seeds of benevolence can be sown for others and for ourselves.

Investing in Your Capacity to Be Kind

Whether you are planting a garden or exercising a muscle, the key is that you are investing the effort now, not because you expect immediate results (however much any of us might like that instant gratification), but because you have some faith that it will pay off over time to cultivate lovingkindness (or "boundless friendliness") in this way. This is the essence of why we practice lovingkindness meditation: to tap into and develop a deep inclination of the heart toward kindness, joy, and satisfaction.

Lovingkindness meditation has a long and rich history and was mainly brought from Asia to the West by meditation teacher Sharon Salzberg. The practice is a way of training the mind to be more loving and compassionate through a variety of means, especially the use of language, as the "vehicle" of the meditation. Words have particular power over us and our way of thinking about and being with our experiences.

We all learned to respond to people who said mean things (in a sing-song voice): "Sticks and stones will break my bones, but words can never hurt me." Sadly, as is the case with many platitudes, it sounds good but is entirely wrong. Think about it. Have you ever experienced a broken bone in your life? Has it healed? Now think about times when you have been deeply hurt by words that were spoken by someone else. Do you still feel the sting of that injury? Words matter. There is a saying, "Be careful what you say to yourself because you're listening." Words can often hurt us, which is why schoolyard bullies are often so skilled in finding just the right thing to say to push your buttons.

REMEMBER

If words can leave lingering pain and distress, then the good news in this is that we can use other words to promote healing and ease. We can bring words over from the dark side to the light side and gently but firmly cultivate an attitude of kindness and warmth if we are consistent and persistent in our practice.

Mixing together the power of words plus a dollop of imagery (for those among us who are visual learners), a sprinkling of concentration, a pinch of connection, and a dash of good old-fashioned human caring, lovingkindness meditation manages to become a rich stew for us to marinate in and coax out our natural juices of goodwill. Are you getting hungry just thinking about this practice? Time to give it a try.

Practice: Lovingkindness for a Loved One

This practice is drawn directly from the Mindful Self-Compassion program and is called Lovingkindness for a Loved One.

Begin by settling yourself into a comfortable position for your body, either sitting or lying down. You may even set the stage for this practice by offering yourself some soothing or supportive touch and allow yourself to really feel the kindness in the warmth of your hand touching your body. Let yourself feel supported and soothed by yourself.

When you are ready, call to mind a person or other living being who naturally makes you smile when you think of them. Choose someone with whom you have an easy, uncomplicated relationship, such as a child, a grandparent, perhaps your pet — any being that naturally brings happiness to your heart. See if you can settle on just one if more than one appears.

With some patience, allow yourself to pause and feel what it is actually like to be in the presence of this beloved being. Allow yourself to enjoy the good company by creating a vivid image of this being in your mind's eye.

After a few moments, reflect on the fact that this being wishes to be happy and free from suffering, just like you and every other living being. Repeat softly, slowly, and gently, feeling the importance of your words:

> May you be happy.
>
> May you be peaceful.
>
> May you be healthy.
>
> May you live with ease.

TIP

You may even want to repeat these phrases again. If at any point you notice your mind wandering, you can simply return to the words and the image of the loved one that you have in mind. Take the time to appreciate any warm feelings that may have arisen. Linger and savor this precious being.

Now, when you are ready, gently usher yourself into your circle of goodwill and create an image of yourself in the presence of your loved one, visualizing the two of you together. Feel your way into this connection and take your time. Eventually offer these phrases:

> May you and I be happy.
>
> May you and I be peaceful.

May you and I be healthy.

May you and I live with ease.

Again, take your time and possibly repeat the phrases.

Now, when it feels right, let go of the image of the other, maybe even briefly thanking your loved one before moving on. Then let the full focus of your loving attention rest upon yourself, just for now. You may want to again offer yourself some form of soothing or supportive touch. Take the time to visualize your whole body and scan from head to toe, noticing any stress or uneasiness that may be lingering within you at this time, and offer yourself the phrases:

May I be happy.

May I be peaceful.

May I be healthy.

May I live with ease.

Let the words and the kind intention wash across and through you, possibly repeating them again and again and feeling them land in your experience.

And, when you are ready, just take a few breaths and rest quietly in your own experience, allowing yourself to feel whatever you are feeling without needing anything to change. Meet yourself just as you are in this moment, with kindness, warmth, courage, and affection.

Take some time after concluding this practice to simply settle, reflect, and perhaps take a few notes about your experience, what you noticed, and how things unfolded for you. Don't be too quick to judge your experience, but take note of it and let it settle.

Inquiring: What was it like to cultivate kindness?

After having reflected a bit, consider what you noticed in your practice of loving-kindness. Whether it was the first time you've tried this or if it is a part of your regular meditation routine, what came up in *this* meditation today?

It may be helpful to consider what you noticed in each of the three components of the practice:

>> What was it like to call to mind a beloved being and to wish them these good wishes?

>> What was it like to include yourself alongside your loved one and to wish both of you good wishes?

>> How did it feel to let go of the other and let your "circle of goodwill" rest solely on yourself?

After people encounter this meditation, it is not unusual for them to enjoy the first part of it, be a little uncomfortable when they slip themselves into the mix, and have a harder time when the spotlight of lovingkindness rests solely on them. If this approximates your experience, you're not alone. We are not accustomed to being kind to ourselves (for a variety of reasons that are explored later) and we get twitchy when we're in the spotlight — even our *own* spotlight.

In general, people have one or more of three different experiences with this practice: They enjoy it, they feel neutral about it, or they find it uncomfortable. None of them is a reflection on you or your ability to practice lovingkindness, and each is explored briefly later in this chapter. Each time you practice this meditation your experience will vary, sometimes a little bit and sometimes a lot.

REMEMBER

Just like working out at the gym, you have good workouts, you have neutral workouts, and sometimes you have unpleasant workouts. But in the end, the important thing is that you *worked out,* and you kind of knew that working out was not necessarily going to be consistently enjoyable anyway.

LIFTING THE HEAVIEST WEIGHTS IN THE GYM

Traditionally, the lovingkindness meditation is practiced with a large cast of mental characters that customarily begin with those who are presumed to be the easiest and proceed to more challenging ones, almost like you might begin at the gym with the lightest weights you can lift and, as you get stronger, you move on to the heavier ones. Interestingly, the sequence that evolved in Asia from the Buddha's teachings tended to begin with directing the wishes to oneself, which was presumed to be the easiest starting place. What teachers like Sharon Salzberg and others discovered in the early days of presenting the practice in the West was that many people really struggled with directing these wishes inward toward themselves, mainly because so many people felt undeserving of this kindness and very uncomfortable wishing it for themselves. Thus, the practice in the West tends to start with a beloved being to kind of "jump-start" the process or warm up the heart so that you can move on to yourself and then others. If you struggled a bit in the Lovingkindness for a Loved One practice here, that may have been a manifestation of this phenomenon.

(continued)

(continued)

For our purposes here (and in the Mindful Self-Compassion program), we confine our focus to just two beings: the beloved other and ourselves, as a preparation for more focused practice related to self-compassion and being able to direct this goodwill toward ourselves specifically. But as noted earlier, typically lovingkindness meditation is practiced with a variety of beings. The whole idea, consistent with this parallel of working out in the gym, is that you are "trying out" a variety of different "weights" to slowly build strength or capacity to access your lovingkindness. The sequence is often something like this: beloved being, self, friend, neutral person, difficult person, all beings. (You can find quite a number of lovingkindness meditations, referred to as *metta* in the Pali language, online and in books. And if you are interested in pursuing this as a regular practice, it's highly recommended.)

You may be an ambitious person (perhaps "perfectionistic"?) and you may wonder about the potential value of challenging yourself even more by trying to direct lovingkindness wishes to neutral people, difficult people, or whole groups of people. In the spirit of self-compassion, if you decide to explore this further, be willing to cut yourself some slack and meet yourself in the practice with kindness.

Especially when you begin to direct lovingkindness wishes toward a difficult or challenging person in your life, it will be like walking over to the heaviest barbell in the gym. This being is included in the practice precisely because they are challenging, and you might even question why you would want to wish goodwill for someone you dislike or may even hate. The rationale is embedded in the common humanity practice of Just Like Me from Chapter 3 in Book 2. This is an opportunity to see that, below the ill will and bad feelings, you can still recognize that this other person wishes to be happy and free from suffering, just like you. This person suffers at times, is afraid at times, has had hard times and joyful times, has succeeded and failed at times, and through it all they are genetically 99.9 percent the same as you. When you can see through your feelings to this essential reality, and your heart can remain warm and open in the practice, you are truly practicing lovingkindness in its most transformative form.

But please be willing to go slow. Perhaps if you are going to identify a difficult person to work with (a heavy weight to start with), you may want to choose one at first that is less challenging and easier to work with and then work your way forward to the more challenging ones as you feel more adept at meeting this challenging practice and remaining kind.

What if you practiced and felt absolutely nothing?

Good for you in noticing your experience, even though nothing stood out or seemed noteworthy. It's not easy to notice the absence of thoughts, feelings, or emotions. You may be thinking of this as a failure, but in fact it is a glorious success of mindfulness. Take a moment to take that in. You noticed the absence of something, which is equally noteworthy and important as noticing the presence of something.

Think of all the times you have felt sick and thought to yourself, "I don't appreciate being well often enough, because this is terrible." Does this sound familiar? We so often overlook feeling well because we expect things to be that way, and then we kick ourselves when we realize how good we had it when we weren't sick. So, noticing the absence of something is a great skill akin to acknowledging when we are feeling well.

But perhaps your observation comes with a concern that perhaps you did something wrong or that you were *supposed to* feel something. Perhaps you thought if you did a lovingkindness meditation, you would actually *feel* lovingkindness. A reasonable and logical expectation to have, but look back and reread what we say earlier about the practice. Were you ever promised that you would *feel* lovingkindness? No, because this practice is not about cultivating *good feelings* but instead about cultivating *good intentions,* a warm inclination of the heart toward kindness.

When we exercise, we are cultivating physical fitness, but often when we exercise (or shortly thereafter) we don't feel physically fit at all. We continue because we know that persistence and consistency will lead to our desired goal of fitness. It is the same with lovingkindness, and perhaps why we call it "practice."

We practice and practice and practice lovingkindness (using various images of beings in our lives like weights at the gym), and ultimately, we incline our hearts and tap into our natural leanings toward kindness and warmth. Jon Kabat-Zinn refers to mindfulness practice as akin to weaving a parachute, and this applies to lovingkindness as well.

REMEMBER

The time to start weaving your parachute is not right before you have to jump out of the plane. You begin early and often, weaving your parachute (practicing lovingkindness), over and over, day after day, week after week, so that when you need it, it is there for you. In a moment when you want to tap into your natural loving human heart qualities, if you've been practicing, kindness is more readily available to you and it becomes more often your default stance toward experience.

What if you practiced lovingkindness and felt great?

You probably don't see this outcome as a problem, but it is important to be clear on what feeling something positive or pleasant or enjoyable in some way means. Don't get your heart set on having this experience all the time. It doesn't mean you've mastered lovingkindness (or failed at it, for that matter), and having a good feeling wasn't really the point of the practice. But that doesn't mean you can't take a moment to simply revel in the warm feelings of lovingkindness, to savor them and to let them register in your mind ("taking in the good" as Rick Hanson likes to say). Just don't get attached.

One of the sneakier aspects of pleasant experiences is that they can be seductive. We do something like practicing lovingkindness, and a pleasant feeling arises while we are doing it or shortly thereafter. We pat ourselves on the back for having conjured such a nice feeling, and then we're off in the pursuit of the next pleasant experience. When it's put like that, it's almost like an addiction, which it probably is, as we go about our days craving the pleasant, trying to avoid the unpleasant, and even seeing the neutral experiences as unpleasant because they are boring. On the latter point, we are finding boredom to be particularly uncomfortable these days, and we carry around an easy distraction to these moments: a smartphone. This accounts for why so many of us find ourselves checking our phones while we are sitting in the bathroom.

So when we meditate and then have a pleasant experience, our amazing human brains begin to wire those two experiences together and very subtly, over time, we begin to act as if doing one (meditation) will bring the other one (bliss). But note that we are not meditating to conjure a feeling but to practice being present to whatever comes up, and the same is true for lovingkindness. We are inclining the heart so we can access our loving intentions more readily, regardless of the situation.

REMEMBER

Encountering the felt sense of lovingkindness as a result of the practice is a welcome but seductive and unpredictable outcome. Enjoy it for what it is . . . and let go when it passes.

Chapter **5**

Discovering Core Values: Your Inner Compass

Well, if you've read Book 2 up to this point, you now know pretty much everything anyone ever needed to know about self-compassion. Practice mindfulness, embrace and appreciate your common humanity, and offer yourself kindness when you struggle or suffer. Simply treat yourself the way you would treat a dear friend when *they* have a hard time, and you're good to go. You're all loaded up on all the necessary supplies for the self-compassion adventure, and you're being dropped off at the trailhead. Happy trails and best of luck!

"Wait!" you may be thinking. "That's it? But just because I know all this stuff and I've dabbled in accessing my inclination for goodwill doesn't mean I know what to do with it, where I'm actually headed, or really why I want to embark on this journey at all. What about practical skills and applications of what I've been learning?"

Ah, you are beginning to see the challenge to this work. Knowing it and doing it are two entirely different things. Okay, you've talked us into sticking around and walking you through the tricky territory of self-compassion in daily life that lies ahead. Over time you will get accustomed to becoming your *own* best guide.

No good journey begins without a clear map of the landscape ahead, and that is what the preceding chapters provide you. But even with a map in hand, you still need a good compass and a healthy dose of motivation to propel you out on the trail and to sustain you when you hit the inevitable rough spots. This sense of tuning into your guiding intentions and finding a deeper purpose in this work is what this chapter explores.

Most importantly to your point of not *really* knowing what to do with the knowledge you've gained so far, it's important to emphasize here that self-compassion is a practice or a way of being and not an intellectual pursuit. Up until this point the emphasis has been on teaching *about* self-compassion, but as you proceed forward, you will be focusing much more on *learning* self-compassion itself, from the inside. Imagine the difference between reading a travel book on Morocco and actually being there, tasting the food, seeing the views, meeting the people. The actual practice of self-compassion will come alive as you explore how to make changes in your life, how to work with challenging emotions and people, and all sorts of other human endeavors that are better when we are kinder to ourselves. Time to get moving and see where this trail leads and why you may want to explore it with self-compassion.

Core Values Guide Us and "Re-Mind" Us

As Chapter 1 in Book 2 establishes, the quintessential question of self-compassion is, "What do I need?" The thing is, this is a pretty deep question with a lot of layers when you consider it. If someone were to strike up a conversation with you at a party and ask you, "What do you need?" you might be at a loss to answer it. You would most likely respond by saying something like, "What do you mean? Like what do I need right now? Like would I like another beer, or do I have another party to go to?" Another possibility would be that you would take it as a deeply philosophical question: "Do you mean, what do I, as a human, really *need* in life?" And of course, there all the other layers of "need" in between these two extremes.

There is also the issue of deciding what "need" actually means relative to wants. If you are a parent, you have undoubtedly had this discussion with an insistent child at some point, perhaps many times. You find yourself explaining that your child does not *need* the latest toy or version of the video game, but instead they actually really *want* it. Tuning in to the fundamental role of needs in your life allows you to disentangle them from your more fleeting and insubstantial wants. In fact, you might say that wants come from the neck up and needs come from the neck down.

Finding meaning through core values

As you begin to plumb the depths of the layers of need, you encounter not only basic human needs but also core values. Human needs are most commonly associated with physical and emotional survival, such as the need for security, connection, or health. In most cases, we share a fairly similar set of human needs with all our fellow humans. We all need food, clothing, and shelter, for example.

Core values, on the other hand, relate more directly to meaning in life and tend to vary a bit more from person to person. For example, someone might enjoy creative pursuits more than you do, but you may find social connection and friendship to be more important than that person does. Each value (creativity or social connection) may exist for each of us, but to differing degrees. Your values inform your sense of meaning in your life. This variation has a lot to do with how you choose to spend your time, who you are drawn to, and what you may seek in a career or hobby. And of course, values and human needs do overlap to some degree. A life devoid of meaning may not feel worth living, so meaning is no less crucial to our survival than are food, clothing, and shelter.

Because core values vary from person to person, they are big factors in what makes each of us unique and special in spite of our similarity to each other. When we say, "They march to the beat of a different drummer," we are often just saying, "They're kinda weird." But really what we mean is that something different motivates them, that they have different core values from ours, and we just acknowledge it by naming it in this way. We recognize that, despite our common humanity, we also each possess a relatively unique set of core values that determines how we show up in the world.

This is all well and good, but it also suggests that perhaps we can all hear our own "inner drummer" and are largely going about our lives fully in sync to that drumbeat in a world that is a kind of chaotic cacophony of various core values and different drumbeats. To some extent this may be true (although the mental image is pretty jarring), but nobody was ever handed a list of their core values and a set of instructions about how to align with them. Most of us operate on a felt sense of what moves us combined with life circumstances that may facilitate us living in alignment with those values.

We muddle along, like a paramecium under the microscope, drawn in by some things and repelled by others and just trying our best to find our way in the world with some degree of ease and peace. Paramecia probably don't have core values, but like you, they "know" in their core what they like. Our human needs and abilities are more complex, and that is why we are exploring this topic here.

You see, core values are a bit like an internal compass. A real-world compass is attuned to the earth's magnetic poles and gives the adventurer a constant guide as to which way is north, and therefore, which direction to walk if one wants to go in a particular direction. Our core values are like our own unique inner compass that is attuned to what is most important to us (instead of to the North Pole).

REMEMBER

The challenge for us is to find a way to tune into our core values and to be able to sense the position of the needle on our inner compass, to detect when it is aligned with our core values and when it is not. Bluntly speaking, when we are living in alignment with our values, we are happier than when we are not.

What this means is that our core values are intimately intertwined not only with our life satisfaction but also with our suffering. In fact, one could say that our suffering largely arises out of a conflict between our actual life circumstances and our deeply held core values. If you deeply value human connection, then you will be disappointed when a friend cancels a visit, but if you really value your "me time," then the same cancellation could be an unforeseen gift instead.

Your core values determine your experience

The view of core values described in the preceding section also helps explain why things that seem objectively to be good things may not be seen so by some people. For example, if you are a social worker who values making a difference for individuals in their lives, then your recent promotion to agency manager may not make you that happy. Perhaps the promotion means more money or prestige or freedom (all of which may be valuable to you too), but if this takes you away from the joy you derive from working one-on-one with people, the new role may be a hollow achievement in some ways. Another social worker, with a desire to bring about system-wide changes and transformation in the community may find the same promotion from the one-on-one work to be a dream come true. How the promotion is experienced is driven by the core values of the one who has been promoted. Being laid off from your job may be a disaster if you value security and supporting your family, but it may be a godsend if you really treasure adventure and new horizons.

REMEMBER

We're speaking specifically about core values here, and not goals. In other words, core values speak to valued *directions* whereas goals speak to valued *destinations*. Other ways in which these two concepts are different include the following:

>> Goals can be achieved, but core values guide us even after we achieve our goals.

>> Goals are something we do, but core values are something we are.

>> Goals are set by us, while core values are discovered.

>> Goals can be visualized, while core values are more often felt.

A few examples of core values are more stable across human beings and are related to how we treat other people, such as compassion, generosity, honesty, and loyalty. At the same time, many of our core values tend more to our own personal needs and desires that are deeply relevant to us but may not have the same importance to others. Some examples of personal core values are personal growth, creativity, tranquility, nature, and busyness.

The relationship between core values and suffering

Because we are not routinely aware of exactly what our core values are, we can often find ourselves in situations (relationships, jobs, geographical locations) that do not support us in fulfilling those values, and thus lead to us feeling dissatisfied, unfulfilled, unhappy, or even anxious or depressed. Complicating matters further, we have a tendency to see the blame for our discomfort or dissatisfaction as due to the circumstances (an insensitive boyfriend or a crummy job) rather than the mismatch between those circumstances and our core values.

This unfortunate situation often leads us to re-create these unsatisfactory situations over and over again. If you decide that you are unhappy in your factory assembly job, so you quit and then go find another factory assembly job, you may be overlooking the very real possibility that your original dissatisfaction had to do with the type of job it was and not the specific one you had.

This is not to say that you may not have a lousy boyfriend (or job), for example, but rather than pinning everything specifically on him, you might consider what you value in relationships that is not being honored in this particular one. This way you can come away from the relationship with a better sense of what is meaningful and important to you, and seek out that quality in your next boyfriend. And if you reverse this situation and have a partner you love and enjoy very much and that relationship ends, you may be heartbroken. But if you can identify what you loved about your ex-partner, it can help you find someone new who makes you happy.

Practice: Uncovering your core values

If you are willing to explore self-compassionately within yourself to identify your inner compass and what *you* are living for and what is getting in the way, then the exercise in this section is for you.

This exercise is extensively drawn from an exercise called Discovering Our Core Values in the Mindful Self-Compassion program, and *that* exercise is adapted from Acceptance and Commitment Therapy and the work of Hayes, Strosahl, and Wilson (2003). The process is intended to take you a bit deeper to discover the core values that are already a part of who you are and see where you can better align with them, as well as how self-compassion may support you in that shift.

TIP

Even if you aren't a person inclined to follow and do multi-step exercises like this one, there is a "short form" that may be helpful. Take the time to look around at your particular situation (your home, your partner, your job, your hobbies and activities, your friends and family, your house of worship, and your community). Take each one in turn and ask yourself, "What is it *about* this person or thing that brings up my joy and satisfaction, or my discomfort and dissatisfaction?" In other words, look below the particular features of meaningful things to the *essence* of what they bring (or don't bring) to your life. This will provide clues to your core values and a rudimentary map for the road ahead (and maybe inspire you to do this full exercise too!).

TIP

To prepare for this reflective exercise, it would be helpful to have paper and pencil nearby, or a keyboard to record your thoughts and observations. Once you have this, take a moment to "clear the decks," close your eyes, and settle yourself in to this moment. Maybe even give yourself a little warm inner smile of welcome to this moment and this exercise on what is most important to you. You might remember that this is just a continuation of your life, in which you have sought happiness, joy, and satisfaction all along, sometimes with more or less awareness of what brings that joy, but always with a good, warm heart that simply wants to be happy and free from suffering.

Looking back on a life well-lived

Take a few moments now to imagine yourself in your later years. You are in a comfortable place, feeling relaxed, safe, and content, and you are contemplating your life. As you look back on the period of time between that later date and now, you feel a deep sense of satisfaction, joy, and contentment. Even though life has not always been easy, you managed to chart a course for your life that kept you true to yourself and your values the best that you could.

What core values were expressed or followed in that life? These could be values such as meaningful work, adventure, tranquility, loyalty, service, or compassion. Take some time to write down some of the core values that were represented in your life. You may also take the time to write down the activities that you engage in that align you with these core values, the things you do that bring you joy, contentment, and satisfaction in your daily life.

Considering where you are not aligned with your values

When you are ready and feel you have identified at least a few key core values for yourself, drop back inside and pause to settle and reflect on something different. Ask yourself whether there are any ways in which your life seems out of balance with your values, especially the more personal ones. Maybe your leisure time activities are too full of pressing demands for you to indulge in more creative pursuits, even though creativity is a great love in your life.

If you have more than one value that feels out of balance, for now just choose one that feels most important to focus upon and write it down. You can always come back to this exercise again and again and explore other values as well.

Identifying the obstacles you face

We all have obstacles that prevent us from living totally in alignment with our core values. Take a moment to consider first what *external obstacles* may be getting in the way. These obstacles may be not having enough money or time, or having other more pressing obligations or responsibilities to tend to. These are often the first things that come to mind when we realize we are out of accord with our values. Take some time to reflect on these obstacles that you face and write them down.

Also consider that, in addition to *external* obstacles that you may face, there may well be some *internal* obstacles as well. Often these are a bit less obvious and may take some time and patient reflection on what they are and how they are pulling you out of alignment with your core values. Maybe you have a fear of failure, or maybe you doubt your abilities, or perhaps you have a particularly vocal inner critic that gets in the way of you moving in valued directions.

Cultural obstacles are an insidious form of internal obstacle, where you may doubt your ability due to a prevailing cultural narrative about your identity that is limiting in some way. It is even possible, from a cultural perspective, to realize that your internal obstacle is sheer exhaustion from feeling pulled to stand up for yourself all the time. Whatever the obstacle, take your time and make note of any internal obstacles you face.

Finding a place for self-compassion

Give yourself some time now to consider whether self-compassion (in either its yin or yang form) may help you live more in accord with your deeply held core values. Following are some examples:

>> See if you can find a compassionate alternative to your inner critic, one that motivates you out of a desire to align with your values rather than out of a fear of failure.

>> Perhaps self-compassion may help you feel safe and confident enough to take new (maybe even bold) actions.

>> Tap into the yang energy of self-compassion to see whether you can find enough inner safety and bravery to risk failing at something that is meaningful to you.

>> Pause to look around to see whether you are clinging to anything that isn't serving you anymore, and if so, consider self-compassionately letting that thing go so you can move on.

Give yourself plenty of time to explore how self-compassion can support you in this inner work of connecting to your core values. Try things on for size, test them, and be willing to be creative, patient, and kind with yourself in this process.

If you identify some obstacles that are truly insurmountable in this moment, can you give yourself compassion just for the fact of that particular hardship? Maybe just pause here, if this is the case for you, and give yourself a few words of appreciation for even doing this work and respecting your core values, even if your obstacles are just too big or imposing right now. You may even consider exploring *other* ways that you can express your values in some way, even if that expression feels somewhat incomplete. For example, if nature is a great value but your family responsibilities get in the way, perhaps you can find time to simply gaze at photographs or videos of nature in the meantime until other opportunities arise.

And finally, if the absolutely insurmountable problem is that you are imperfect, as all human beings are, can you forgive yourself for that fact as well?

Inquiring: What was it like to discover your core values?

Did you uncover any core values in this exercise? If you discovered a few, did one in particular rise to the top as you reflected upon it? If one did, how did it feel to name it and consider it? Were you aware of any feelings that arose as you did that?

Please note that sometimes people identify a core belief in this exercise that they feel has been overlooked or ignored for large portions of their life for a variety of reasons (both within and outside of their control).

REMEMBER

The purpose of this reflection is to identify these important values, not to assign blame for not living in alignment with them or to feel any amount of shame or embarrassment for losing track of them along the way.

If difficult feelings came up as you contemplated a core value, see whether you can simply comfort yourself because sometimes discoveries can be painful at first. This is understandable, but see whether you can be patient with yourself, as most of us live much of our lives without much conscious awareness of our values. The good news is that once these things are in your consciousness, then, and only then, can you begin to make changes, to make amends with yourself and to find your way into alignment with what is important to you deep down.

How did it feel to name the obstacles, both internal and external, that you face in trying to live in accord with your core values? Were there any surprises or any apparent obstacles that perhaps turned out to be less formidable than you had assumed? Sometimes an obstacle in one area can loom so large in a person's awareness that it seems like it prevents them from pursuing any of their values. Often people who have a physical disability let that challenge prevent them from engaging socially with others or finding meaningful work, but when they look a bit closer they realize that it need not be an obstacle to these activities.

Most relevant to your purpose here, did you find any way that being more self-compassionate could help you to align better with your core values?

TIP

This is not a "one and done" sort of exercise. Many people find that returning to this reflective process over and over can be very helpful to periodically "recalibrate" and focus on what is most important, as life can often cause us to drift off course. A patient who was previously in the military referred to becoming "OBE." OBE stands for Overcome By Events, and life can feel like one incident of OBE after another. We can often feel like a ship being tossed about by stormy seas and can easily be blown off course through no fault of our own. The good news is that values work is like the North Pole or the stars above, always available to support us in navigating back to our intended course.

Translating values into action

Exploration of our core values is often a very fruitful exercise and stirs up a lot of feelings for people. We may feel bad for not having lived up to our core values in the past, but it's important to view this practice as a potential turning point instead. As mentioned earlier, once you are more acutely aware of your core values, *then* you are actually able to do something about them.

Quite often, based on the experience of this exercise, people resolve to take action on what they discover and try to figure out ways to make the changes that they see as crucial for realignment with their values. It's good to really cement these values in your awareness so that you are more conscious of them and they're available to you when you make decisions in your life.

If life is like a long boat journey where you are the captain, each moment when you make a decision is like a tiny turn of the wheel on your boat. It may seem small at the time, but if you stay on course it can lead to a very different destination over time. Only when you have your direction firmly in mind can you steer the ship of your life in a steady, consistent direction, making course corrections now and then when you drift off course, and always keeping your eyes on the prize.

TIP

The following hints can help you stay aligned with your values and keep them in your awareness as you go about your life:

>> Write down your core values and post them someplace where you will see them daily, such as your bathroom mirror, the refrigerator door, or the wall of your cubicle at work. (Tattoos are good, but perhaps a bit too permanent and public for your taste.)

>> Create a little vow for yourself. A simple statement that is much like a lovingkindness wish can be quite powerful if you return to it on a regular basis, almost as a kind of small sacred ritual for yourself.

For example, turning a core value such as social justice into a vow might look like "I vow to seek justice whenever the opportunity arises." Repeating it each morning, or lighting a candle and reciting it each evening, can slowly embed it in your consciousness and guide you like the north star.

Dark Nights and Dark Clouds: Wisdom Gleaned from Life's Challenges

Perhaps it has slowly dawned on you that much of the practice of self-compassion is focused on the benefits of being able to kindly accompany ourselves through the challenges of life and the suffering that each of us experiences as a human being. Maybe your initial motivation for exploring the practice and buying this book was to see whether there was a way you could tiptoe around the suffering in your life (or possibly simply banish it) and simply be happy (or at least happier) all the time. Sorry about that, but you have probably begun to realize that this is not actually realistic, and frankly it would be a relatively dull life if everything always went smoothly.

You're probably rolling your eyes at that last statement and thinking, "I would be more than happy to have a nice long stretch of smooth sailing and happy feelings. That whole 'suffering builds character' is highly overrated, and I already have more than enough character, thank you." That's understandable, but think of the richness of your life when you look at it in its entirety.

REMEMBER

The joys and sorrows, the pleasures and the pains all blend together into a complex stew of experience that makes up where you have been and partially determines who you have become (the nurture part of the age-old "nature versus nurture" discussion).

Seasoning in the stew

A stew is made up of a lot of ingredients and spices. Each life is like a rich stew, with a variety of intense experiences (flavors) that all blend together to create the experience that you call "me." These experiences don't define you, but they do contribute to who you are.

You shouldn't necessarily love or treasure all the painful or challenging things you have experienced, but the experiences you have had all blend together to contribute to where and who you are. And of course, the past is behind you and your challenge is really to give up all hope of a different yesterday so that you can show up fully for today, where you *can* make a difference. This can take the form of realigning yourself to your core values, as we just explored, or seeing what deeper lesson can be learned from your past experiences to enrich your future.

REMEMBER

It's important to clarify that some painful and traumatic experiences are hard to acknowledge and embrace as ingredients in the stew of your life. If you have had this sort of experience, you may feel as though it has poisoned the stew or at least made it incredibly distasteful. We're not discounting this possibility at all. Rather, we ask that you continue to go slow and explore how you can engage in what psychologists call *post-traumatic growth* to see if you can find a way forward that makes some meaning out of your terrible experiences and eventually transform your history into a foundation for some freedom from this particular suffering.

REMEMBER

Quite often, the simple fact that you survived a terrible, painful, or traumatic experience is the most important takeaway message you can glean from these things, and that is more than enough. Again, please be kind to yourself, go slowly, and let your own experience be your guide as to what you need and what you may learn if you are gentle but brave in touching these experiences only as much as you are willing. Be curious and kind and see what you might discover when you listen in this self-compassionate way.

How failure and hardship teach us

None of us seeks to flop when we try things, and we don't usually seek adversity to overcome, but nonetheless these things happen. The challenge to living our lives to the fullest is not figuring out how to eliminate these inevitable things from happening, but seeing if we can learn lessons from them when they do.

Often the lessons that you learn or the silver linings you discover inside the dark clouds of your hardships are things you never would have realized otherwise. Even infants and toddlers learn from unexpected and unfortunate experiences. When the toddler pushes his sippy cup off the edge of the table, they learn about gravity (and what not to do if you are thirsty). Often our hard lessons are much more painful than spilt milk, but they are nonetheless potential teachers. The poet Jane Hirschfield says, "Suffering leads us to beauty the way thirst leads to water."

REMEMBER

Challenges often force you to go deep inside and uncover resources or capacities that you never knew you possessed or never dreamed you would have to tap into. Self-compassion plays an important role here because it helps you to create that brave and safe inner space that gives you courage to turn toward this suffering and see what it may have to teach you.

Exercise: Silver linings and golden gifts

This reflective exercise is drawn from the Mindful Self-Compassion program and is intended to support you in discovering first-hand what is possible when you look at life's failures or hardships in a different light.

This reflection is best done with a way to make notes, either on pencil or paper or on a keyboard. Once you have prepared yourself to write a few things, allow your eyes to close and your body and mind to settle. Perhaps take a few slow, deep, relaxing breaths to allow your attention to drop inside and out of your thinking mind.

When you are ready, call to mind a struggle in your life that seemed very difficult or even impossible to bear at the time, but that in retrospect, taught you something important. Be sure to choose a situation that is far enough in the past and has been *very clearly resolved* such that you have already learned whatever you needed to learn from it. Please, do not choose a traumatic event that could be re-traumatizing if you recall it now.

REMEMBER

Not every dark cloud has a silver lining, and sometimes there is nothing to be learned from suffering, except that simply having returned (or tried to return) to ordinary life is a triumph in itself. But for *this* reflection, choose an event that did have a silver lining.

Call to mind the situation in question, what the challenge was, and how it felt to go through it at the time.

Pause to really take some time to honor yourself for the difficulty you endured and how you struggled with it at the time. This is not about reviewing how you handled the situation, per se, but how it was to be in it, doing your best to navigate through it.

Make a few notes about the situation for yourself, what the experience was like. Also, take some time to add some kind words to offer yourself that validate what you went through. These may be the kinds of words you would offer a friend telling you a similar story of their own struggles. You might have words like: "That was hard!"; "You were so brave to get through that!"; or "There was no way you could have anticipated that, but you got through it."

As you are ready, give yourself some time to reflect on what *deeper lesson* this challenging situation taught you that you may not have learned otherwise. Write that lesson (or lessons) too. Consider how that lesson has resided within you ever since, perhaps guiding you through other difficult situations or helping you avoid some hardships as a result. This is the golden gift of the silver lining: a lasting legacy of wisdom gained in the midst of a challenging experience of suffering.

Inquiring: Were you able to identify a silver lining?

Like many of the reflective exercises in Book 2, this one can be returned to over and over, and new discoveries can be made. Also as with the other exercises, you would be wise to take your time and let these practices, reflections, and ideas linger and mellow and transform over time. Don't be too quick to formulate a concrete lesson learned, but instead entertain possibilities, like a scientist entertains hypotheses. Hold it in mind, test it, see how it withstands the test of your patient scrutiny, and see what emerges. As always, patience, persistence, kindness, and curiosity are the keys to discovering the transformative power of reflecting on silver linings.

REMEMBER

We don't have just one core value, but many of them, and they can be related to important dimensions of being human, such as your relationships, your culture or community, your spiritual life, your work, your family, and so on.

3

Facing Challenges with Resilience

Contents at a Glance

CHAPTER 1: **Embarking on the Journey to Resilience** 175

Noting That Resilience Is for Everyone. 175
Figuring Out the Factors That Determine Resilience 176
Understanding What Resilience Is Not. 180
Breaking the Victim Cycle. 185

CHAPTER 2: **The Basis of Resilience: Harmony Versus Stress**. 187

Understanding the Perpetual Quest for Harmony. 188
Examining the Stress Response Feedback Loop. 189
Living in Disharmony: The Real Stress 191
Expecting a Good Outcome Is the Key. 192
Coping to Adapt, or Not 193
Harmonizing Stress and Becoming Resilient. 195

CHAPTER 3: **Developing Mental Toughness and Clarity** 199

What Kind of Mindset Do Resilient People Have?. 200
Fixed Versus Growth Mindsets When It Comes to Resilience. . . . 201
Developing Mental Toughness 202
Accessing Mental Clarity. 208

CHAPTER 4: **Achieving Emotional Equilibrium** 211

Emotions Exist for a Very Good Reason. 211
How Emotions Influence Perception and Coping. 213
Evaluating Your Feelings. 214
Choosing to Manage Your Emotions 215
Calming Your Emotions By Calming the Stress Response. 217
Shifting to Positive Detachment and Reappraisal 218
Enhancing Your Self-Awareness and Willingness to Grow 219
Always Choosing Love. 220

CHAPTER 5: **Improving Your Relationship with Yourself** 221

Connecting Resilience with Self-Worth. 222
Believing in Your Worth 223
Noting Self-Criticism 224
Evaluating Your Self-Value 225
Starting to Take Action 227
Taking Care of YOU. 233
Allowing Love In. 237

» **Examining factors that determine resilience**

» **Knowing what resilience is not**

» **Stopping the victim cycle**

Chapter 1

Embarking on the Journey to Resilience

ontrary to what many people think, resilience has nothing to do with avoiding stress, hardship, or failure in life. Instead, it's about knowing that life is filled with both joy and adversity and that when hardship happens, you'll be prepared to take it on, learn from it, and become stronger as a result. Resilience confers the ability to bounce back easily and thrive in the face of life's *many* inevitable challenges. This chapter describes the factors that determine resilience, explains how it's possible to develop resilience even if your genes aren't wired that way, and sets the stage for how you can embark on the journey to building your bounce-back muscle and becoming stronger, wiser, and feeling more fulfilled.

Noting That Resilience Is for Everyone

It's true that some people are naturally more resilient than others. These folks see challenges as opportunities, maintain a positive outlook, find meaning in the struggle, and successfully adapt to adversity. The good news is that even if it doesn't come naturally to you, you can build your bounce-back muscle. It comes down to choosing not to let adversity get you down and instead work toward using the situation to become stronger and wiser. Here are your options:

>> **Stay broken:** Succumb to stress, fall apart, and stay that way — you're unable to recover normal functioning and feel helpless.

>> **Stay weak:** Succumb to stress, get injured, and partially recover — you're weak and your functioning is still subpar.

>> **Get back to baseline:** Manage the stress and bounce back to baseline, whatever that may be.

>> **Become stronger:** Reckon with the stress and grow stronger, wiser, and fitter as a result.

REMEMBER

You can choose to feel victimized by life's hardships or choose to accept them and make the most of every situation. You'll have to make some effort to build your resilience muscle, but it's absolutely possible, especially if your choice is to thrive rather than dive.

Figuring Out the Factors That Determine Resilience

At some point, most people incur some form of suffering, whether it's the death of a loved one, illness, injury, divorce, job loss, or another difficult life event. Not everyone copes with adversity in the same way, though, because it's influenced by multiple factors. Some of these factors you have no control over, such as your genes, the culture you grew up in, or critical life events that may have occurred in your past. Some of these factors are within your control, such as your beliefs, behaviors, attitudes, and chosen networks of support. The question is, which of these determinants carries the most weight when it comes to resilience? Is it up to nature, or is it a result of nurture?

REMEMBER

Though genetics does play a role, it appears that people have the ability to develop resilience despite genetics. According to a study conducted by the National Institutes of Health's National Institute of Nursing Research, led by Heather Rusch, two critically important factors associated with resilience are in your control to change:

>> **Self-mastery:** The degree to which you perceive yourself as having control and influence over circumstance.

>> **Social support:** The degree to which you perceive you are cared for and receiving help from other people.

The stronger these two factors, according to the research, the higher the likelihood that an individual will be resilient in the face of trauma or stress. The following sections describe the different factors that determine resilience and see how it all works.

Your genes

Though it hasn't been established that a single gene or gene variation confers resilience, it has been found that genetic factors can influence how you respond to stress and deal with adversity. A range of genes has been identified that are associated with resilient *phenotypes* (how a gene expresses itself physically). Genes or variations of genes, for example, can influence the stress response, nervous system, immune system, and pathways that produce feel-good neurotransmitters such as serotonin and dopamine and determine your biological response to stress. The bottom line is that science is showing that although genes play a role in determining resilience, they're only part of the story because it's now widely known that nature and nurture go hand in hand.

Your life experiences — especially early life, culture, and behaviors — influence the expression of genes and the neurobiological systems that enable adaptation to stress and resilience. Meditation, exercise, healthy nutrition, and social support are examples of lifestyle changes that can effect such neurobiological changes and, possibly, genetic expression. In short, you can influence your genes and still achieve better self-mastery and social support.

Childhood development

Early childhood experiences can positively or negatively affect the development of the stress response and how individuals subsequently learn to cope with adversity. Trauma and abuse can lead to changes in central nervous system circuits, a hyperactive stress response, more anxious behavior, and vulnerability to stress from learned helplessness, as people learn to believe that they have no control to change their circumstance or situation.

It has also been shown that when individuals realize that it's possible to change behaviors — even in the face of adversity — and feel better, learned helplessness doesn't happen. Examples might include when a child suffers bullying at school and receives a lot of love and support from family, friends, and counselors and is provided with effective coping tools. Children who gain the ability to adapt to stress develop better self-esteem, prosocial behavior, and more immunity to stress as they age.

As such, neither your genetics nor your past necessarily blocks you from being resilient. Either of these may support a tendency to adapt to stress more effectively or less effectively, but neither seals the deal on your ability to become stronger and more positive and have a better sense of self-mastery.

Culture

Individual behavior and coping styles are influenced by cultural patterns of beliefs, values, commitments, resources, and expected behaviors. Culture, therefore, can predict resilience as it shapes how people might see themselves and how they relate to others. The culture of a family can especially shape how a child develops a sense of self-concept and self-esteem. For example, a culture might value the woman's role as being quiet and docile, and subject to a man's authority, whereas another culture advocates for gender equality. Children growing up in either of these households will likely grow up to have very different self-concepts.

Culture refers not just to your ethnicity or religion but also to the culture of your family or your workplace. Cultures that promote respect, collaboration, reliance, open communication, and strong core values promote resilience within the community as well as individual resilience.

Psychological outlook

Your upbringing and environment can influence your outlook and how you see yourself and the world at large. A positive outlook has been found to be protective in the face of adversity and associated with better coping behaviors, quicker recovery times, improved health and wellbeing, and a better sense of self-mastery. The reverse is true for a negative outlook, as a negative view of oneself and the world increases the perception and magnitude of stress and reduces the sense of self-mastery and belief that challenges are manageable. A negative outlook is associated with limiting beliefs, negative self-talk, narrow thinking, and less effective coping habits.

A myriad of traits are associated with a positive outlook. Those most associated with resilience are believing that success is possible (optimism), viewing difficulties as opportunities for growth and learning, having the willingness to push forward, being able to accept change, and being open to making mistakes and learning from failures. All these traits can be cultivated with practice and also aren't purely dependent on upbringing and genetics.

Coping habits

Coping habits are habits you have developed that have helped you get through challenges or difficulties. In general, there are two types of coping habits:

>> **Adaptive** habits are the behaviors that help you cope with stress that are also healthy for the mind and body.

>> **Maladaptive** habits are behaviors that might reduce anxiety and therefore help you cope but are themselves destructive to your health.

Confronting your fears head-on, appraising situations realistically, calming your emotions, and maintaining healthy behaviors — such as good sleep hygiene and a balanced exercise-and-nutrition regimen — are examples of adaptive coping habits. Choosing to avoid dealing with fear and drinking alcohol, binge eating, or throwing yourself into work so that you aren't sleeping, exercising, or eating appropriately are examples of maladaptive coping habits.

Some adaptive coping habits that improve resilience are exercising (see Book 4), eating a healthy diet (see Book 5), meditating (see Book 1), accessing social support, connecting to spirituality, learning to reappraise thoughts and beliefs, regulating emotions, and partaking in altruistic activities. These habits can be learned and cultivated, even when maladaptive coping has been the norm.

Social support

Support comes in the form of family, intimate partners, colleagues, neighbors, friends, spiritual community members, and others. The presence of strong networks of support and the seeking of social support are both associated with resilience. Both invigorate psychological hardiness and the ability to thrive in the face of adversity. Studies show that stronger social bonds can improve quality of life, wound healing, and life expectancy. In contrast, the lack of support is correlated with more depression and a weaker sense of control.

The ability to forge healthy social bonds, be able to communicate effectively, and show value and compassion are traits that a resilient person exemplifies, enabling them to have a truly viable social support system in times of need. With help, anyone can learn to improve their ability to form healthier relationships and stronger networks of support.

Humor

Sometimes, you have to laugh to literally keep yourself from crying, and when you do, it can make you more resilient. Humor helps you release stress, and it's a conduit to strengthening social bonds while being protective against stress. A study of sojourn students from mainland China attending school at a Hong Kong university, for instance, found that the students who used humor to adjust to the new culture were able to thrive best, and that humor acted as a buffer against stress.

Humor and laughter are wonderful resources when coping with hardship, because they lighten the load emotionally as well as physiologically. Laughter especially can relax the stress response, give you more energy, and soothe tension. It has also been found that laughter can improve your immune system, relieve pain, improve your mood, and enhance a sense of wellbeing. You always have the option to make use of your funny bone during times of stress.

Spirituality

The internal belief system that guides values, ethics, social behaviors, and psychological outlook also influences resilience. Individuals who have a strong sense of purpose, a feeling of connection to a greater whole, or a feeling of connection to spirituality are more resilient. Studies show that purpose in life is a key factor in helping individuals manage traumatic events, and that low spirituality is a leading predictor of low resilience. Whether it's because you have a sense of purpose, belong to a spiritual community, partake in healthier behaviors, or have a more optimistic outlook, science confirms that spirituality confers better health.

It doesn't matter what pathways you choose to connect to spirituality, because it comes in many forms. You can follow a particular faith or religion, feel connected to a higher power, spend time in nature, read uplifting literature, or be driven by a higher purpose. How spiritual you are today may be influenced by your upbringing and culture, but it's also a factor that can be cultivated in order to build your resilience.

Understanding What Resilience Is Not

Until I (coauthor Eva) was in my late 20s, I believed that if I worked hard, good things would come my way, which drove me to complete medical school and a challenging residency. I also believed that my value was wrapped up in my accomplishments. Whenever I was praised or succeeded in an endeavor, I felt confident and good about myself. If I did not succeed or did not receive praise, my sense of value plummeted. I blamed myself for not being good enough and, as a result, worked even harder — at the expense of my own health. When I finally took the time to self-examine my behavior, I came to understand that unless I succeeded or received praise, I had a pattern of feeling unworthy and victimized by the universe. I realized that I needed to work on myself, reach the source of my negative thinking, and find ways to correct it if I wanted to be a healthier and more resilient person.

REMEMBER

When you take responsibility for your behavior and learn to overcome feelings of victimization, helplessness, low self-worth, or hopelessness, you're truly on the path to resilience. I don't mean that you don't experience periods of fear, worry, or upset. Of course, you do! You're human. The key is that you don't stay in these negative states for too long because you're able to shift your perspective and use the situation to learn and grow.

The victim mindset

Life can be hard, and when it knocks you down, it's normal to fall and even to cry. *Staying* in a state of pity for too long, though, can lead to a victim mindset, where you feel you're powerless to effect change and that life is totally out of your control.

When you have a *victim mentality,* you believe that life is happening to you rather than for you or with you. It's a mindset that usually develops over time, after experiencing multiple setbacks or hurts or the loss of love and support. Eventually, you decide that you have no control over life and that you're helpless to change it. As a result, you may avoid taking responsibility for yourself or your life and avoid taking risks, embracing change, improving yourself, or making hard decisions. Instead, you may live in fear, complain a lot, and tempt other people to feel sorry for you.

WARNING

This list describes some of the signs that indicate you're on the verge of having a victim mentality:

>> **You feel powerless.** When bad things happen to you, you believe that you have no control over the situation and that you're helpless to effect change. You believe you have no power and are therefore a victim of life's circumstances. Powerlessness can manifest as a lack of self-esteem, feelings of failure and incompetence, and low motivation.

If you find that you're feeling helpless or powerless, ask yourself, "What is it that I do have control over? Is the belief that I am powerless true?"

>> **You put yourself down.** Feeling powerless often goes hand in hand with negative self-talk and self-doubt. You question your abilities, feel you aren't worthy of success, believe you're incapable of succeeding, and often end up self-sabotaging your efforts. You regularly put yourself down and, in so doing, paint yourself as a victim.

If you find that you're putting yourself down, ask yourself, "Am I really that terrible? Is this belief even true? Can I think of times when I was successful?"

>> **You overgeneralize the negative.** When a negative event happens, you overgeneralize and view it as part of a continued pattern of negativity and ignore evidence to the contrary — that many aspects of your life, and even similar situations, have been positive. You may use the words *never, always, all, every, none, no one, nobody, or everyone* to support your belief that you don't, and never will, have or be enough or that a situation will forever be bad. Examples of statements you might make are "I can never win," "I am always the last to know," and "You never listen to me."

If you make these kinds of statements, ask yourself, "Are there times when this doesn't happen?" and "Is this statement really true?"

>> **You catastrophize.** When you exaggerate the importance of a problem, making it bigger than it necessarily is, you're *catastrophizing*. For instance, you might tell yourself that you absolutely cannot handle a given situation when the reality is that it's just inconvenient. In other words, you believe that even the smallest inconveniences are the end of the world. A tendency to make such problems important can indicate your underlying fears of being inadequate, unimportant, or dispensable.

If you find that you catastrophize and make mountains out of a molehill, ask yourself, "What is the worst thing that could happen? Is this statement really true?"

>> **You feel paranoid.** You regularly feel that the world is out to get you and inflict misery on you. You believe that no matter what you do, life will be miserable and always unfair and you can't count on anything, least of all other people. Life is not only happening to you but also against you.

If you find yourself feeling like life is against you, ask yourself, "Are there times when things went my way? Is this belief really true?"

Learned helplessness

Most people vacillate between feeling optimistic and feeling victimized, depending on what is happening in their lives and how they're feeling about themselves at that particular juncture. Though people don't start out feeling victimized as children, for the most part, they can eventually learn to feel this way as they incur hardships, traumas, or other difficult life events that may cause them to feel more helpless about affecting change in their lives. For some people, as they face continuous negative and uncontrollable hardships, and their efforts fail at effecting change, they eventually stop trying and give up believing that they have any power to improve their circumstances.

Ask yourself the following: Is there something in your life you have tried to do and regularly failed, so you gave up trying? How did that failure make you feel?

TECHNICAL
STUFF

The term *learned helplessness* was coined by the psychologists Martin Seligman and Steven Maier in 1967, when they were studying how dogs behaved when experiencing electric shocks. Seligman and Maier discovered that dogs who realized that they couldn't escape the shocks eventually stopped trying, even when it was possible for them to avoid the shock by jumping over a barrier. In later experiments, Seligman studied human subjects and their response to loud and unpleasant noises. Subjects had the option to use a lever to stop the noise. Subjects whose lever was ineffective at stopping the noise gave up trying after one round.

Learned helplessness can show up in all aspects of your life. You can see it all around you if you look. People are discouraged about politics and decide not to vote, or they're discouraged about losing weight because nothing has worked, or their best friend won't leave a bad relationship because they believe that no one better is out there, or their child has decided not to study because they believe that they will fail anyway. You or someone you know might be depressed, emotionally unpredictable, unmotivated, and unwilling to change healthy habits. When you learn over time that you have little to no control over your life and life circumstances, no matter what you do, you give up hope and give up trying. It may keep you in an abusive relationship or a stressful job or keep you physically ill, even though you have options available to you to get out and change.

WARNING

Here are some common signs of learned helplessness:

>> Mental health problems, such as anxiety, depression, or post-traumatic stress disorder (PTSD)

>> Inability to ask for help

>> Easy frustration and willingness to give up

>> Lack of motivation and desire to put in effort

>> Low self-esteem and lack of self-belief in success

>> Passivity in the face of stress

>> Procrastination

Hopelessness

When you feel *hopeless,* you lack hope in the possibility of a better future. This belief negatively affects how you see the world, yourself, and other people. It can lead to feeling depressed, as though darkness has descended on your life and there's no point in doing anything. You're devoid of inspiration and you have no interest in going out, seeing people, working, or engaging in normal activities. The scarcity of social connection and poor motivation to seek help then adds to feelings of isolation or abandonment, exacerbating the feeling of hopelessness.

Hopelessness is often associated with mental health issues such as anxiety, depression, substance dependency, suicidal ideation, eating disorders, post-traumatic stress, and bipolar disorder. It can also show up intermittently during periods of difficulty and eventually pass when life lets up a bit. The problem is that when you fall into hopelessness, it can feel like a trap so that you lose the motivation to find help and get out, even though you have plenty of pathways to do so.

Many people who have complained of depression have described feeling this way. Feeling hopeless was a symptom of feeling defeated, dissatisfied, and beat up by life events and feeling too exhausted to gather the energy to fight back. With time, love, and support, and reappraising core beliefs and improving self-care, hopelessness was eventually turned back into hope.

REMEMBER

If you're having difficulty getting out of the trap, it's important to seek help from a therapist, counselor, or trusted friend. You aren't on this journey alone, and you have available options to feel better.

WARNING

Here are some signs that you're starting to feel hopeless:

>> Your situation will never improve.

>> It's too late for you to change.

>> No one can help you.

>> You will never be happy again.

>> You will never find love.

>> You have no future.

>> Success isn't possible.

Breaking the Victim Cycle

The first step to breaking the victim cycle is to first accept that you're human and that it's normal to feel stress, fear, anxiety, grief, and loss. You want to accept that when you feel negative emotions and are overcome by stress, it's natural for your brain to trigger a fight-or-flight response and to cause you to feel more fear or overwhelm. The next step is to *choose* not to stay there.

REMEMBER

When you make the choice to shift your mindset away from the victim mentality, you choose to remember that you have the ability to view yourself and your life differently; you have the ability to access resources to not only survive difficulty but also to come out better and stronger. Once you have made the choice to shift, you can then access the tools that will support you to attain a more resilient mindset and eventually stay there.

You can find out how to recognize negative and self-sabotaging thoughts and then take responsibility for them, realizing that you have the power to shift them to a more positive narrative. You can see how to connect with and regulate your emotions, develop positive beliefs and a more optimistic outlook, uphold behaviors that will support you to thrive, and cultivate strong social support networks. Embarking on this journey ultimately requires that you take responsibility for your life; take ownership for your actions, thoughts, and feelings; and do a bit of work to design your life in a way that empowers you to be at your best. When you make the choice to do so, you break the victim cycle.

Chapter **2**

The Basis of Resilience: Harmony Versus Stress

Resilient people have the ability to think clearly and find solutions to complex situations, even under duress. They are able to maintain adaptability and flexibility in the midst of change, stay open to support and learning, cultivate optimism, dedicate themselves to person renewal, and, ultimately, thrive in the face of adversity. Resilient people not only resist succumbing to stress but also find a way to adapt to it and become stronger, wiser, and get better at a given task as a result.

In this chapter, you can find out what stress is, how the stress response affects the mind and body, why perception is half the battle, and how it's possible to improve your ability to not only manage the stress in your life but also use it to your advantage on your path to resilience.

Understanding the Perpetual Quest for Harmony

Stress is part of life. You can't get around it. You actually *need* stress to live. Stress can manifest as mild feelings of discomfort about real-life threatening challenges or hidden stressors such as having the gene for breast cancer, harboring low feelings of self-worth, or discovering mold in your bedroom. The brain doesn't care, because the brain simply wants harmony. Anything that challenges your state of harmony (or *homeostasis,* in scientific terms) qualifies as stress. The brain doesn't care whether it's physical, psychological, or environmental; real or imagined; microscopically small in your body; or a major event happening in the world. If it's challenging your state of harmony, it's also challenging your livelihood — or your value as a human being, according to your brain.

In response, your brain activates a series of responses to motivate action in an attempt to adapt to the stress and regain your harmony. The process of achieving harmony or stability by way of change or adaptation is *allostasis.* The brain drives this process until it finds harmony, and as far as you're concerned, this happens when you feel better.

When you're uncomfortable, what do you do? You shift positions. You go from feeling achy to feeling at peace. When you don't understand something, what do you do? You "google it." You go from feeling confused to feeling smart. When you're anxiously awaiting a call after a job interview or a date, how do you feel when you finally receive the call and it's good news? You're relieved and happy!

And there you have it — every one of your actions, habits, or behaviors is built on the desire to find relief and happiness.

REMEMBER

Take a moment to think about why you're driven to make more money or maintain the perfect relationship or become thin or eat your favorite meal. What do you receive at the end? Satisfaction? Peace? Joy? Happiness? No matter what you believe is driving you, in the end, deep within the wiring of your brain, you're driven to feel at peace and be happy. This desire is hard-wired into your nervous system and driven by the stress response.

Examining the Stress Response Feedback Loop

The stress response, or the physiological response to stress, exists for good reason: It gets you out of bed in the morning, to meet your nutritional needs, to prepare your body to fight infections and heal wounds, to maintain blood pressure and survive traumas, to solve difficult problems, and to allow energy to be expended in response to a wide range of signals so that you can adapt to an ever-changing environment and survive.

Fight-or-flight

Walter Cannon, a Harvard physiologist, coined the term *fight-or-flight* in the 1930s to describe the inborn defense response to threat or danger that ultimately ensures survival. When faced with danger, we humans are catapulted into action by stress hormones such as adrenaline and cortisol. As we became heavily focused and hyperalert, our pupils dilate and our peripheral vision is blocked, forcing our focus on reaching safety. Our muscles tense, our heart rate increases, and we breathe faster to economize on oxygen consumption. Energy stores from the liver, fat cells, bones, and muscles are released into the bloodstream, and our digestive system shuts down so that this energy can be dedicated toward fighting like mad or running like there's no tomorrow (literally because, if you die, there will be no tomorrow).

Here's a rundown of the stress response and its effect on your body:

>> The **pupils** dilate.

>> **Blood vessels** constrict in the hands and feet and gut.

>> The **gastrointestinal tract** shuts down, causing slower movement of the colon and other organs.

>> The **reproductive system** shuts down.

>> **Muscles** become tense, especially the back, neck, jaw, and shoulders.

>> The **immune system** suffers more inflammation, clotting, and allergic reactions (over time, causing poor immunity against infections or cancers).

>> The **cardiovascular system** experiences an increase in heart rate and blood pressure.

>> The **respiratory system** experiences an increase in breathing rate and inflammation.

>> The **metabolic system** shifts to *catabolism,* or breakdown. The liver releases glucose stores. Fats are broken down to fatty acids. Proteins from muscle stores are broken down into amino acids. Bones are broken down for minerals.

>> The **brain** experiences less complex thinking, and more fear-related behaviors are initiated, causing hyper-alertness and arousal.

>> Your **mood** is affected by a loss of serotonin, and other neurotransmitters cause depression, anxiety, and other mood disorders.

>> In your **mind,** higher-thinking centers are shut down, as are big-picture thinking and judgment to enable focus (causing more myopic thinking).

The feedback loop

Once out of danger, the built-in turn of the switch in your brain turns off the stress response. Stress hormone levels drop, your heart rate, blood pressure, and breathing slow down, your muscles relax, your digestive system starts working, and blood flow resumes to your fingers and toes, as the parasympathetic nervous system (the one that creates calm) is activated, and the sympathetic nervous system (the one that creates hyperalertness and hyperactivity) is turned down. Happy chemicals, such as dopamine and morphine-like substances, fill your brain as adrenalin levels wear off, giving you the feeling of euphoria and calm. This is considered a *positive feedback loop*, or when the message is received by the brain that the outcome is positive (stress gone), so it turns off the stress response switch.

Here's an example, which shows how you go from hangry (the combination of *h*ungry and *angry*) to happy:

1. Your blood sugar drops.

2. The body picks up the imbalance and sends an alert to the brain.

3. The stress response is activated, stress hormones are released, the heart rate increases, and the intestines contract.

4. You notice the aches in your belly — that you're feeling a bit weak and dizzy and that you're irritable.

5. Your conscious brain understands that you're hangry.

6. Your conscious brain remembers that eating food will help you feel better.

7. You eat.

8. Your blood sugar goes back to normal.

9. The message travels to the brain.

10. The brain turns off the stress response as dopamine, serotonin, and endorphins flood your brain.

11. The result of all this activity is that you now feel happy and satiated.

To continue with this scenario, if you can't manage to find food, the stress of having low blood sugar doesn't get fixed. In fact, the problem grows worse, as do your symptoms, so the stress response keeps firing. This causes your blood pressure and heart rate to remain high, as stress hormones fly through your body and muscles remain tense. And, this is in addition to the fact that you're starving. This is considered a *negative feedback loop*.

Aside from your dying of hunger, an unchecked stressed response that results from a perpetual negative feedback loop can also be problematic. If left unchecked, physiological responses that are meant to be beneficial in the short term can become harmful as they rage on. Heightened blood pressure can turn into heart disease; muscle tension, into fibromyalgia; negative mood, into dysphoria and depression; heightened inflammation, into a wide variety of immune disorders; and focused thinking, into myopia and an inability to make sound decisions.

WARNING

This negative feedback loop, and an unchecked stress response, happens *all* the time and most people don't even realize it. They don't realize that they're living in constant disharmony until one day they find that their body has to fight a virus, recover from an accident, or withstand the stress of moving homes — and their body can't handle it. They get sick.

Living in Disharmony: The Real Stress

You might be starting to understand the real problem with stress: It's not just the stress that is problematic but also the stress response itself. Disharmony breeds more disharmony, which leads to a bigger stress load, which weakens the mind and the body.

To make matters worse, the brain can't tell the difference between one stress and another. It can't distinguish between running for your life and running late to work or between having your life threatened and your self-esteem challenged.

In the 1950s, Hans Selye expanded on Walter Cannon's work and explained that you don't have to be chased by a raging animal for the fight-or-flight response to be mounted and that this heightened reaction occurs regardless of whether the challenge at hand is life threatening. You might be physically ill or worried about paying your bills, getting fired, or surviving after your spouse leaves you. You might worry about an event that is happening now or one that might happen in the future. The physiological response is the same.

When a threat is ongoing — such as a constant worry, a deep feeling of unworthiness, the presence of an abusive family member, or chronic pollution exposure — the negative feedback loop persists and the stress response doesn't shut down. As a result, an overactive stress response can lead to a host of physical problems as well as a negative state of mind, belief, and mood. Ultimately, when your brain perceives that you're continually under threat and that there's no end in sight, feelings of helplessness or hopelessness can take over.

REMEMBER

In other words, if you frequently worry, get upset, feel anxious or frustrated, or become wracked with self-doubt, your brain receives messages that your world is extremely threatening and that you're weak and lack the capacity to handle it, which makes the brain continue firing the stress response. The more the response fires, the more stress hormones rage, while happy chemicals such as serotonin drop and fear-related and nonsocial behaviors are activated, causing you to lash out or withdraw socially.

In contrast, when you see your world as manageable and any stress as not threatening but rather as a challenge to be reckoned with, the stress response is activated for short periods that motivate you into action, positive feelings and moods are maintained, and resilience is assured.

Expecting a Good Outcome Is the Key

The key to keeping the stress response under control is expecting good, or the belief that a positive outcome is possible. If your brain perceives a particular situation to be manageable, it fires the stress response only long enough to motivate the necessary action, such as an athlete who is motivated to compete and win a race.

Positive expectation reflects a state of inner certainty or trust in success or manageability of a particular endeavor or challenge. Negative perception, in contrast, indicates a mental state of lower self-appraisal and a negative worldview. The brain sees this negative perception as disharmony and a stress in itself, which triggers the stress response and the associated response or reactions.

For example, you may agonize over what to do about a work project. You worry that you'll make the wrong decision, one that your boss will disapprove of. You worry that if you make a mistake, you'll be raked over the coals. You agonize night and day over this issue. You worry about getting fired, even though you have never given your boss reason to fire you. You worry about it anyway. You lose sleep. You drink too much coffee during the day and too much alcohol at night, in an attempt to calm your nerves. You can feel your heart rate increase and your blood pressure rise. You feel tired and achy and overwhelmed now by the demands of your life, and you simply don't think you can handle much more. You argue with your spouse and honk the car horn repeatedly at the driver in front of you. You dislike the way you're behaving, but you can't seem to help it. Your life is falling apart and so are you. A negative expectation has bred a negative outcome.

If you were able to change your mindset to believe that whatever choice you make, you would be okay, the scenario would likely play out quite differently. You might, for instance, feel confident about your ability to make choices and truly believe that there's no such thing as a wrong choice because every choice brings opportunity for growth and learning. You might expect a good outcome no matter the situation, which in turn influences how your body responds. You have that much control!

Coping to Adapt, or Not

Generally, coping means we have managed to adapt to a given stress and feel better. If you're hungry, you cope by eating. If you're tired, you cope by sleeping. Or maybe you don't? Maybe you drink caffeine instead so as not to be tired. Hm. Does this latter scenario count as coping?

In a way, yes, it does count as coping. It's just not *adaptive,* which means it's not good for you. And, rather than support your body to ultimately thrive, it's more likely to cause you to dive — at some point, anyway.

All of our human behaviors and habits are learned ways of coping with stress. We developed them early in life, when we learned that doing something in a certain way leads to feeling good. We also learned to avoid doing other things, because they caused us to feel badly.

The problem is that feeling better doesn't necessarily translate into managing a given stress or the body actually being in harmony. For example, you may have learned that asking for help leads to being rejected, so you avoid doing so. Working hard and getting a job done yourself makes you feel valued and accomplished, so you keep doing it, and at 150 percent effort. You may have learned to cope with sleep deprivation by drinking caffeine and to cope with your anxiety by eating ice cream.

What's wrong with this picture? All these actions, behaviors, and habits help you cope and temporarily feel better, and probably enable you to be more successful at your job, but in reality you aren't fully addressing all your stress. You have neither addressed your fear of rejection nor listened to your body and taken care of its needs. You're coping, but it's *maladaptive.* Adaptive coping would involve you addressing your fears, creating work–life balance, sleeping when you're tired, and nurturing your body with the right kind of fuel or food.

Maladaptive coping

WARNING

Maladaptive coping usually has negative consequences and is often counterproductive, working in the short term but causing trouble in the long run. Here are some examples:

>> Avoidance

>> Substance use

>> Addictions

>> Emotional eating

>> Workaholism

>> Impulsive decision-making

>> Rumination (continuously thinking the same thoughts)

>> Risk-taking

>> Self-harm

Adaptive coping

Adaptive coping has positive consequences and enables a more resilient body and happy life. Here are some examples:

>> Facing difficult situations head-on

>> Asking for support or advice

>> Meditating

>> Regulating emotions to find calm

>> Addressing negative beliefs and hurtful memories from the past

>> Exercising

>> Fueling the body with nutrient-rich food

>> "Sleeping on it" to clear your mind

>> Being patient

>> Maintaining a positive outlook and looking for meaning and opportunities for learning and growth

How do you cope when life throws you curveballs, and it feels like you're being punched in the gut? Do you ruminate, avoid the situation, drink yourself silly, binge-watch TV, or stuff your face with food? Or, do you face the situation head-on and see it as a chance to learn and grow, gather advice, meditate on the problem, give it some time to unfold, and take good care of yourself because you know you'll need it?

REMEMBER

In life, you'll invariably experience hardship or negative emotions, be stressed by life's curveballs and by relationships, and face decisions that are hard to make. You'll also always have the power to make choices that will support you to function at your best at all times — choices that enable you to be truly resilient.

Harmonizing Stress and Becoming Resilient

The environment is constantly changing, and so are you, which means that you can influence any change in a positive or negative direction by the choices you make. You have the power to transform your mind and improve the functioning of your body, if you choose.

If you do make the choice, the work is logical and involves three foundational steps that follow the belief that the quieter your mind is, the calmer you are, the more open you can be to learn and take in new information. With this information, you can be better equipped to create a framework for yourself and your life that supports you to thrive:

1. Quiet the stress response.

2. Remain open to learn and understand.

3. Build and restore your supporting infrastructure.

Quieting the stress response

When you quiet the mind and limit the stress response, you reduce negative chatter and gain better access to your intelligence, and your rational and positive mindset, while helping keep in check the physiology of your body. Whether you choose to take deep breaths, meditate, take a mindful walk, or stretch, quieting the stress response helps you

>> Think more clearly

>> Make wiser decisions

>> Listen attentively

>> Maintain a positive outlook

>> Encourage positive expectation and a belief in a good outcome

>> Keep the stress response effects beneficial rather than harmful in that the stress response is only active for short periods

>> Be more social and friendly, enabling you to seek support when necessary

>> Shift out of a negative mood or state

Being open to learn and understand

When you view difficult challenges as opportunities for learning, growing, and gaining wisdom, you stay curious, ask questions, and remain open — traits that are consistent with emotional resilience. The desire to seek a better understanding and to see everything as a mystery for you to unfold can give you a better sense of control, which invariably also better keeps the stress response in check. Being open, therefore, helps you

>> Make more informed decisions

>> More easily solve problems and find solutions

>> Become curious and playful

>> Feel more in control

>> Seek help or advice

>> Examine your motivations and behaviors more deeply

>> Develop better self-awareness

>> Be more positive, more imaginative, and more likely to believe in new possibilities

Building and restoring

Who supports you, what supports you, where you feel most supported, and how you support yourself all influence the stress response and your physical, psychological, mental, and spiritual health. This infrastructure of support includes such factors as your social support network and relationships, the physical environment where you spend most of your time, and your self-care practices, such as restful sleep, exercise, a nutrient-rich diet, meditation, time spent in nature, play, and being involved in spiritual practices of one kind or another. Building and restoring your infrastructure helps you

>> Enhance physical and mental health

>> Maintain a strong social support network

>> Recognize that you belong to a community

>> Improve your sense of spirituality or your sense that you belong to something even greater than you can imagine

>> Keep the stress response in check by ensuring that needs are met

>> Support a positive self-image and self-belief

REMEMBER

You have the ability to create a life and a mindset that support you to thrive and live your best possible life. You can do so by improving your physical health, balancing your emotions, developing a resilient mindset, enhancing your sense of spirituality, cultivating quality relationships, and building a resilient community. Read on and learn more!

Chapter **3**

Developing Mental Toughness and Clarity

Your thoughts — positive and negative — also serve as fuel for your body and mind. When you're under duress, positive beliefs, confidence, and the ability to think clearly can falter, largely a result of fear and anxiety taking over, along with a cascade of stress hormones such as adrenaline and cortisol. This doesn't happen often to the resilient person. Studies show that resilient individuals are more likely to remain confident, optimistic, and open in the face of change. They have a certain mental toughness that enables them to push through hardship, knowing that they will come out stronger and wiser.

This chapter explores the why's and the how's of a pillar of resilience: mental clarity and toughness.

What Kind of Mindset Do Resilient People Have?

If you were to take two objects, one made of rubber and the other made of glass, and throw them on the ground, what would you expect to happen? The glass breaks, the rubber bounces. One you can glue back together, but it's never quite the same, and the other is as good as new.

Resilient people manage adversity in the same way. They bounce back as good as new, if not stronger and better. As a result, they possess a confident mindset, one that is self-assured, optimistic, tenacious, and mentally tough. Bouncing rather than breaking, they're flexible and adaptable — and usually calm under pressure — and they embrace change and challenges.

A resilient mindset isn't always easy to come by. Life has a way of knocking people down, and it hurts. Once hurt, people tend to shy away from being hurt again, believing that they're weaker than they truly are.

The truth is that the human brain and body are quite resilient — and you have the ability to develop a mindset that sees hardships as challenges to be reckoned with and as opportunities to grow and learn. You can cultivate a resilient mindset by first recognizing the traits that make people resilient.

REMEMBER

Resilient people

>> **Foster a growth mindset.** They believe that life constantly provides them with opportunities to learn and grow, even when challenging. They don't feel victimized by life's circumstances; in other words, they believe that they're the co-creators of their destiny.

>> **See failures as opportunity.** They refuse to give up after failing. Rather, they view setbacks as opportunities to innovate, create, and grow.

>> **Avoid taking things personally.** They don't see failures as a representation of their value, and they don't blame or shame themselves when situations go awry.

>> **Embrace change.** They're excited about change, seeing it as a chance to learn something new, gain new perspectives, and challenge themselves.

>> **Choose to commit and persevere.** They're committed to achieving their goals, purpose, relationships, and beliefs, and they persevere despite obstacles.

>> **Maintain a positive self-image.** They know their value and don't feel victimized by their circumstances or seek value externally, such as worrying about what other people think.

>> **Think optimistically.** They believe that a positive outcome is possible.

>> **Keep an open and objective mind.** They stay open to opportunity and remain level-headed to enable better decision-making.

>> **Envision success.** They have insight and vision that enables them to respond to challenges decisively and often quickly.

Fixed Versus Growth Mindsets When It Comes to Resilience

Carol Dweck, in her book *Mindset: The New Psychology of Success*, identifies two mindsets: fixed and growth. A *fixed* mindset is "believing your qualities are carved in stone," and a *growth* mindset is "the belief that your basic qualities are things you can cultivate through your efforts."

With a fixed mindset, your beliefs in your own abilities are self-limiting, and you see the road ahead filled with negativity, hardship, and challenges. You tend to feel more victimized by life, believing that life is happening *to* you. You often feel self-doubt and feel easily discouraged or defeated, letting your insecurities, failures, or negative beliefs define you and hold you back from learning and growing.

With a growth mindset, on the other hand, you perceive opportunities for growth and learning everywhere. You view failures not as defeats but rather as chances to learn and develop new skills. You see the silver lining in difficult situations and maintain an optimistic attitude. You keep moving no matter the setback, adapting to change and believing in the myriad of possibilities ahead. You believe that life is happening with you and that you're the co-creator of your destiny.

Most people vacillate between mindsets depending on the situation and sometimes the day. Take this example: John was an astute businessman who ran a successful company. He felt confident about his work and didn't blink an eye if he had a difficult client or was called away to solve a big problem at the office. He wasn't working on managing his stress with work, however. Insecure when it came to relationships, he was 48 years old and still single, and he pretty much threw himself into work and avoided intimacy. His belief was, "I fail at relationships. It will never work. I don't know why I bother."

If you break down this sentence, you can pick out the negative terms that reflect a fixed and limited mindset, like "I fail" and "It will never work" and "why bother?" None of these phrases motivate action or reflect openness for growth. The statements reflect a fixed mindset.

Having said that, John was seeking help to work to overcome whatever was blocking his ability to be intimate. That act of seeking help showed that he was indeed interested in learning and changing. He tried changing his words this way: "I have had challenges with intimate relationships in the past, and I am hoping to learn more about why this has been the case so that I can heal and grow as a person. I am looking forward to having a healthy relationship someday." After stating these words, he felt less defeated and more confident about his future.

Perhaps you can repeat John's two statements to yourself. Do you notice the difference? Which motivates, and which defeats? Which opens the door to new opportunities, and which slams the door in your face?

REMEMBER

You might feel confident in one area of your life and insecure in another. No matter how you feel, when you decide that all experiences present chances to learn and grow, you begin to adopt the resilient mindset.

Developing Mental Toughness

When you let go of your limiting assumptions and the fixed mindset, setbacks don't keep you from pushing forward. The most resilient people don't drop out when the going gets hard. Rather, they have grit, so they push back just as hard and keep going. They're mentally tough.

Wikipedia defines *mental toughness* as a measure of individual resilience and confidence that may predict success in sport, education, or the workplace. Achievers and high performers face setbacks all the time — from failure to fatigue, stress, and burnout — yet they keep going and don't stop until their goals are met. They have grit, meaning they can sustain interest in an effort toward long-term goals. Their grit is their drive.

REMEMBER

Ian Turner and his colleagues developed a scale called MTQ48 Psychometric Tool to measure mental toughness. They described *the 4Cs*, which are the four important traits on the scale that, when combined, form mental toughness:

>> **Control:** Addresses how much control you feel you have in your life and how much self-control you have over your emotions. It reflects your inner confidence and self-value as well as your ability to remain calm during trying times.

>> **Commitment:** Looks at how committed you are to achieving your goals. When you're fully committed, you delay gratification, stick with your plan, and work hard, no matter the obstacles.

>> **Challenge:** Assesses the degree to which you embrace change and challenges as opportunities to learn and grow rather than see them as threats. When you embrace challenges, you're more willing to take risks and push way beyond your comfort zone.

>> **Confidence:** Involves your self-belief, in your own abilities to manage through adversity and in knowing that, come what may, you have the strength to stand your ground and succeed.

REMEMBER

Resilient people don't take falls or failures personally. They don't define their value according to their successes, either. Rather, they have an inherent confidence in their value, worth, and ability to reach their goals.

Getting in control

People who are resilient are able to weather hardships because they are certain in their life's purpose and feel that they have a sense of control in their life and their emotions. They don't feel victimized by circumstances — rather, they believe that they have a role to play in their destiny and therefore have the ability to effect change. They're comfortable with who they are, and they don't allow negative thoughts or feelings to run them over. Rather than fall prey to anxiety or fear, resilient people remain calm and objective, able to listen to their gut instincts, weigh in on information as it unfolds, and make sound decisions.

The opposite of this is someone who lacks a sense of self-control over emotions and feels like they aren't in control of their life. They feel more victimized by life circumstances, believing that they are trapped and have no ability to create change. More prone to being overrun by fear and anxiety, they're less capable of making decisions under duress. Indeed, science indicates that difficulties in decision-making are associated with both anxiety and depression.

How do you rate when it comes to feeling or being in control? Are you confident in your ability to influence change? Can you rein in your emotions and stay calm when you're nervous, angry, or frustrated?

Everyone has had to face uncertainty and instability at some point, whether it's a pandemic, an unstable economy, the loss of a loved one, or global warming. It's not so unusual to feel anxiety, helplessness, or hopelessness. It's up to you to decide how you want to respond to life's events. You can lose your cool or stay calm, withdraw or stay engaged, argue to prove your point or have an open discussion to gain clarity. Neither response is wrong or right. One of the responses is simply more conducive to a resilient life, and it's your choice to make.

The good news is that it's possible to develop these four components of getting in control to feel more in control of your life and your emotions:

>> **Quieting your mind:** Calming your mind allows you to feel a better sense of control and gain a bigger perspective. People who are able to achieve this sense of calm are better able to gain insight, wisdom, and a positive outlook; maintain their sense of wellbeing; and stay clear-headed regardless of the situation. You too can find calm through a variety of techniques, including meditation and mindfulness practices, physical exercise and other movement, or sleeping and journaling, to name a few.

>> **Regulating your emotions:** You can also use a variety of methods to better regulate your emotions to find your sense of calm, and they all involve improving your self-awareness and being attuned with the beliefs and thoughts that are exacerbating your feelings of helplessness or hopelessness, and anger or resentment. When you lessen the emotional charge, your stress levels diminish and you're better able to detach from the situation and remain objective and clear-headed.

>> **Building your self-worth:** As you build your resilience, you develop a strong sense of self-value and self-belief. You rarely experience the self-doubt that disables your ability to move forward, because you believe in your inherent capacity to adapt and be at your best. You don't look outside of yourself to feel worthy, and you don't assess your value according to accomplishments or failures. It is this knowing of your value that allows you not to judge yourself when you fail or make mistakes.

>> **Being optimistic:** The ability of resilient people to bounce back from hardship and maintain their emotional balance is predicated on the ultimate belief that a positive outcome is possible and that, invariably, they are valued and worth having this outcome. They're optimistic, in other words. Optimism enables them to transform negative feelings and thoughts into positive ones. A fascinating study evaluating the longest-detained American prisoners of war in Vietnam confirmed this finding and confirmed which factors most influenced that ability to exhibit intact psychological functioning despite the trauma, or *resilience*. After analyzing psychological variables and their ability to repatriate, the research showed that dispositional optimism was the strongest variable in determining resilience. The authors concluded that optimism was protective and discussed the need to train individuals to increase it — *which is possible.* Indeed, it's possible for you to learn ways to maintain a more positive outlook and stay optimistic.

Making a commitment

When a resilient person makes a commitment, they're setting goals and making promises to work toward achieving those goals, without wavering or being distracted. They are consistent with their actions and intentions, and they establish routines and habits that ensure success. Setbacks and failures don't stop them in their tracks. They may slow down to learn from their mistakes and reevaluate their processes, but then they bounce back and head back on the path toward achieving their goals.

You can be committed to your self-improvement, a relationship, a sport, or a purpose.

Can you think of a commitment that you wavered from or lost interest in after a setback? Are you easily distracted or unable to prioritize your targets enough to be able to make the long haul and then wait to collect the final reward? How many times have you lost your commitment to start exercising or lose weight?

REMEMBER

Being committed to making a change isn't easy. If it were, everyone would be successful at it all the time. You can better commit to change by developing these four elements:

>> **Connecting with purpose:** The more aligned you are with a strong sense of purpose, the more likely you will stay committed to your path. The purpose is the reason you want the change. Why do you want to lose weight, become a successful lawyer, or run a marathon? When you discover the purpose and don't lose sight of it, you're more likely to stay on the path, because you have a stronger emotional attachment to it.

>> **Aligning with your heart:** Regularly align your purpose with your heart's desires. The more passionate you are, the more drive and commitment you will have to stay the course.

>> **Delaying gratification:** You need to be willing to delay gratification, or reaping the benefits of the reward. If it's challenging, that means it takes time. Being patient and reminding yourself that a payoff will happen — but not overnight — helps you stay committed for the long haul.

>> **Being willing to sacrifice:** When you're clear about your purpose, aligned with your passion and heart's desire, and ready to wait it out to collect the payoff, you're also willing to make the necessary sacrifices to get there. You may have to give up something or make an uncomfortable change, but the pros outweigh the cons, and you make the sacrifice anyway.

Embracing challenges

Resilient people are open to learning and growing, and they see challenges and change, including making mistakes or failing, as opportunities rather than threats. When faced with a challenge, they are excited and feel driven to work hard to achieve their personal best and are better able to adapt and be flexible. They perceive life as a journey, filled with new opportunities, and they believe that they're the co-creators of their life, so change and challenge are opportunities to be creative and innovative.

Many people, alternatively, fear change and prefer not to be challenged, or at least not in a way that will lead to failure or pain. They avoid taking risks and often lose out on having new experiences. How open are you to experiencing change? Do you welcome challenges, or do you prefer to keep life as it is?

You can become better at embracing challenges. Here are the four basic components:

>> **Learn to be okay with uncertainty.** Whatever picture you have in your head of how life should be or a situation should turn out, erase it. Embracing challenges involves keeping on open mind about what the future may hold and enjoying the journey you're on now, in the present moment. This doesn't mean you don't make plans but rather that you realize that the best-laid plans often go awry, and that's okay.

>> **Be curious.** Though they experience failures and setbacks like everyone else, resilient people don't let the negative experiences stop their drive to learn and create; they instead use these same experiences to stimulate them to discover, understand, create, and investigate. Resilient people don't stop being curious. This attribute supports them in feeling happier and maintaining a more positive outlook, motivating them to embrace change rather than resist it. Indeed, research shows that curiosity, whether in the young or old, is associated with less anxiety, higher life satisfaction, positive emotions, and psychological wellbeing.

Continue to wonder about life, how things work, why things happen, where things go, or if something can be done in a different way. Enjoy asking questions.

REMEMBER

>> **Look for creative solutions.** Rather than focus on the negative, or what you don't have, or ruminate on problems, focus instead on igniting your creativity and see the challenges as opportunities to find new solutions and problems to solve.

>> **Get support.** Remember, challenges aren't happening to you, but for you, with you and other people who can rally by you and support you. When you turn to other people and lean on them to help you through, challenges become more manageable.

Being confident

Resilient people have a strong sense of self-value and navigate their life with a lot of confidence. They believe in their ability to perform, adapt, and influence others to support them. They believe in achieving what others might think impossible, which drives them to forge ahead with determination and assuredness. They remain resolved despite failures, learning from their mistakes and not skipping a beat.

How often have you felt total confidence in your ability to accomplish a hard task? How often do you find yourself riddled with self-doubt? You might feel confident in one area of your life and full of self-doubt in another. Low self-confidence unfortunately, undermines your ability to take risks, move forward, and be open to embracing and learning from challenges.

REMEMBER

The more confident you are, the more committed and motivated you will be to stay on your path and bounce back from setbacks, and the more pleasure you will gain by simply living your life. Confidence comes from building your skills and competency, having a more positive outlook, improving your wellbeing, and accepting yourself. This list describes the basic elements you can develop to improve your sense of confidence:

>> **Don't compare yourself to others.** You're a unique individual and no one is like you, nor are you like anyone else. Your success isn't measured according to the success or failure of another person. Focus on yourself and how you can improve and grow. Comparing yourself to other people to determine your value is a reflection of low self-worth and lack of belief in your own journey and ability to achieve greatness on your own terms.

>> **Develop your competency.** Rather than put yourself down or compare yourself to others, work on developing skills, knowledge, and self-mastery. Practice and practice until you feel adept and competent. Hone your strengths and fix your weaknesses. The more you do, the more your confidence will grow.

>> **Set attainable goals.** If you set a goal that feels like a mountain you have to climb, you may become easily defeated and lose your confidence. Break the bigger goals into smaller, attainable goals. Each time you succeed, you inch closer to achieving the larger goal while also building your confidence in your ability to get there.

>> **Celebrate your wins.** Avoid dismissing your successes, especially when they're small. Every achievement deserves celebration. The more islands of success you create, the higher your confidence will climb.

Accessing Mental Clarity

A calm and open mind is a clear mind. A confident and competent person who knows their value is more likely to be decisive and clear when faced with challenges. Conversely, a person whose mind is filled with self-doubting thoughts and fears has a hard time seeing their way through hardships and making good decisions.

Anytime you believe you're not enough — whether it shows up as self-doubt and thoughts of being inadequate, feelings of overwhelm, worries about what others may think, angry feelings at someone or something else for taking away your power, or beliefs that you're not deserving of good or success — you sabotage your ability to think clearly, solve problems, think creatively, and make good decisions. Especially when you're negatively emotionally charged, the stress response is activated so that your brain actually shuts down, making complex and rational thinking difficult. (See Chapter 2 in Book 3 for more about the stress response.)

Have you ever made a good decision when you were upset or anxious or angry? Was it hard to think clearly? Are you able to communicate your needs or be clear about what you want?

You can access better mental clarity in the very same ways you can build up your mental toughness, and this includes, first and foremost, quieting your thoughts and regulating your emotions so that you can become more detached and objective in your view of any given situation.

Here's an example: Melissa was extremely anxious about her upcoming performance review with her boss to see whether she qualified for a raise. Admittedly, Melissa was a hard worker, dedicated and passionate, and even put in long hours at the expense of her personal life. She was worried, though, because she had never received any praise, was convinced she had done something wrong, and believed that her boss didn't like her, though she had no proof either way. Her anxiety was keeping her up at night, causing her to overeat and make mistakes and to be unable to think clearly, all of which made her more stressed and question all of her work.

Melissa said she knew she was good at her job and spoke of all of her accomplishments. So she was asked, "So why are you so anxious about this meeting? You're good at what you do. Why don't you believe in yourself right now?"

Melissa realized there was a disconnect between what she knew was true, or her own recognition of her competence and abilities, and the beliefs that her negative emotions and anxiety were leading her to think, which was that her competency and worth were predicated on being recognized by her boss.

The next step, therefore, was to guide Melissa to quiet the negative thoughts and emotions and see whether her heart and mind could join together. She learned a simple breathing technique aimed at lowering stress response activity and increasing relaxation, by turning down the sympathetic nervous system and turning on the parasympathetic nervous system. She was also instructed to be present with her emotions and the feelings in her body, to observe them, accept them, and allow them to come and go with the movement of her breath, and not to judge them or hold on tight, but simply to watch them move with her breath, like a curtain that moves with the breeze.

Within a couple of minutes, Melissa felt calmer and said her mind was quiet, and her body felt relaxed and free of tension. When she reflected again on her upcoming meeting, she said she no longer felt an emotion other than being ready for it and, come what may, knowing her value, no matter the outcome. She felt clear about how to present herself, and better yet, she felt focused.

Melissa discovered how to quiet her mind, regulate her emotions, and access her mental clarity. You, too, can develop the ability to have a resilient mindset, be mentally tough, remain mentally clear without confusion, and feel more in control of your life, even in the face of the unknown.

REMEMBER

You can't control the unknown — that's why it's the unknown! You can be in control of yourself, your emotions, and your responses, however, and choose to make peace with the unknown and embrace it as life unfolds. You can be confident in yourself, your abilities, and resources to handle uncertainty and commit to taking on challenges to enhance your growth, learning, and fulfilling your heart's desires.

Chapter **4**

Achieving Emotional Equilibrium

E*motional equilibrium* or balance occurs when you can objectively observe and accept your emotions without judging yourself, feeling the need to suppress them, or being overwhelmed by them, and instead use your emotions to heal, learn, and achieve growth. Emotionally resilient people are able to manage painful or difficult emotions, feel them without being consumed by them, and stay balanced despite the hardships they face.

This chapter helps you understand why emotions exist, how they influence your perception and behavior, and why achieving emotional equilibrium is necessary when working to achieve true resilience.

Emotions Exist for a Very Good Reason

Emotions are part of human nature. You have them for a reason. In the same way that the sensory fibers in your hand can tell you that the stove is hot or the bones in your ear tell you that the vibration of a sound is too loud, your emotions act as sensory signals, letting you know when you're safe and when you're being threatened. They serve the purpose of motivating you into action to warn others to back off or urge them to come close. Emotions inform your mind, letting it know it's okay to stop and smell the roses and see the big picture of life — or focus and get the heck out. As such, your emotions are intricately intertwined with your stress response (see Chapter 2 in Book 3), influencing stress hormones, and all bodily functions, including your heart rate, blood pressure, gastrointestinal system, muscles, and immune system — as well as the behaviors that ensue.

REMEMBER

To summarize, emotions have the following roles:

>> **Signaling you:** They signal you to act when you need care or when you or someone you love is in danger or when you want to bond and connect with others.

>> **Signaling other people:** They signal other people to come closer or back off.

>> **Motivating behavior:** How you feel influences how you act.

>> **Influencing your body's physiology:** They influence your body and stress physiology, leading your pupils to dilate when you're scared and your muscles to tense, heart rate to increase, digestive system to shut down, or inflammation to increase.

>> **Motivating you to engage or disengage:** Positive emotions tend to encourage you to engage with your environment, including other people, and forge relationships; negative emotions encourage you to fight like mad, run like heck, freeze in place, and, sometimes, tend and befriend.

>> **Prompting your thought-to-action inventory:** Your emotions activate thinking patterns that are either broad (open-minded or rational, for example) or narrow (myopic or concrete).

This fact that your emotions are directly intertwined with your stress response and the ensuing behaviors is what can get you into trouble. When the negative emotional charge is high, your brain assumes that your life is being threatened and triggers the fight-or-flight response. It doesn't know the difference between being affected by your child's misbehavior, being late on a deadline, or being chased by a mugger. If you're emotional (negatively), it fires the stress response, which motivates the behavior that helps you feel better. You might scream, withdraw, stuff your face with food, or ruminate all night so that you don't sleep.

WARNING

The problem is, in short, that negative emotions can consume you and dictate your perceptions, behaviors, reactions, and decisions, and therefore your ability to stay clear-headed, communicative, mindful, and compassionate; enjoy balanced and loving relationships; and, ultimately, be resilient.

How Emotions Influence Perception and Coping

When you experience a particular emotion, your brain recalls any other time you felt the same way. It pulls forward the behaviors you used to feel better along with the assumptions or beliefs you came up with at the time. These assumptions and beliefs pertain to how you see yourself, as enough or not enough, and how you see your world, as safe or threatening or as happening to you or with you.

Take this example: Clara repeatedly experienced rejection from her mother. Nothing was ever good enough for her mother, and if Clara didn't come home with good grades, she didn't get to have dessert with dinner. Without knowing it, Clara developed a belief that she wasn't worthy of being loved unless she did well in school. It showed up in her behaviors as she avoided intimate relationships and threw herself into her work, which never let her down, and eating sweets, which were always a comfort. At 46 years old, she was a successful businesswoman, and likely a workaholic, and she had a weight problem because she rewarded herself at the end of each day with a pint of ice cream. Anytime she went on a date, felt a semblance of rejection or feelings of failure, or had to deal with her mother, she would go to the bakery, buy a pie and eat it. The thing is, Clara knew rationally that she was a funny, loving, intelligent, smart, and worthy person. She also knew that her coping habits of overworking and eating too many desserts was unhealthy. The problem was that when she felt nervous, anxious, or any other negative emotion, she fell back into old patterns. Her emotions got the better of her.

REMEMBER

Your emotions thus influence your perception of yourself and the world, both positively and negatively, and subsequent coping behaviors, which influence your ability to be resilient. Negative emotions tend to encourage you to feel victimized and negatively impact resilience, whereas positive emotions boost you to feel empowered, like a co-creator of your life, and to improve the following traits that reflect better resilience:

>> **Self-esteem or self-value:** Positive emotions are strongly linked to higher self-esteem.

>> **Flexibility and adaptability in the face of change:** People with positive emotions versus negative ones show less resistance and more openness to change.

>> **Clear judgment and broad thinking patterns:** Positive emotions prompt a more open and broad mindset, with better access to rational and creative thinking as well as better decision-making.

>> **Supportive relationships:** Positive emotions direct you to improve social bonds and to collaborate and communicate with others rather than fight with them or avoid them.

>> **Access to personal resources:** Positive emotions allow you access to physical, psychological, intellectual, and social resources.

>> **Coping under duress:** Positive emotions improve coping under stress.

Evaluating Your Feelings

Emotions are part of your human makeup, so you will experience them, often, and you may even experience multiple emotions at the same time. Can you recall a time when you felt angry, sad, elated, relieved, and guilty — all at the same time? It can be extremely unpleasant and distressing to feel this way, not to mention confusing. Being resilient doesn't mean you don't feel emotions, but rather that you're able to identify and evaluate them, which enables you to understand yourself better, heal negative beliefs, develop compassion and empathy, grow as a person, and improve mental clarity and decision-making abilities.

When you evaluate your emotions, you take the time to identify exactly what you're feeling, and why, so that you can gain a clear understanding of what it is you really need and want.

Here's an example: Julie was upset with her boyfriend because she felt he was ignoring her needs. Her boyfriend, meanwhile, claimed he was trying to understand Julie's needs, but she kept changing her mind, and he was ready to give up. I (coauthor Eva) worked with Julie to evaluate her feelings and understand the source of her anxiety. When she was growing up, she told me, both her parents had to work evenings, and she recalled having to fend for herself most days and take care of her siblings. Julie realized that what she was craving was a sense of security.

Together, we figured out ways she could help herself feel more secure and then thought of some ways her boyfriend could support her to feel that way. Julie later communicated how she was feeling, and why, and told her boyfriend exactly what she needed, and he was easily able to comply. By taking care of herself, Julie was able to forge a stronger and more loving relationship.

REMEMBER

The process of evaluating your emotions to gain better insight entails following these action steps:

1. **Pause.** Take the time to pause and slow down your thoughts. Your best ideas and realizations come when you're relaxed or at peace (such as in the shower or on a mindful walk).

2. **Validate.** It's important that you validate the way you feel. You aren't wrong, good, or bad for feeling the way you do. Validating prevents you from suppressing or numbing your emotions.

3. **Stay calm.** Use your breath or another relaxation technique to slow down the stress response to give you access to a calmer and more open mind. Your emotions are intertwined with your physiological responses such that there is a feedback loop. Your emotions influence physiology, and physiology influences emotions. By calming the stress response via relaxation techniques, you change physiology and improve access to positive motions and broader thinking.

4. **Reflect.** Ask yourself questions that will bring you some clarity around what you're actually feeling, why you're feeling a certain way, when you have experienced this feeling in the past, and whether there's an explanation for it all.

5. **Express.** Rather than keep inside the answers and reflections that arise, express them by writing them down or talking them out.

6. **Uncover.** Once you can better see what your emotions are and why you're experiencing them, you can then figure out the assumption, belief, and core need that's provoking them. Examples of core needs are safety, security, comfort, support, love, connection, recognition, respect, and growth.

Choosing to Manage Your Emotions

You've probably had times when you lost your temper (such as when dealing with an automated phone tree when you have limited time). You have the choice of deciding whether to feel angry or frustrated or to pause and manage your emotions. When you decide to manage your emotions, you experience an emotional equilibrium, where you feel balanced and effective in managing problems and setbacks. The trick is realizing that you have this option in the heat of the moment. That's what the "pause" is for.

TIP

Once you have paused, you have several options to manage your emotions. Whichever you choose, you will find that you feel calmer and gain better insight into yourself. These are some of your options:

» **Identify.** Choose to be curious about your emotions, such as being curious about a butterfly or a bee. Identify and label it. You might say, "Oh, look at that. I am feeling anger." Identifying and objectifying emotions diminishes their charge.

» **Assess the pattern.** Reflect on the emotion and the impact it might have on you physically and psychologically, on your behaviors, and on other people (and therefore on how they affect your relationships or professionalism). You might notice that anger makes your face hot and that fear makes your heart race and muscles tighten in your neck. You might notice that fear makes you want to eat more or hide under the covers. Look for the patterns and the triggers associated with the emotion to give yourself insight into your behaviors and coping methods. Regularly assessing your emotions for patterns empowers you to be more in control of your emotions rather than let the emotions be in control of you.

» **Nurture yourself.** Whether you have uncovered the core need in an evaluation process, you can safely assume that your negative emotions are telling you you're in need of nurturance, security, respect, value, or love. You don't have to know what it is to decide to nurture yourself with self-loving acts and thoughts of kindness.

» **Accept what is.** Accept your feelings, your reactions, and the situation and feelings of others, without judgment. Avoid repressing, suppressing, shaming, or blaming. Allowing your emotions to be present without judging or pushing them away enables you to gain some distance from them, maintain positive detachment, and ultimately be able to let them go.

» **Let it go.** Emotions have a charge. That charge normally needs to be released and expressed. You want to be able to release and express the energy in a way that isn't harmful to you or others. A variety of techniques enable you to release pent-up energy, whether it's some type of movement such as karate or hitting a pillow, writing, exercising, screaming at the top of your lungs (in private), painting, laughing, crying, meditating, or engaging in creative activities.

» **Redirect to the positive.** You can also choose to redirect your thoughts and attention to memories of positive experiences that remind you of times you felt the opposite, more positive feeling. If a situation causes you to experience feelings of being disrespected, for example, you can remind yourself of a time when you felt valued and honored. Positive memories enliven positive associations, emotions, and memories, expanding your point of view so that you align with more positive beliefs and expectations.

>> **Shift to gratitude.** When you feel grateful and lucky, you're more likely to feel more forgiving and able to stay open and positively detached. Another way to redirect your attention is by intentionally shifting your focus to gratitude. You can contemplate the reasons you feel fortunate in your life, find appreciation in the given situation, and find reasons to be thankful that you have been given this opportunity for growth and healing.

>> **Reappraise.** Ask yourself a series of questions that can provide you with answers and insights into a more logical, true, and less stress-provoking viewpoint, allowing you to restructure your thoughts and, ultimately, change how you feel.

Calming Your Emotions By Calming the Stress Response

When negative emotions run high, the stress response is activated (see Chapter 2 in Book 3), provoking more fear-related behaviors and more narrow-minded thinking. When you develop your self-awareness, you gain the ability to listen to your body's signals, aware of the stress response when it's activated and aware of techniques you have access to that will calm and regulate the stress response. It's so cool: You can calm the stress response by managing your emotions, and you can manage your emotions and calm the stress response.

Often, you don't need to do a deep dive and evaluate why you feel a certain way. You simply just need to know that you don't like the way you feel or the way you're behaving, which takes self-awareness. Once you have assessed that you're experiencing a negative emotion and you want to feel differently, you have at your fingertips some tools that can help you easily shift out of the negative state that involve paying attention to the body rather than to your thoughts or emotions and calming the stress response.

You can achieve this effect by employing relaxation techniques. These techniques help you control emotions by

>> Activating the parts of the brain that control the autonomic nervous system

>> Inhibiting the adrenalizing sympathetic nervous system

>> Stimulating the calming parasympathetic nervous system

>> Slowing down brain waves to create a state of relaxation

>> Reducing the production of stress hormones

>> Improving emotional processing

Examples of such techniques are progressive muscle relaxation, mindfulness, guided imagery, and movement meditations such as yoga and tai chi. You can use these techniques to help you achieve relaxation while also improving your concentration and attention so that you're relaxed and alert, a state that is optimal for problem solving, self-awareness, and self-control.

There's no single right way to regulate the stress response, other than the one you actually do.

REMEMBER

Shifting to Positive Detachment and Reappraisal

When you manage your emotions, you discover better ways of expressing yourself, gain insight into yourself and a given situation, communicate more effectively, and make better decisions. The key is to be able to detach from negative emotions so that you can experience them without being overwhelmed by them.

Also known as *positive detachment,* this state of mind enables you to loosen your grip on your thoughts and emotions and instead gives you space to breathe so that you can move toward accepting yourself as you are and the world as it is. Positive detachment does *not* involve suppressing or pushing anything away. It does *not* mean distancing yourself or creating a wall that separates you from something or someone because of your negative feelings and emotions. Rather, with positive detachment, you create some space between you and your emotions so that you're better able to perform cognitive reappraisal, a trait that emotionally resilient people possess.

Cognitive reappraisal represents the ability to change and reframe the way you think about a situation to better regulate emotions and lessen their impact. The opposite of this process is *suppression expression*, whereby you suppress, hide, or reduce your emotions by way of behavior (such as changing your facial expressions or purposefully hiding your anger). People who are able to partake in cognitive reappraisal versus people who suppress their emotions

>> Experience and express more positive emotions

>> Have better interpersonal functioning

>> Enjoy a greater sense of wellbeing

WHAT DO YOU DO WHEN SOMETHING UPSETS YOU?

If and when something happens to you that upsets you, do you express your emotions or stifle them?

- Are you able to detach from the situation and see all points of view?

- How fixated on the story do you become?

- How long does it take for you to let go of the story and achieve some peace of mind?

With the process of positive detachment and reappraisal, you decide to focus on the present moment and disengage from habits of thinking and negative emotions that usually don't serve you. Instead, you focus on being in the now, on your thoughts or emotions as they come and go, and on being completely true to yourself and your true nature so that you become more peaceful and more self-aware and become liberated from your past and your limiting beliefs.

Enhancing Your Self-Awareness and Willingness to Grow

Self-awareness is a precursor to resilience. First defined in 1972 by Shelly Duval and Robert Wicklund, self-awareness involves being able to focus attention on yourself to objectively examine whether, and then how, your behavior is in coherence with your values and standards.

With better self-awareness, you're able to reflect and understand that your actions, words, and even energy impact your body, your life, and the lives of those around you. You're able to be honest and accountable with yourself, your strengths, and your weaknesses. By seeking to understand yourself better, through your own eyes and the eyes of others, you enhance your ability to achieve self-control, especially over your emotions. How self-aware you choose to become depends on how strong your willingness is to grow as a person.

REMEMBER

Let's face it: Negative emotions can be extremely unpleasant to experience, and it's often easier to repress or suppress them than to go ahead and feel them. The result is that you lose your sense of self-awareness. To override this reaction, you need to be okay admitting that you may have been or done something "wrong" or made a mistake. You need to be wanting and willing to change and grow.

Always Choosing Love

The ability to bounce back from hardship and maintain emotional balance is predicated on the ultimate belief in a positive outcome and that, invariably, you're valued and loved. When negative emotions become all-consuming, people tend to shift away from feeling valued to feeling more victimized. A way to counteract this process is to enhance the feeling of being loved and connected.

The neurobiological changes that occur during the experience of love reflect in many ways the changes that occur during meditation. Levels of stress hormones fall, reward centers in the brain are activated, and feel-good neurotransmitters such as dopamine, hormones, endorphins, and morphine-like substances course through your brain, helping you feel euphoric and full of positive expectation.

Interestingly, the experience of love seems to have an even more powerful effect, likely because love induces feelings of pleasure and security, leading to further feelings of trust and positive belief, resulting in motivation of positive behavior and further positive expectation. Love also stimulates *oxytocin*, a hormone that reduces stress response activity, lowers cortisol levels, protects dopamine neurons, and reduces anxiety. Less anxiety and less stress mean more access to your positive memories, positive emotions, higher cognition and thinking, healthier behaviors, and healthier memory.

Love comes in many forms — in your relationships, your self-care, and your spirituality. The more loving and balanced your relationships, the better your self-care; and the more spiritually connected you feel, the bigger your love reserves. The bigger your love reserves, the less likely you are to shift into a victim mindset, and if you do, the more likely you are to shift out of it.

REMEMBER

Negative emotions aren't bad, and you're better off not suppressing or repressing them. Rather, you should understand that they're signaling to you that you're in need of care and that you have a choice to learn from your emotions and manage them to find your calm — or to let them control you so that you lose control.

Chapter **5**

Improving Your Relationship with Yourself

Resilient people take responsibility for their actions and attitudes and are constantly working toward self-improvement. They have a positive self-image that enables them to hit their stride and keep moving to achieve their goals, despite setbacks or failures. Their positive self-belief allows them to forge healthy relationships and maintain a strong sense of self-mastery. Studies show that high self-esteem is associated with psychological resilience and that low self-esteem is associated with psychological maladjustment.

This chapter spells out how self-worth and a positive self-image support resilience and gives you tools to help strengthen self-belief by improving the relationship you have with yourself.

Connecting Resilience with Self-Worth

Truly resilient people have a positive self-belief and self-image no matter what is happening in their lives — whether life is moving along smoothly or throwing them curveballs, whether they succeed or whether they fail. These folks are able to celebrate their successes and still remain positive when they falter, viewing setbacks as opportunities to learn and grow. In other words, resilient people don't look outside of themselves to feel valued — they already know their value at their core.

What do you believe? Do you believe, at your core, that you are a valued and unique individual? Can you hold that belief without comparing yourself to the successes or failures of others? Is your worth dependent on your marital status, your weight, your looks, your income, or whether you win or lose?

REMEMBER

Most resilient people share several traits that reflect a positive self-image, which invariably enables them to get through hardship. These include the following:

>> **Avoiding being affected by others' opinions:** You don't let others' opinions affect your own self-image or value.

>> **Recognizing their uniqueness:** You recognize what you have to offer that makes you special.

>> **Taking pride in achievements:** You feel proud about all your accomplishments, big and small.

>> **Risking rejection:** You risk rejection to show your true self.

>> **Having a desire to grow:** You aspire to become better as a person.

>> **Showing self-compassion:** You are more kind, rather than critical, to yourself when you make a mistake or fail.

>> **Learning from mistakes:** You see mistakes as opportunities to learn.

>> **Self-reflecting:** You take time to reflect on your emotions and try to understand your feelings.

>> **Practicing gratitude:** You feel a strong sense of gratitude and regularly count your blessings.

Everyone has situations or times in their lives when they feel confident and worthy and others when they feel the opposite. The question is, are you confident of your worth at your core?

Believing in Your Worth

When you believe in your worth, you don't look outside of yourself to feel worthy or validated. You feel empowered and confident in the face of challenges and problems. You don't take things personally, you don't compare yourself to others or seek external approval, and you aren't defined by life's events. When you believe in your worth, you can then

>> **Feel free to make mistakes.** You won't judge yourself or negate your efforts when you make mistakes. Instead, you welcome mistakes as opportunities to learn and grow and then accept them as a part of being human.

>> **See everything as fodder.** Along with your mistakes, you perceive everything that occurs around you as holding opportunity for learning, growing, and deepening your awareness and sense of self.

>> **Persevere.** Because you avoid viewing mistakes as failures and because opportunities abound, you persevere and push through setbacks. Your self-belief gives you the courage and drive to persist and keep going.

>> **Stay open.** You lack any fear of being judged or of making mistakes, so you're curious, open, and receptive to learning — to advice and seeing how life unfolds.

>> **Believe in the possible.** You don't take things personally, and you believe in yourself and your ability to find solutions and achieve a positive outcome.

>> **Remain true.** You never lose sight of yourself, your values, and your goals by comparing yourself to other people and worrying what other people might think. You stay true to yourself.

>> **Attract support.** You believe in yourself, and your conviction influences other people to believe in you as well so that they're willing and wanting to help and support you.

>> **Take care.** You value yourself and believe that your body is a temple. No matter the challenges in your life, you take time for self-care, nurturing yourself so that you're more fit to handle anything that pops up.

>> **Maintain healthy boundaries.** You feel whole within yourself, so you know when to give to others and when to take care of yourself. You're clear about your values and priorities and you can express your needs clearly.

Cultivating resilience means developing most if not all these traits. The more positively you view yourself, the more capable you will feel about overcoming challenges, believing in your ability to succeed despite setbacks, and the likelihood that you will choose the right people to be part of your close network of support. As you read on, you will be asked to evaluate your relationship with yourself and use this information to guide you toward what needs strengthening.

Noting Self-Criticism

Most people can be their own harshest critics. Think about it for yourself. When you're wracked with self-doubt, how do you respond to your boss criticizing your work? When you don't believe in your abilities to be alone, how likely are you to leave an unhealthy relationship? Do you forgive yourself when you make a mistake, congratulate yourself when you succeed, or accept yourself with your imperfections? Do you take good care of yourself?

Think of the number of times you've heard people make these statements:

"I can't believe I did that. I'm such an idiot."

"I'm so stupid."

"I'm never going to understand this."

"I'm a failure."

"Why can't I ever learn?"

WARNING

These statements may seem innocuous, but in reality they convey a lack of confidence in oneself and in one's abilities, strengths, resources, and support. They reflect negative self-talk and self-criticism. In many ways, self-criticism can motivate you to learn more and grow, and to enhance self-awareness. On the other hand, it can also block growth and negatively affect your self-esteem. You can use self-criticism to learn from your mistakes as a way to develop better behavior, for example, or use it to shame yourself and feel less valued.

A friend named Jocelyn called me (coauthor Eva) once in a panic. She had clicked Reply All to a work email meant to be private and to be sent only to the sender, who happened to be a friend. Jocelyn was worried because the language she used was personal and a bit inflammatory. As she spoke, she kept beating herself up and saying, "I can't believe I did that! I am such an idiot, and I am so embarrassed. I am going to need to avoid everyone for a while."

After letting her vent for a bit, I asked her whether she wanted to keep venting or get some help, and she chose the latter. We did some deep breathing together to calm her emotions and help her find her center. Then I said, "You made a mistake. You weren't paying attention. You're human and you make mistakes, and you especially make them when you're stressed. What is in this situation for you to learn?"

Jocelyn self-reflected and said, "I need to take a timeout for myself and be more mindful. I am going to practice being more mindful. I may need to apologize to the others and will do so as I am accountable for my actions. It will work out in the end."

In this situation, Jocelyn was able to shift out of her negative self-talk by calming her emotions and using self-reflection. She was able to see that, in a negative state, her self-criticism was leading her down a path of low self-worth. When she was able to shift into a more positive state, she was better able to be accountable for her actions without denying her value.

REMEMBER

Self-criticism can thus be a reflection of how you relate to yourself. Do you accept yourself as you are, as a valuable human being who makes mistakes while acknowledging a desire for growth and further development, or do you admonish yourself for failures or not being good enough? Read on and evaluate your self-value.

Evaluating Your Self-Value

How you relate to yourself — especially with regard to your imperfections, failures, or mistakes — reflects your self-value. Your self-value, in turn, informs your behaviors, decisions, and self-confidence, and the stronger it is, the better you're capable of forging ahead and believing in yourself during hard times.

The following is a self-value inventory checklist that helps you evaluate your relationship with yourself and your self-value. Pick the answer that best applies.

1. I know I am valuable.

Never true   Rarely true   Not sure   Sometimes true   Always true

2. I think positively about myself.

Never true   Rarely true   Not sure   Sometimes true   Always true

3. I don't need validation from other people to feel good about myself.

Never true   Rarely true   Not sure   Sometimes true   Always true

4. I am not afraid to ask for what I want or need.

Never true   Rarely true   Not sure   Sometimes true   Always true

5. I don't worry about rejection. I accept myself anyway.

Never true   Rarely true   Not sure   Sometimes true   Always true

6. I do not think I am inferior to other people.

Never true   Rarely true   Not sure   Sometimes true   Always true

7. I don't feel like a failure.

Never true   Rarely true   Not sure   Sometimes true   Always true

8. I am confident that if I can't do something, I will figure it out.

Never true   Rarely true   Not sure   Sometimes true   Always true

9. I can accept criticism without getting upset.

Never true   Rarely true   Not sure   Sometimes true   Always true

10. I don't berate myself when I make mistakes.

Never true   Rarely true   Not sure   Sometimes true   Always true

11. I am able to say no to people when I know I need to take care of myself.

Never true   Rarely true   Not sure   Sometimes true   Always true

12. I treat my body as a temple, no matter what happens in my life.

Never true   Rarely true   Not sure   Sometimes true   Always true

13. I eat food that is healthy and nutrient-rich.

Never true   Rarely true   Not sure   Sometimes true   Always true

14. I exercise frequently throughout the week.

Never true   Rarely true   Not sure   Sometimes true   Always true

15. I make sure I get restful sleep.

   Never true   Rarely true   Not sure   Sometimes true   Always true

16. I take time to relax and take care of myself.

   Never true   Rarely true   Not sure   Sometimes true   Always true

Take your time evaluating each question and your answers. Sometimes people think they have a better relationship with themselves than they actually do. Do you know of any areas that need strengthening?

REMEMBER

Building your self-value means learning to think about yourself more positively and taking good care of yourself physically, emotionally, and spiritually.

Starting to Take Action

At times you may feel good about yourself, and at other times you may feel more self-critical and less confident. The goal is for you to know, on the deepest level, that you're valued no matter what you do or what happens, and that it's normal for you to sometimes feel badly or negatively.

The first step is to simply be *self-aware* — aware of what you're feeling at any particular moment. Once you know, you can consciously choose in which direction you want to go: toward beating yourself up or toward lifting yourself up.

Practicing self-awareness

REMEMBER

When you start paying attention to your behavior, thoughts, feelings, or beliefs, you begin to notice how often you put yourself down, look for validation, compare yourself to others, or engage in other self-defeating or self-deprecating ways. Self-examination is an ongoing process. The way you react and behave is never wrong. It's not right, either. Whatever you notice is fodder, enabling you to learn more about yourself and why you have negative beliefs in the first place.

You can begin the process by posing these questions to yourself:

>> When do I put myself down?

>> When do I compare myself to others? What is it usually related to? What are my insecurities? When do they show up?

>> How often do I doubt my decisions? Is it about certain subjects or most of the time?

>> When do I believe in myself? What are the situations? How does it feel when I do?

>> How well do I take care of myself?

>> When I am stressed, what are my habits? What do I choose to do?

>> When did I start behaving this way?

>> Where did I learn this self-doubt? What is the limiting belief?

Making a conscious choice

The observations you accumulate for self-examination should also reveal to you the times you feel confident or successful. Being more self-aware alerts you to how both positive and negative mindsets can coexist. The goal is for you to make a conscious choice to feel positively about yourself more often than not. You choose not to empower and give credence to the negative self-talk and choose instead to focus on your value.

TIP

You can take action by following these steps:

1. **Think about a situation when you felt confident, powerful, worthy, or another positive feeling.**

2. **Describe the feeling and how you felt about yourself, as if you're writing your story of victory.**

   Write down as many positive adjectives as you can think of.

3. **Close your eyes and contemplate each adjective, allowing the feelings associated with each word to fill your body.**

   Allow yourself to relive your story of victory. Tell yourself to remember this feeling for other times.

4. **Examine your notebook (if you have one) containing observations of your negative statements, actions, or beliefs.**

   See how you might reframe the situation from the standpoint of feeling positively about yourself.

5. **Watch your step in the future.**

   If you catch yourself putting yourself down, ask yourself how you can restructure this thought, statement, or action to one that is constructive and representative of who you truly are at your best.

Celebrating yourself

When you move into self-doubt and limiting beliefs, you tend to forget the good stuff. You forget your wins, all the times you did feel confident or valued, and the belief that you are indeed capable of success or feeling good. It happens to the best of us. When the stress response is highly activated, the tendency is to focus on the negative and only the negative. When you make a conscious effort to remember your wins, you're less likely to fall into the trap of self-deprecation while also better regulating the stress response. Celebrate yourself every day for big or small accomplishments, recognizing your worth, strengths, abilities, and value.

TIP

These are some actions you can take now:

>> **Keep a separate notebook.** Mark down the times when you feel good, victorious, and valued.

>> **Note during these times the sources of this feeling.** Did the sense of value come from you or from someone or something recognizing you or validating you?

>> **Remember the positive.** If you notice that your sense of accomplishment or values is ignited because someone else recognized you, focus on the positive feeling and see whether you can reframe the situation to feeling valued first and then being happy about the accomplishment.

>> **Celebrate with self-loving actions as well as words.** Perhaps you buy yourself some flowers or take yourself out to a fine dinner or write yourself a thank-you note or love letter and then mail it to yourself.

Keeping an inventory

As you recognize and validate yourself, start identifying your strengths, abilities, and qualities, especially ones that are unique to you. Look for qualities that you bring to every situation in your life, whether it's work, home, or friendships, for example.

For instance, a client of mine (coauthor Eva) was asked by his boss to create a succession plan, or how he envisioned himself succeeding and what his goals for the future might be. My client felt overwhelmed by the task as he stated, "I don't like to promote myself. I just do my job and hope that I will be recognized and then promoted to whatever is next. I worry about pointing out my weaknesses because then I might be viewed as inadequate."

Can you see how his self-doubt or insecurities were limiting him from looking forward and planning and taking responsibility for his own learning and growth?

I instructed him to approach the task as an exercise that could help him learn more about himself. I told him to list and review his abilities and accomplishments and to also look at his weaknesses to figure out what he might need to learn to move forward. His team, for example, trusted him, and he was extremely adept at listening and helping them feel at ease in speaking to him. He was able to realize that his ability to forge strong relationships with trust and communication is an amazing quality. He also came to understand that one of his weaknesses was understanding some of the technical issues that often arise in the company. So he made a list of ways that would help him gain more technical knowledge.

REMEMBER

Keeping an *inventory* of your strengths and weaknesses is not an exercise where you judge yourself for being good or bad — it is instead a list that's meant to support you to know your value because you're confident in your abilities and you're motivated to learn and grow.

You can start to keep an inventory by taking these actions:

>> **Take an ongoing inventory.** Throughout the day, create an ongoing inventory of your qualities, competencies, and accomplishments.

>> **Pause to reflect.** When you feel good about something you have done, take a moment to reflect and elucidate your qualities or abilities that enabled you to accomplish this feat.

>> **Count everything!** Whether you have managed to always get to work on time (quality of being punctual), managed to pull off a surprise party (resourceful and discrete), or were able to resolve a conflict between employees at the office (effective communicator, empathic, and so on), everything counts.

>> **Review your positive qualities.** Regularly read over your list, and remind yourself of your positive qualities and ways you're valued.

>> **Note areas of your life where you want to grow and improve.** Look for weaknesses, note setbacks or situations where your efforts were not successful.

>> **Do your research.** Research ways to learn the skills you need to improve on your weaknesses.

Accepting and being your unique self

Knowing your value means understanding that you're human and therefore imperfect. You are, however, perfectly imperfect and one-of-a-kind. Your imperfections aren't cause for putting yourself down, but are rather manifestations of ways you can lift yourself up. They can be road signs that urge you to grow and learn something new or reflections of your own individual uniqueness.

Your goal is to learn to fully accept yourself as the unique individual that you are — imperfections and all. Here are some guidelines to help you get there:

>> **Avoid comparing yourself to others when noticing a perceived imperfection.** Someone else will always perform better or worse than you, and neither makes you more or less valuable.

>> **Get the right focus.** Rather than focus on what is wrong, focus on what is right.

>> **Give your imperfection a new job description: a representation of your perfection as a unique individual.** Always remember that your imperfections add to your uniqueness, of you being you.

>> **Use your mistakes as opportunities for growth.** Learn and develop new skills and knowledge. Use the situation as an opportunity to become stronger and smarter.

>> **Live and act with integrity.** No one can make you feel badly about yourself — only you can do that. When you live your life with integrity, you start believing in your own integrity. Be authentic, truthful, and ethical. If you find yourself wanting to lie or hide or pretend to be someone you're not, examine the reasons you're feeling compelled to act this way, and then align with your worth and integrity. Act from this place.

You're perfectly imperfect! There is no one like you anywhere.

Holding on to your vision

Wherever and however you find yourself at any particular moment, accept yourself and your behaviors, thoughts, or actions while holding in your heart the vision of your true value. You are human. You will make mistakes. Your limiting beliefs will show up in your life. On some days you'll feel positively, and on other days, negatively. There is no right or wrong. What exists is a vision of who you are from a lens of value. Hold on to it.

This list describes some actions you can take today to hold on to the vision of your value:

>> **Take time to contemplate and meditate on your story of victory.** Allow yourself to see yourself as confident, strong, loving, and compassionate, for example.

>> **Create a vision board.** Write down positive statements, add photos and magazine cutouts, and use markers and crayons to create the picture of your

vision. Refer to this "story" anytime you need reminding, by either reading the story or closing your eyes and remembering the vision.

>> **Have a few of your loved ones evaluate your strengths and positive qualities.** Sit opposite at least one person who absolutely adores you — or as many as five or six. Each person takes a minute or more to look into your eyes and speak from their heart, listing your positive qualities and what they admire about you. You listen, receive, and write down what you hear. Keep this list in your purse or wallet to refer to any time you need.

>> **Find opportunities to accentuate your competencies and abilities.** Then you can continue affirming this vision.

Being loving toward yourself

If you love and believe in yourself, you can forgive yourself for being human and making mistakes. Be kind toward yourself, treating yourself as if you were your own best friend, and find gratitude even in the smallest actions or deeds. When you feel special, you forgive and accept yourself for other imperfections. The key is to love yourself and treat yourself with loving kindness.

TIP

Here are some actions you can take now to love yourself more:

>> **Avoid self-critical or derogatory statements.** Especially avoid using words like *should* or *can't*.

>> **Speak lovingly.** Ask yourself what you might say to someone you love, and use those words instead.

>> **Give thanks.** Focus on what you have rather than on what you don't have. Keep a gratitude journal and reflect on ways you're lucky and grateful.

>> **Accept compliments.** Rather than deflect or rebuff, simply say "Thank you." Receive the compliment even if you feel uncomfortable.

>> **Honor your body.** Believe that your body is the temple that houses your magnificence. Without a healthy body, you cannot let your light shine in this world.

>> **Pamper yourself.** There's nothing wrong with a little love-me gift every now and then, which may be a physical object or simply giving yourself some Me Time to relax and take care of yourself.

Taking Care of YOU

Between exercise, healthy nutrition, meditation, and a good sleep regimen, you can nurture your body to stay strong and vibrant. When you feel strong physically, you have energy, and this energy supports your mental attitude and bandwidth to handle challenges. The problem is that many people let go of positive self-care habits when they're under stress or when they feel that their care is needed elsewhere. The truth is that everyone has value, but no one and nothing has more value than you or your wellbeing.

When you take care of yourself, you have the energy and bandwidth to care for others or do great work. According to researchers, individuals who make conscious healthy-lifestyle choices feel more masterful about themselves and their accomplishments, feel confident spending time among people who are younger, and uphold a positive mental attitude while tending to live longer and happier lives.

REMEMBER

What does this mean for you? It means choose *you*. If you don't take care of you, who will? Rather than look outward for people, places, or things to complete you, focus on people, places, or things that can support you to be at your best. You want to ask yourself whether it fuels you to really feel good about yourself and within yourself. Ultimately, you want to learn to have a deep connection with yourself, your desires, and your passions, and to do what you can to support yourself to thrive.

The following sections are a guide for taking care of you.

Nourish yourself with nutrient-rich food

Eat foods that fuel your mind and body to be healthy and strong. Foods high in fat and sugar content may comfort your anxiety initially, but they also cause inflammation, fatigue, and more depression or anxiety.

REMEMBER

Food is neither reward or punishment. It's *fuel*. It provides your brain and body with energy, energy that comes from fiber, proteins, fats, vitamins, and minerals. Check out Book 5 for details on eating clean and giving your body the best fuel possible.

Exercise and stay active

Find ways to keep your body fit and strong. If it's an activity you enjoy, you're more likely to stick with it. You can jog, dance, or do yoga or weight training and build movement into your everyday routine. (See Book 4 for details on improving your physical fitness.) Here are some different types of exercise to help you stay active:

>> **Metabolic conditioning:** In this type of conditioning, you get your heart rate up at least three times a week.

>> **Resistance training:** Use weights or your own body weight at least two times a week.

>> **Walking:** Walk as often as you can instead of driving.

>> **Nature:** Being in nature will help you feel more energized and less focused on discomfort.

>> **Exercise buddy:** Working out with a friend can help you stay accountable and also ensures that you enjoy the activity.

Connect with support

Turn to other people to support you to feel good about you. In other words, surround yourself with other individuals who can help you reflect and stick to training, a healthy diet, and positive emotions and outlooks.

>> Choose the right people from your friends and family who you know can support you to be at your best.

>> Let go of, or spend as little time as possible with, people who criticize you and bring you down.

>> Seek counseling or support from a coach, therapist, or healer.

>> Join a support group for extra care of reciprocity.

>> Join a spiritual community where you share positive beliefs and meditation practices and display acts of compassion and gratitude.

Quiet your mind

TIP

The mind is a wonderful tool, but negative thinking hinders your ability to connect with your value. Take time to quiet the mind and find peace to enable relaxation and reflection. Here are a few tips to help you quiet your mind (and see Book 1 for more guidance):

>> Choose from a variety of meditation practices.

>> Take a mindful walk in nature, focusing on the beauty and wonder around you.

>> Regularly take time to do a mindful breath focus, shifting your awareness away from your thoughts and simply focusing on the movement of the breath and the sensations you experience in your body.

>> Practice visual imagery. For example, you can imagine that when you exhale, your thoughts dissolve into the sunlight and that when you inhale, the sunlight enters your mind. As you continue this process, the light eventually moves throughout your entire body, filling you with a sense of peace and joy.

Heal through your negative emotions

Quieting the mind and building self-awareness enhances your ability to catch your negative emotions before they gain momentum, and then you can use the opportunity to take better care of yourself. Here are some suggestions for healing:

>> Pay attention to how you feel from moment to moment.

>> If and when you feel negatively, don't judge yourself — simply be aware and honor your feelings, knowing that your emotions are signals telling you you're in need of care.

>> Notice how your body reacts to these emotions. Where do you feel the energy show up in your body? What does it feel like?

>> Breathe into the area in your body where you feel the emotion. Gently breathe love and compassion into your body.

>> Reflect as you want with regard to why the emotion is there, in what way it's serving you, and how it's a reflection of your feeling hurt, ineffective, or undervalued.

>> Reflect on your value and your positive story.

Have fun!

TIP

Wake up in the morning and choose to have a luxurious and adventurous day. According to science, you live a longer and healthier life when you're happy. Here are some suggestions for having fun:

>> Find ways to be more playful. For clues, observe a child at play.

>> Go out with friends and enjoy yourself. (This book was written during the COVID pandemic. If it's still happening when you read this, make sure you practice social distancing and wear masks if required.)

» Sign up for a dance class, even if you have two left feet, so that you can laugh at yourself, or watch a funny movie.

» Discover new ways of being that put a smile on your face and a laugh in your heart.

Appreciate all that you have and all that you are

When you're filled with gratitude, you're more likely to see any situation as an opportunity for growth and meaning rather than as bad, or even as a curse. You're more likely to feel happy.

TIP

Here is an exercise named I Am a Miracle, which you might find helpful, especially in those times that you cannot seem to find anything to be grateful for:

1. **Think about the definition of a miracle: "a surprising and welcome event that is not explicable by natural or scientific laws and is therefore considered to be the work of a divine agency."**

2. **Close your eyes and repeat, "I am a miracle."**

3. **Smile.**

4. **Say it again.**

5. **Smile even wider.**

6. **Say it again.**

7. **Open your eyes.**

It's okay to rest

Resting and recovery are just as important for your wellbeing and reaching your goals as being active. Here are some suggestions:

» **Take the time.** Give yourself time and space to meditate, relax, and take some Me Time.

» **Say no when you need to.** It's okay to say no and choose to take care of yourself. You aren't being selfish; rather, you're taking care of yourself so that you can give later.

>> **Set boundaries.** Set them in your relationships and with yourself to allow time for you to take care of yourself so that you can be fully present in your life.

>> **Get restful sleep.** Turn off electronics in the bedroom, relax a couple of hours before sleep, and make sure your bed and bedroom are comfortable and quiet.

REMEMBER

Whatever you choose to do, set the intention to be on the path to loving yourself. Believe in your own ability to create and have joy, ease, comfort, and love. Do what you need to do to feel alive, vibrant, and healthy. When you feel good, you radiate goodness and you attract more of the same.

Allowing Love In

At the core of low self-value is the belief that you aren't worthy of being loved. For most people, over the course of their lifetime, they have experienced hurt, betrayal, neglect, or abandonment that has led them to believe that they aren't important or worthy of love. As a result, people have closed their hearts so as to avoid getting hurt, which has led to a disconnection from themselves and the ability to let the right people in.

I (coauthor Eva) had this realization after a relationship ended in my 20s. I felt betrayed, hurt, and taken advantage of by my former boyfriend. I kept asking myself, "Why?" and "Why doesn't he love me?" and "Why am I not good enough?" and "What did I do wrong?" When I realized that I was berating myself for someone else's actions, I took the time to sit with my emotions, my negative beliefs, and the pain in my heart to try to answer those questions truthfully and with compassion.

The truth was, I realized, that my value was not predicated on whether he loved me; that I did nothing wrong other than trust someone I knew wasn't trustworthy (the signs were there before), which happens to the best of us; that I was guilty of loving and nothing else and was therefore forgiven; and that just because someone doesn't love me doesn't mean that I am not loveable. I understood that I was looking outside of myself to feel loveable when I had the ability to provide that love to myself. It was then that I started embarking on my journey to understanding love better, to love myself better and let love in.

Do you let love in? Do you accept compliments, allow people to help you or make sure you take care of yourself?

You don't have to wait for other people to give you love to have it. You can do it yourself by opening your heart to love itself and by taking the myriad action steps and techniques that involve taking care of you. You can start now to allow love in by

>> Being vulnerable and asking for help from your support people

>> Practicing gratitude and appreciation

>> Allowing yourself to feel, even negatively, and seeing all of yourself as valuable

>> Intentionally nurturing yourself through your self-care practices (nutrition, exercise, and sleep, for example)

>> Spending time in nature and feeling a sense of connection and awe

>> Engaging in meditation practices that build self-compassion, love, and forgiveness, like the following meditation for opening the heart

Meditations to open the heart have been done by many a healer and meditation practitioner in a myriad of variations. There is no right way — just the way of opening your heart to receiving some form of love, whether it's gratitude, compassion, or awe, for example.

TIP

The following is a meditation exercise that guides you to open your heart so that you can fully receive love:

1. **Find a comfortable position.**

   Make it somewhere quiet where no one will disturb you.

2. **Close your eyes and bring your awareness to the center of your chest.**

   This area is known as the *heart center.*

3. **Gently breathe into and out of the heart center, counting 1-2-3 as you breathe in and 1-2-3-4-5-6 as you breathe out.**

4. **As you breathe in and out, observe any sensations or feelings that you're experiencing in your chest.**

   Does it feel open, closed, relaxed, tight, heavy, or light? What emotions do you notice? Observe without judgment. There's no right or wrong. You're just observing energy.

5. **Be aware that you're observing energy in your heart and noticing what it feels like.**

6. **Allow your breath to start moving the energy in your chest, like a curtain that moves with the breeze.**

   It's effortless. Just let it move in and out with your breath.

   The energy in your chest is gently moving with your breath like a curtain that moves in the breeze.

7. **As you breathe in, imagine that you're breathing in unlimited love and infinite intelligence from the universe into your heart, and that when you exhale, you're simply letting go of everything else.**

   Breathe in unlimited love and infinite intelligence, exhaling and letting go of everything else.

   With every breath, your heart fills with unlimited love and infinite intelligence until it's so full that this love and intelligence begin to overflow.

8. **Observe that there is no separation between your heart and the heart of the entire universe, because you're connected by unlimited love and infinite intelligence.**

   You may want to say to yourself, "Our hearts are one heart."

   You may want to see other hearts as your heart connects with other hearts, unlimited love, and infinite intelligence flowing freely.

   "Our hearts are one heart."

9. **Stay in this state as long as you want.**

10. **When you're ready, give thanks for the fullness of your heart and the fullness of your being.**

4

Feeling Better with a Bit of Fitness

Contents at a Glance

CHAPTER 1: Cardio Crash Course: Getting the Right Intensity 243

Comparing Aerobic and Anaerobic Exercise 244

Understanding the Importance of Warming Up and Cooling Down 245

Using Simple Methods to Gauge Your Level of Effort 246

Measuring Your Heart Rate 248

CHAPTER 2: Exercising Outdoors 255

Walking for Fitness 256

Running: Get Up and Go 258

Bicycling Around 261

Exercising in Water 263

CHAPTER 3: Strengthening and Lengthening Your Muscles 269

Why You've Gotta Lift Weights 270

Flexibility Training: Getting the Scoop on Stretching 273

Exploring Stretching Techniques 276

Still Life: Doing Static Stretching 278

CHAPTER 4: All about Yoga 289

Looking at What Yoga Can Do for Your Body 289

Finding a Yoga Style That's Right for You 290

Getting Started 292

Trying a Yoga Routine 294

CHAPTER 5: Choosing an Exercise Class or Virtual Workout 303

Getting Through When You Haven't a Clue: Taking an Exercise Class 304

Working Out with an Onscreen Instructor 311

IN THIS CHAPTER

» **Comparing aerobic and anaerobic exercise**

» **Warming up and cooling down**

» **Using simple methods to gauge your intensity**

» **Measuring your heart rate**

Chapter **1**

Cardio Crash Course: Getting the Right Intensity

f you hang around people who exercise, you're going to hear the word *cardio* or *aerobics* pretty often. Someone may say, "I do cardio four days a week," or, "My gym has awesome cardio equipment." *Aerobics* — a term coined in the 1960s by fitness pioneer Dr. Kenneth Cooper — refers to *cardiovascular exercise*, the kind that strengthens your heart and lungs and burns lots of calories.

There are all kinds of reasons to pursue this sort of exercise — everything from lowering your risk of dementia and diabetes to trimming that spare tire to experiencing the glory of a personal best in a 10k run. This chapter explains what it takes to reap those benefits — in other words, what type of exercise counts as cardio. It introduces you to terms such as *aerobic, anaerobic,* and *target heart-rate zone.*

REMEMBER

After you read this chapter, you may be very excited about all the information and want to put it — and your feet — into action. On the other hand, with all this talk of maximum heart rate, anaerobic threshold, and heart-rate monitors, you may wonder whether cardio exercise is just too darned complicated to bother with. It's not! This chapter provides all this information so that you understand the basics of how to determine your exercise intensity and set goals for your program. All this science is pretty simple to put into action.

Comparing Aerobic and Anaerobic Exercise

Aerobic exercise is any continuous, repetitive activity that you do long enough and hard enough to challenge your heart and lungs. To get this effect, you generally need to use your large muscles, including your butt, legs, back, and chest. Walking, bicycling, swimming, and climbing stairs count as aerobic exercise.

Movements that use your smaller muscles, like those leading into your wrists and hands, don't burn as many calories. Channel surfing with your remote control can certainly be repetitive, sustained, and intense — particularly when performed by certain husbands — but it burns very few calories.

Aerobic means "with air." When you exercise aerobically, your body needs an extra supply of oxygen, which your lungs extract from the air. Think of oxygen as the gasoline in your car: When you're idling at a stoplight, you don't need as much fuel as when you're zooming across Montana on Interstate 90. During your aerobic workouts, your body continuously delivers oxygen to your muscles.

However, if you push yourself hard enough, eventually you switch gears into using less oxygen: Your lungs can no longer suck in enough oxygen to keep up with your muscles' demand for it. But you don't collapse, at least not in the first three minutes. Instead, you begin to rely on your body's limited capacity to keep going without oxygen. During this time, your individual muscles are exercising *anaerobically*, or without air.

Anaerobic exercise refers to high-intensity exercise like all-out sprinting or very heavy weight lifting. After about 90 seconds, you begin gasping for air, and you usually can't sustain this activity for more than three minutes. That's when your body forces you to stop. You may still use large muscle groups, but you do so for only a short burst of time, and then you need to take a break before starting the next burst. Running a 30-minute loop around the neighborhood is aerobic, whereas doing all-out sprints around the track with a 2-minute break between them is anaerobic. Both count as cardio because they challenge your heart and lungs and burn lots of calories. You also may do hybrid activities referred to as "stop-and-go" sports, such as basketball, soccer, and tennis. These activities involve long periods of slow, sustained movement with some short bursts of high-intensity activity mixed in.

Understanding the Importance of Warming Up and Cooling Down

Automobiles are built to go from 0 to 60 miles per hour in mere seconds and to stop practically on a dime if necessary; humans aren't. With any type of physical activity, whether it's walking, playing basketball, or cross-country skiing, you need to ease into it with a warm-up and ease out of it with a cool-down. (Weight-training workouts also require a warm-up, although they typically don't require a cardio cool-down.)

Warming up

REMEMBER

A *warm-up* simply means 3 to 15 minutes of an activity performed at a very easy pace. Ideally, a warm-up should be a slower version of the main event so it works the same muscles and gets blood flowing to all the right places. For example, runners may start with a brisk walk or a slow run. If you're going on a hilly bike ride, you may want to start with at least a few miles on flat terrain. Be aware that stretching is not a good warm-up activity.

People who are out of shape need to warm up the longest. Their bodies take longer to get into the exercise groove because their muscles aren't used to working hard. If you're a beginner, any exercise is high-intensity exercise. As you get more fit, your body adapts and becomes more efficient, thereby warming up more quickly.

WARNING

Many people skip their warm-up because they're in a hurry. Cranking up the elliptical machine or hitting the weights right away seems like a more efficient use of time. Bad idea. Skimp on your warm-up, and you're a lot more likely to injure yourself. Besides, when you ease into your workout, you enjoy it a lot more. A trainer we know says, "If you don't have time to warm up, you don't have time to work out!"

What exactly does warming up do for you? Well, for one thing, a warm-up warms you up — literally. It increases the temperature in your muscles and in the tissues that connect muscle to bone (tendons) and bone to bone (ligaments). Warmer muscles and joints are more pliable and, therefore, less likely to tear. Warming up also helps redirect your blood flow from places such as your stomach and spleen to the muscles that you're using to exercise. This blood flow gives you more stamina by providing your muscles with more nutrients and oxygen. In other words, you tire more quickly if you don't warm up because this redirection of blood flow takes time.

Finally, warming up allows your heart rate to increase at a safe, gradual pace. If you don't warm up, your heart rate will shoot up too quickly, and you'll have trouble getting your breathing under control.

Cooling down

REMEMBER

After your workout, don't stop suddenly and make a dash for the shower or plop on the couch. (If you've ever done this, you've probably exited the shower with a hot red face or dripped sweat all over the couch.) Ease out of your workout just as you eased into it, by walking, jogging, or cycling lightly. If you've been using a stationary bike at Level 5 for 20 minutes, you can cool down by dropping to Level 3 for a couple minutes, then to Level 2, and so on. This *cool-down* should last 5 to 10 minutes — longer if you've done an especially lengthy or hard workout.

The purpose of the cool-down is the reverse of the warm-up. At this point, your heart is jumping and blood is pumping furiously through your muscles. You want your body to redirect the blood flow back to normal before you rush back to the office. You also want your body temperature to decrease before you hop into a hot or cold shower; otherwise, you risk fainting. Cooling down prevents your blood from pooling in one place, such as your legs.

WARNING

When you suddenly stop exercising, your blood can quickly collect, which can lead to dizziness, nausea, and fainting. If you're really out of shape or at high risk for heart disease, skipping a cool-down can place undue stress on your heart.

Using Simple Methods to Gauge Your Level of Effort

REMEMBER

To reap the benefits of cardio exercise, how much huffing and puffing do you need to do? Not as much as you probably think. Sure, you don't burn many calories from walking on the treadmill at the same pace that you stroll down the grocery store aisles; they don't call it *working out* for nothing. On the other hand, exercising too hard can lead to injury and make you more susceptible to colds and infections; plus, you may get so burned out that you want to set fire to your stationary bike. Also, the faster you go, the less time you can keep up the exercise. Depending on what you're trying to accomplish, you may gain just as much, if not more, from slowing things down and going farther.

To get fit and stay healthy, you need to find the middle ground: a moderate, or aerobic, pace. You can find this middle ground in a number of different ways. Some methods of gauging your intensity are extremely simple, and some require a foray into arithmetic. This section looks at the two most basic ways to monitor your intensity.

The talk test

TIP

The simplest way to monitor how hard you're working is to talk. You should be able to carry on a conversation while you're exercising. If you're so out of breath that you can't even string together the words "Help me, Mommy!" you need to slow down. On the other hand, if you're able to belt out tunes at the top of your lungs, that's a pretty big clue you need to pick up the pace. Basically, you should feel like you're working but not so hard that you feel like your lungs are about to explode.

Perceived exertion

If you're the type of person who needs more precision in life than the talk test offers, you may like the so-called *perceived exertion* method of gauging intensity. This method uses a numerical scale, typically from 1 to 10, that corresponds to how hard you feel you're working — the rate at which you perceive that you're exerting yourself.

REMEMBER

An activity rated 1 on a perceived exertion scale would be something that you feel you could do forever, like sit in bed and watch the Olympics. A 10 represents all-out effort, like the last few feet of an uphill sprint, about 20 seconds before your legs buckle. Your typical workout intensity should fall somewhere between 5 and 8. To decide on a number, pay attention to how hard you're breathing, how fast your heart is beating, how much you're sweating, and how tired your legs feel — anything that contributes to the effort of sustaining the exercise.

The purpose of putting a numerical value on exercise is not to make your life more complicated but rather to help you maintain a proper workout intensity. For example, suppose you run 2 miles around your neighborhood, and it feels like an 8. If after a few weeks running those 2 miles feels like a 4, you know it's time to pick up the pace. Initially, you may want to have a perceived exertion chart in front of you. Many gyms post these charts on the walls, and you can easily create one at home. After a few workouts, you can use a mental chart. Table 1-1 shows a sample perceived exertion chart.

TABLE 1-1   **Perceived Exertion**

Scale	Description
10 Maximum effort	It's nearly impossible to continue. You're completely out of breath, your heart is pounding, you're sweating profusely, and you're unable to talk.
9 Very hard effort	It's very challenging, though not impossible, to maintain activity. You're breathing hard, your heart is pounding, you're sweating a lot, and you can barely talk.
7–8 Vigorous effort	You're on the edge of your comfort zone. You're short of breath, your heart is beating hard, and you're sweating, but you're able to speak short sentences.
4–6 Moderate effort	It feels like you can keep moving for quite a while without having to stop. You can have short conversations even though you're breathing heavily, your heart is beating fast, and you're sweating.
2–3 Light effort	It feels like you can keep moving with very little effort for a long time. Your heart rate is somewhat elevated and you may be sweating lightly, but you can breathe easily and hold a conversation.
1 Very light effort	You're doing something that requires virtually no physical effort — sedentary activities such as watching TV, riding in a car, or working on a computer.

Measuring Your Heart Rate

The talk test and the perceived exertion chart (see the preceding sections) are both valid ways to make sure that you're exercising at the right pace. But there's a numerical way for those of you who like concrete numbers: measuring your *pulse*, or *heart rate*, the number of times that your heart beats per minute. You can determine this number either by wearing a gadget called a *heart-rate monitor* or by using your fingers and counting the beats manually. This section discusses both methods and also explains why you want to measure your heart rate and how to determine your own target heart-rate zone.

Looking at what heart rate tells you

Keeping track of your heart rate, by whatever method, sounds like an incredibly advanced thing to do — something way beyond a beginner's needs. But especially when you're just starting, heart-rate monitoring is immensely effective. Here are three reasons to follow your heart rate:

>> **You find out whether you're working too hard.** When you're just starting to exercise, you may not have a good sense of how hard to push yourself. And with all that "no pain, no gain" propaganda, you may be exerting yourself more than is good for you. For example, running 9-minute miles on a hot, humid afternoon takes a lot more effort than running at the same pace on a cool, overcast morning. If you rely only on your stopwatch, you may push yourself to run 9-minute miles in the heat, when that pace may put excess stress on your body. If you pace yourself according to your heart rate instead, you know when you need to back off.

The same goes for when you're tired. Without checking your heart rate, you may force yourself to walk up an 8-percent grade at 4 miles per hour, when on that particular day, your body isn't up to the task. If you monitor your pulse, you may find that, to keep up with Level 4 on the bike, you have to exceed the high end of your training zone — a signal to drop down a notch or two.

>> **You have another way to track your progress.** When you start exercising on a regular basis, your cardio respiratory system gradually becomes more efficient. Suppose when you started, Level 1 on the exercise bike used to get your heart up to about 140 beats per minute; now, two months later, your heart rate is 125 beats per minute. This drop means that you need to step up the difficulty of your workout.

TIP

Another way to see how much your fitness level is improving is to watch how fast your heart rate drops after a workout. Measure your heart rate immediately upon finishing your exercise session and then one minute later. The better shape you're in, the faster your heart rate drops. Ideally, your heart rate should plunge at least 20 beats in the first minute. People in really good shape drop 40 beats or more. Keep track of this measure. You'll see a gradual improvement over a period of weeks and months.

REMEMBER

Taking prescription or over-the-counter medication may affect the way your heart and blood pressure respond to exercise. Check with your doctor about this.

Yet another measure of your progress is your *resting heart rate,* the number of times your heart beats per minute when you're just sitting around.

>> **You see how well you've recovered from your last workout.** You can use your resting heart rate to follow your recovery from day to day. Keep your monitor by your bed and strap it on first thing in the morning. Or take your pulse manually. If your heart rate is 10 beats higher than usual, you probably haven't recovered from yesterday's workout. Consider easing up or taking a day off.

Understanding your target zone

How do you know what heart rate to aim for? There's no magic number. Rather, there's a whole range of acceptable numbers, commonly called your *target heart-rate zone.* This range is the middle ground between slacking off and knocking yourself out. Typically, your *target zone* (as it's called for short) is between 50 and 85 percent of your *maximum heart rate,* the maximum number of times your heart should beat in a minute without dangerously overexerting yourself.

TECHNICAL
STUFF

The top end of your target zone — somewhere between 80 and 90 percent of your maximum heart rate — is the point at which your body switches from using oxygen as its primary source of energy to using stored sugar. The point is referred to as your *anaerobic threshold.* Lactic acid builds up in the blood vessels of your muscles during especially high-intensity (or very long bouts of) exercise. As soon as more lactic acid builds up in your muscles than they can flush out, you begin to feel a burning sensation. Your muscles start to slow down, and moving becomes difficult. Fortunately, after you slow back down or stop, lactic acid clears your system within minutes. (It's not responsible for the soreness you feel for several days after a hard workout session.)

When you're in poor physical shape, your body isn't very efficient at taking in and utilizing oxygen and food sources, so you hit your anaerobic threshold while exercising at relatively low levels of exercise. As you become more fit, you're able to go farther and faster yet still supply oxygen to your muscles. If a couch potato tries to run an 8-minute-mile pace, he's going to go anaerobic pretty darned fast. An elite runner can run an entire marathon at about a 5-minute-mile pace and stay primarily aerobic.

TIP

At the low end of your zone, you're barely breaking a sweat; at the high end, you're dripping like a Kentucky Derby winner. If you're a beginner, stick to the lower end so you can move along comfortably for longer periods of time and with less chance of injury. As you get fitter, you may want to do some of your training in the middle and upper end of your zone.

Finding your maximum and target heart rates

So how do you know what your maximum heart rate is? Well, you shouldn't run as hard as you can until you keel over and then count your heartbeats for one minute. A safer and more accurate way is to have your max measured by a professional such as a physician or exercise specialist. You can also use a number of mathematical formulas to estimate your max.

THE KARVONEN METHOD FOR TARGET HEART RATE

One of the problems with the standard formula for finding your target heart rate is that it takes only your age into consideration. This is a valid consideration because your recommended maximum heart rate declines as you age. However, the following formula, called the Karvonen method, is somewhat more accurate because it also factors in your *resting heart rate,* the number of times your heart beats when you're sitting still. Typically, as you become more fit, your heart rate drops.

The Karvonen method requires a bit more math, but don't let that intimidate you. This example uses the case of a 40-year-old man who has a resting heart rate of 60 beats per minute and who wants to work at between 50 percent and 85 percent of his maximum heart rate. Grab your calculator and follow these instructions:

1. **Subtract your age from 220 to find the estimated maximum heart rate.**

   220 – 40 = 180

2. **Subtract your resting heart rate from your estimated maximum.**

   180 – 60 = 120

3. **Multiply the number you arrived at in Step 2 by 50 percent. Then add your resting heart rate back in to find the low end of the target zone.**

   120 × 0.50 = 60

   60 + 60 = 120

   The low end of the man's target zone is 120.

4. **Multiply the estimated maximum from Step 2 by 85 percent. Then add your resting heart rate back in to find the high end of the target zone.**

   120 × 0.85 = 102

   102 + 60 = 162

   The high end of the man's target zone is 162.

Okay, now you can compare the results of this formula with those of the traditional formula. Using the age-related formula, this 40-year-old's target zone is 90 to 153 beats. But when you factor in his resting heart rate, this allows him to work up to 162 beats per minute. And he knows that if he drops below 102 beats, he probably needs to pick up the pace.

The best way to understand your max is to have it tested by a personal trainer or a doctor. The tester puts you through your paces on a cardio machine, usually a treadmill, and either makes you work as hard as you can, taking the highest heart rate you can sustain, or takes you to some percentage of your true maximum heart rate. The tester then uses a mathematical formula to get a decent prediction of what your max is.

Using that easy formula to find your max, find your *target heart rate* by calculating 50 percent and 85 percent of your maximum. For instance, for a 40-year-old man, his maximum is 220 − 40 = 180. Take 50 percent of that to get the low end of his target zone: 180 × 0.50 = 90. If his heart beats fewer than 90 times per minute, he knows he's not pushing hard enough. Take 85 percent of the max to find the high end of his target zone (180 × 0.85 = 153). If his heart beats faster than 153 beats per minute, he needs to slow down.

Measuring your pulse

Okay, say you've figured out your target heart-rate zone (see the preceding section). How do you know whether you're in the zone? In other words, how do you know how fast your heart is beating at any given moment? You can check your heart rate in a few ways: using a heart-rate monitor, taking your pulse manually, or making use of your smartwatch health feature.

Checking your smartwatch or fitness band

Aside from providing the time, your smartwatch can provide a lot of health information. Basic features of most health apps include the ability to take your pulse, your blood pressure, measure the oxygen in your blood, and even count your steps.

Fitness bands are designed specifically to monitor your heart rate and movement. You set the band to your particulars and have access to instant information about your heart rate and the number of steps you've taken at the very least.

To get a reading on your pulse rate, you may need to open a specific function, place your finger on the screen, or just look at your screen for the constantly monitored info.

Fitness electronics are readily available and pretty affordable — the smartwatch rated most accurate by one consumer group lists for $59.00. Of course, if you want all the bells and several whistles, you can spend $700 or even more.

Using a heart-rate monitor

The most accurate way to determine your heart rate at any given moment is to wear a heart-rate monitor. The most accurate type of monitor is the chest-strap variety, which operates on the same principle as a medical electrocardiogram (ECG). You hook an inch-wide strap around your chest. This strap acts as an electrode to measure the electrical activity of your heart. This information is then translated into a number, which is transmitted via radio signals to a wrist receiver that looks like a watch with a large face. All you have to do is look at your wrist, and you instantly know how many times your heart is beating that moment, whether it's 92 or 164.

This is much more convenient than taking your pulse manually (see the next section) because you don't need to stop exercising or take the time to count anything. Yes, this convenience will cost you, but a basic model is only about $30.

Most of the cardio equipment in fitness facilities are heart-rate-monitor compatible. The machines pick up the signal from the monitor around your chest, and your heart rate pops up on the display console, so you don't have to wear the wrist watch. Some machines have heart monitor grips as well; however, these generally can't be used while running or doing high-intensity exercise.

WARNING

Chest monitors are very accurate, but some are subject to interference from electromagnetic waves like those given off by some treadmills and stair-climbers. Exercising next to someone else who's wearing a monitor may also scramble signals, a sort of electronic equivalent of getting your braces locked with someone else's when you're kissing. You may need at least 4 feet between users for monitors to function properly, although several companies now offer models with a special device to eliminate interference.

Taking your pulse manually

If you aren't wearing a heart-rate monitor, a manual pulse check can give you some useful information about how hard you're working and what to do with the rest of your workout.

Feel the steady pounding of blood flowing through your arteries. When you're fairly comfortable with the rhythm, count how many beats you feel in 15 seconds. Then multiply this number by 4 — voilà, your heart rate.

TIP

During your workout, take your pulse about every 15 minutes (or do some sort of intensity check) and focus on what you're counting. Otherwise, you may end up counting the number of steps you take on the treadmill rather than the number of pulses in your wrist. You may want to slow down while you take your pulse. True, this is disruptive to your workout, but it's not nearly as disruptive as getting launched off the treadmill.

» **Bicycling on a mountain bike or road bike**

» **Swimming: A total-body workout**

Chapter **2**

Exercising Outdoors

Fresh air: What a concept! With all the super-high-tech indoor exercise contraptions available these days, it's easy to forget you can get an effective workout in the great outdoors, often for no cost other than a pair of athletic shoes. You may even burn more calories per minute in the fresh air because outdoor activities sometimes involve more muscles than their indoor counterparts. For example, when you park yourself on a stationary bicycle, your upper-body muscles basically get a free ride — you can easily flip the pages of a magazine as you pedal away. But when you take your bike out for a spin, your chest, arm, abdominal, and back muscles are all called up for active duty, and you expend extra energy battling the wind.

This chapter covers some of the most popular and invigorating outdoor fitness activities. You discover what gear you need and how much it costs, and there are training strategies and safety tips for rookies and klutzes alike.

TIP

Keep in mind that in addition to trying the activities covered here, such as walking and swimming, you also can have a blast in adult sports leagues, playing soccer, softball, basketball, rugby, and other sports that definitely aren't just for kids. Contact your local parks and recreation department to find out about leagues.

Walking for Fitness

Can you really get fit by walking? Absolutely — as long as you walk long enough, hard enough, and often enough. One study found that among people who are successful in maintaining long-term weight loss, nearly 80 percent walk as their main physical activity.

The beauty of walking is that it's simply a matter of putting one foot in front of the other. Sure, walking burns fewer calories per minute than jogging, but most people last longer on a walk than on a run, so you can make up for the deficit. Plus, compared to runners, walkers enjoy a relatively low injury rate.

However, there is no sugarcoating this: Some exercisers find walking to be a big, fat bore. Some people combat boredom by heading for the nearest nature trail. The change of scenery (not to mention the change of terrain, sounds, and smells) can be very uplifting.

Essential walking gear

Although the rest of the animal kingdom does fine without the benefit of special equipment, human feet don't have adequate padding to meet the demands of walking in the modern world. You need a good pair of walking shoes to avoid foot, ankle, knee, hip, and lower-back problems. Expect to spend at least $50 for good walking shoes.

Walking shoes may sound like a marketing conspiracy hatched by shoe-industry executives. After all, it's only walking — won't any pair of sneakers suffice? Actually, the concept of a walking shoe is a valid one. Walking shoes need to be more flexible than running shoes because you bend your feet more when you walk, and you push off from your toes with more oomph. Also, because your heels bear most of your weight when you walk, you need a firm, stable heel counter, the part of the shoe that wraps around your heel to keep your foot in place. If you walk for long distances frequently, look for a lightweight shoe to reduce stress.

The general distance for replacing walking shoes is after 500 miles. If you walk for 30 minutes a day, shoes can last for six months; if you run, get new shoes every three months. Check your shoes in the meantime for uneven wear patterns or worn tread, which means you need to hit the shoe store sooner.

TIP

If you plan to hike or walk over rugged terrain, look for a walking shoe with treaded soles and added heel and ankle support. If you're focusing on speed walking or high mileage, go for a little more cushioning in the midsole, the area between the tread and the inside of the shoe. If you ultimately plan on graduating to running, you're probably better off buying a running shoe.

Walking with good form

There actually is more to walking than simply putting one foot in front of the other. The biggest mistake walkers make is bending forward, a sure way to develop problems in your lower back, neck, and hips. Your posture should be naturally tall. You needn't force yourself to be ramrod straight, but neither should you slouch, overarch your back, or lean too far forward from your hips. Relax your shoulders, widen your chest, and pull your abdominals gently inward. Keep your head and chin up with your shoulders over your hips and focus straight ahead.

Meanwhile, keep your hands relaxed and cupped gently, and swing your arms so that they brush past your body. On the upswing, your hand should be level with your breastbone; on the downswing, your hand should brush against your hip. Keep your hips loose and relaxed. Your feet should land firmly, heel first. Roll through your heel to your arch, then to the ball of your foot, and then to your toes. Push off from your toes and the ball of your foot.

TIP

Run through a mental head-to-toe checklist every so often to see how you're doing. To find out more about fitness walking (yep, there's plenty more to tell), read *Fitness Walking For Dummies*, by Liz Neporent (Wiley).

Walking tips for rookies

TIP

Although walking is the most basic of all fitness activities, novice fitness walkers can still benefit from the following pointers:

>> Increase your workout time gradually. Most people can start off with five 10- to 20-minute walking sessions a week; after about a month, they can increase each workout by 2 or 3 minutes per week per session until walking 30 to 45 minutes is comfortable. Five days a week may sound like a lot, but an almost-daily walk makes it easier to get in the habit. Plus, for weight control, you probably need to walk at least an hour a day, five or six days a week.

>> Walk as fast as you comfortably can. If you walk very fast — at a 12-minute-mile to 15-minute-mile pace — you burn more calories than when you walk at a 20-minute-mile pace. You may not be able to move at such supersonic speeds in the beginning, but as you get fit, you can mix in some fast-paced intervals.

>> If you're walking on the shoulder of a road, walk against traffic so you can watch cars approach.

>> Add some hills. Walking over hilly terrain shapes your butt and thighs and burns extra calories — about 30 percent more calories than walking on flat terrain, depending, of course, on the grade of the hills.

>> Sneak in a walk whenever you can. Leave your car at home and hoof it to the train station. Take a 15-minute walk during your lunch break. Traverse the airport on foot rather than on that automatic walking belt. It all adds up.

Running: Get Up and Go

Like walking, running is a workout that you can take with you anywhere. You don't need a rack on your car or a suitcase full of equipment; you just open the door and go. Plus, as any pathological runner will tell you, nothing is quite as satisfying as getting a good run under your belt. You work up a great sweat, you burn lots of calories, and your muscles and your brain feel pleasantly invigorated after you finish.

WARNING

But beware: Many runners develop frequent, chronic injuries. Many people have joints that simply will not tolerate all that pounding. If you're not built to run, don't argue with your body. You can get in great condition in other ways. And if you're a beginner, it's probably safest if you start off alternating periods of walking with periods of running. For example, if you can walk for 30 minutes at a reasonably brisk pace and you're raring to go faster, start by alternating 1 minute of running with 3 minutes of walking and gradually decrease the walk intervals as you increase the run intervals.

Essential running gear

Although you can spend hundreds of dollars on spiffy tights, fancy water bottles, smartwatches, and running jackets that do everything but sing and dance, the only equipment that's truly essential for running is a good pair of shoes (although women will want a supportive jogging bra, too). Be prepared to spend at least $80 (and as much as several hundred dollars) a pair, but know that a hefty price tag doesn't always correspond to the best shoe.

REMEMBER

The shoe that's best for you depends on your weight, the shape of your foot, your running style, and any special problems you may have, such as weak ankles or bad knees. Try on several models at the store, and take each one for a test drive around the mall, or at least run a couple laps around the store. Dedicated shoe stores and sports shoe departments usually have knowledgeable salespeople who can take measurements, look at your gait, and use other tools to determine the best shoe for you.

TIP

Bring your current running shoes when shopping for new ones. The wear pattern of your shoes can point to where you need support in your new shoes.

Your running shoes should be fairly flexible, especially across the ball of the foot. Hold the shoe at both ends and bend it; it should break right at the ball of the foot. You want cushioning but not so much that you can't feel your foot hitting the ground. Look for a stable heel counter (the part of the shoe that wraps around your heel to keep your foot in place). If your foot slides around a lot, that can mean trouble down the road.

TIP

Take a week or two to run without indulging in running gear besides shoes and a sports bra. Then, if you're hooked, you may want to splurge on a few items that will truly make a difference, such as a watch, a monitor, or a super-moisture-wicking top.

WHAT'S THE DEAL WITH BAREFOOT RUNNING?

A growing number of runners are shedding their chunky trainers in favor of shoes in a more minimalist category known as *barefoot runners* or *minimalist footwear.* Some of these shoes look like trimmed-down versions of regular running shoes. Others, such as the Vibram FiveFingers, are quite odd, featuring separate compartments for each toe. (Trying to get all of your appendages separated and into the right compartment may remind you of helping a 4-year-old put on gloves.) According to proponents of this running-shoe breed, minimalists prompt you to shorten your stride to a more natural length and land closer to the ball of your foot than you do while wearing a typical running shoe; in theory, your feet and ankles become the flexible shock absorbers they were born to be, and you'll have fewer injuries than when you wear heavier, shock-absorbing versions of running shoes. Some preliminary research seems to support this claim, though only a very few studies have been done.

After testing several brands, we think minimalist footwear is great for speed work and running moderate distances, and they are plenty comfy. But we honestly have no idea how they'd respond by the 25-mile mark of a marathon. Heavier, inexperienced, and injury-prone runners may want to steer clear of this trend. Some runners report feeling sore after the first few runs, which makes sense when you consider that in a way, you're retraining your feet and ankles to fend for themselves.

Running with good form

Runners have a habit of looking directly at the ground, almost as if they can't bear to see what's coming next. Keeping your head down throws your upper-body posture off-kilter and can lead to upper-back and neck pain. Lift your head, keep your shoulders over your hips, and focus your eyes straight ahead.

Relax your shoulders, keep your chest lifted, and pull your abdominal muscles in tightly. Don't overarch your back and stick your butt out; that's one of the main reasons runners get back and hip pain.

TIP

Keep your arms close to your body, and swing them forward and back rather than across your body. Don't clench your fists. Pretend you're holding a butterfly in each hand; you don't want your butterflies to escape, but you don't want to crush them, either.

Lift your front knee and extend your back leg. Don't shuffle along like you're wearing cement boots. Land heel first and roll through the entire length of your foot. Push off from the balls of your feet instead of running flat-footed and pounding off your heels. Otherwise, your feet and legs are going to cry uncle long before your cardiovascular system does.

REMEMBER

If you experience pain in your ankles, knees, or lower back, stop running for a while. Try switching to a lower-impact activity such as walking, cycling, or swimming, or stay off your feet altogether. If you don't, you could end up having to sit on the sidelines for months.

Running tips for rookies

TIP

These tips help you get fit and avoid injury while running:

>> Start by alternating periods of walking with periods of running. For example, try 2 minutes of walking and 1 minute of running. Gradually decrease your walking intervals until you can run continuously for 20 minutes. Of course, sticking with a walk-run routine is fine; you're less likely to injure yourself that way.

>> Vary your pace. Different paces work your heart, lungs, and legs in different ways.

>> Find a running buddy or a running club. Scheduling your runs with someone else keeps you motivated and honest. An experienced runner can share tips and offer ways to avoid mishaps. Most sports stores can put you in touch with like-minded runners.

>> Always run against traffic when running on the shoulder of a road. This allows you to see oncoming cars and dive for the side of the road if necessary. Consider carrying a lightweight cellphone for emergencies, and always let someone know where you're running.

>> Don't increase your mileage by more than 10 percent a week. If you run 5 miles a week and want to increase, aim to do 5.5 miles the following week. Jumping from 5 miles to 6 miles doesn't sound like a big deal, but studies show that if you increase your mileage more than 10 percent per week, you set yourself up for injury.

Bicycling Around

Talk to a group of cyclists and, chances are, you're talking to a group of ex-runners. Cycling is perfect for people who can't take the relentless pounding of running or find the slow pace a real drag. Cycling is the best way to cover a lot of ground quickly. Even a novice can easily build up to a 20-mile ride. Cycling is also a great way to burn calories and spare the environment while you commute to work or get around town doing errands.

On the other hand, cycling can be a hassle. You can't just grab your shoes and head out the door. You need a trustworthy bike that is in good working order and set to your specifications. You also need to pump up your tires, make sure your seat bag has tools and a spare tube in case of a flat, and put on your helmet, gloves, and glasses. And even with all your protective gear, you can never be too cautious. Cycling is a low-impact sport — unless you happen to impact the ground, a car, a tree, a rut, or another cyclist.

Essential cycling gear

If you haven't owned a bike since grammar school, prepare yourself for sticker shock. Mountain bikes, the fat-tire bikes with upright handlebars, are somewhat less expensive than comparable road bikes, the kind with the skinny tires and curved handlebars. Hybrid bikes are — surprise! — a hybrid of the two. With an upright riding position, somewhat hefty frame, and tires of moderate width, hybrids are more comfortable than road bikes, lighter than mountain bikes, and stout enough to withstand potholes and other commuting hazards.

In all three categories, you won't find many decent bikes under $300; many cost more than $2,000. Don't take out a second mortgage to buy a fancy bike, but if you have any inkling that you may like this sport, don't skimp, either. You'll just end up buying a more expensive bike later.

What distinguishes a $300 bike from a $2,000 steed? Generally, the more expensive the bike, the stronger and lighter its frame. A heavy bike can slow you down, but unless you plan to enter the Tour de France, don't get hung up on a matter of ounces. Cheaper bikes are made from different grades of steel; as you climb the price ladder, you find materials such as aluminum, carbon fiber, and titanium. The price of a bike also depends on the quality of the components — the mechanics that enable your bike to move, shift, and brake.

Cheaper bikes come with toe clips (pedal straps) that enable you to pull up on the pedal as well as push down. But you can pull up even more efficiently with clipless pedals, which lock into cleats affixed to the bottom of your cycling shoes. These pedal systems are like ski bindings: you're locked in, but your feet pop out easily if you fall. To clip out, you simply twist your foot to the side. (Beginners usually have an accident or two with clipless pedals because they haven't developed the instinct to twist sideways.)

Find a bike dealer you trust, and know that bike prices are negotiable. Ask the salesperson to throw in a few free extras, such as a bike computer to measure your speed and distance or a seat bag to carry food and tools.

REMEMBER

Don't even think about pedaling down your driveway without a helmet snug atop your noggin. Cycling gloves make your ride more comfortable and protect your hands when you crash. Glasses are important to protect your eyes from the dust, dirt, and gravel.

TIP

Buy a pair of padded cycling shorts and a brightly colored cycling jersey so that you can easily be seen. Unlike cotton T-shirts, jerseys wick away sweat so that you won't freeze on a downhill after you worked up a big sweat climbing up. Plus, jerseys have pockets in the back deep enough to hold half a grocery store's worth of snacks. Always carry a water bottle or wear a hydration pack, a clever backpack-like water pouch. Finally, carry gear to change a flat tire, and learn how to use it. There's no cycling equivalent of the auto club to come save you. Many bike shops offer free demonstrations on changing a flat and basic bike maintenance.

Cycling with good form

To protect your knees from injury, position your seat correctly (ask your salesperson for advice) and pedal at an easy cadence. Cadence refers to the number of revolutions per minute that you pedal. Inexperienced cyclists tend to use higher gears, which forces them to turn the pedals in slow motion; their legs tire prematurely, their knees ache, and they cheat themselves out of a good workout. Set your bike's gearing so you're pedaling comfortably. The faster cadence is easier on your knees.

REMEMBER

Road cycling can wreak havoc on your lower back because you're in a crouched position for so long. Relax your upper body and keep your arms loose. Grasp your handlebars with the same tension that you'd hold a child's hand when you cross the street. Pedal in smooth circles rather than simply mashing the pedals downward. Imagine that you have a bed of nails in your shoes, and you have to pedal without stomping on the nails.

Cycling tips for rookies

TIP

You can learn a lot about cycling — and get faster in a jiff — by riding with a club or friends who have more experience. Here are some pointers to start your cycling career:

>> Remember that you are a vehicle and are required to follow the rules of the road. Ride with traffic, not against it.

>> Stop at all signs and lights, and use those hand signals you learned in driver's ed. Don't trust a single car, ever. Assume that the driver doesn't see you, even if he happens to be staring you in the face.

>> When you go off-road, start on wide fire roads rather than narrow "single-track" trails that require technical skills. And don't think that you're immune to injury because there are no cars. More crashes happen on mountain trails than on the road because there are more obstacles and riders get careless and cocky.

>> Head into a turn at a slow enough pace that you maintain control, and never let your eyes wander from the road or trail. Never squeeze the brakes — particularly the front brake — with a lot of pressure. You'll go flying over the handlebars, a maneuver known as an endo, and go right into a face plant, a maneuver that is self-explanatory.

Exercising in Water

Exercising in the water is truly zero-impact. Although you can strain your shoulders if you overdo swimming, there's absolutely no pounding on your joints, and the only thing you're in danger of crashing into is the wall of the pool. You can get a great aerobic workout that uses your whole body. Plus, water has a gentle, soothing effect on the body, so any exercise you do in the water is helpful for those with arthritis or other joint diseases.

Swimming and other forms of water exercise are great for people who want to keep exercising when they're injured and for people who are pregnant or over-weight. That extra body fat helps you glide along near the surface of the water, so you don't expend energy trying to keep yourself from sinking like a stone.

Lap swimming has the reputation of being drudgery — after all, the scenery doesn't change a whole lot from one end of the pool to the other. The trick is to use an array of gadgets that elevate swim workouts from forced labor to bona fide fun.

Essential water exercise gear

Obviously, a body of water is helpful — preferably one manned by a lifeguard. And in most instances, you must wear a swimsuit. By the way, we said swimsuit, not bathing suit. You don't want a suit that looks good while you're sunbathing but creeps up your butt when you get in the water.

TIP

If you exercise in a chlorinated pool, goggles are a must to prevent eye irritation and to help you see better in the water. Buy goggles from a store that lets you try them on. You should feel some suction around your eyes, but not so much that you feel like your eyeballs are going to pop out. You also need a cap so that your hair doesn't get plastered on your face or turn to straw from the chemicals.

As for the fun water gadgets: Many pools let you borrow equipment, but you can buy a whole set for less than $75. Consider rubber swimming fins, which give you a lot more speed and power when you swim and water jog and give your legs a better workout.

You can use fins when you kick with a kickboard, a foam board that helps you stay afloat. But don't use fins so much that they become a crutch. As you get in better shape, you may want to switch from long swim fins to short fins, which make you work a lot harder. Don't swim with scuba fins; they're too big and too stiff.

Exercising with plastic paddles on your hands gives your upper body an extra challenge. Some paddles are flat and rectangular; others are shaped more like your hand, with a comfortable contour in the palm area. With both styles, you place your hand on top of the paddles and slip your fingers through a thick rub-ber band that secures your hand to the paddles. Paddles can help you perfect your swim stroke technique and increase the intensity of your workout, but use them sparingly; overuse can lead to shoulder injuries. When you swim with paddles, put a pull-buoy (a contoured foam wedge) between your thighs. This keeps your legs buoyant so that you can concentrate on using your arms rather than kicking.

Swimming with good form

If you swim for water exercise, you'll probably spend the bulk of your workouts doing the front crawl, also called freestyle. It's generally faster than the other strokes, so you can cover more distance. Don't cut your strokes short; reach out as far as you can, have your hand enter thumb-first so it slices the water like a knife, and pull all the way through the water so your hand brushes your thigh. Use an S-shaped sculling movement, where your hand moves out, then in, then out again across your body/thigh and out of the water. Elongate your stroke so that you take fewer than 25 strokes in a 25-yard pool. The fewer strokes, the better. Top swimmers get so much power from each stroke that they take just 11 to 14 strokes per length of a 25-yard pool.

TIP

Kick up and down from your hips, not your knees. Don't kick too deeply or allow your feet to break the water's surface. Proper kicking causes the water to "boil" rather than splash.

Breathe through your mouth every two strokes, or every three strokes if you want to alternate the side that you breathe on. You need as much oxygen as you can get. Beginners sometimes make the mistake of taking six or eight strokes before breathing, which wears them out quickly. To breathe, roll your entire body to the side until your mouth and nose come out of the water — imagine that your entire body is on a skewer and must rotate together. Don't lift your head out of the water to breathe — you'll spend a lot of energy doing that, and it'll slow you down in the water.

Swimming tips for rookies

TIP

Even if you're the queen of your kickboxing class or a champion at cycling uphill, you may still tire quickly in the pool at first. More than almost any other cardio activity, swimming relies on technique. The following tips can help you get the most out of your swimming workouts.

>> Take a few lessons if you haven't swum in a while. Beginners waste a lot of energy flailing and splashing around rather than moving forward.

>> Break your workout into intervals. For example, don't just get into the pool, swim 20 laps, and get out. Instead, do 4 easy laps for a warm-up. Then do 8 sets of 2 laps at a faster pace, resting 20 seconds between sets. Then cool down with 2 easy laps, and maybe a few extra laps with a kickboard. Mix up your strokes, too. The four basic strokes — freestyle, backstroke, breaststroke, and butterfly — use your muscles in different ways.

>> Try out a Masters swim club. In this context, "master" means age 18 and over — not expert. You needn't be a fishlike swimmer to join one of these clubs, which are located at university and community pools nationwide and are geared toward adult swimmers of all levels. A coach gives you a different workout every time you swim and monitors your progress. Best of all, you have buddies to work out with. Don't worry about being slow; the coach will group you in a lane with other people your speed. If you have a competitive spirit, you can compete in Masters meets, where you swim against others who are roughly your speed.

>> If you find swimming a big yawn but enjoy being in the water, try water running or water aerobics. Water running is a pretty tough workout because the water provides resistance from all directions as you move your legs. It's an excellent option for injured runners because, even though it's nonimpact and easy on your joints, water running helps maintain cardio conditioning. Don't assume that water aerobics are for little old ladies in flowered caps. With the right instructor and exercise program, you can get a challenging water-workout. Water running can be even tougher.

GETTING YOUR CARDIO IN THE SNOW

In some parts of the country, winter is so blustery that when you see someone walking, running, or cycling outdoors in the dead of January, you can only shake your head and say, "What, don't they have brain freeze?" In these places, your best outdoor cardio options involve snow. We're talking about cross-country skiing and snowshoeing, activities that allow you to enjoy the elements rather than battle them.

Cross-country skiing burns mega calories and comes in two forms: classic and skate. On classic skis, you glide — or, more likely, shuffle — back and forth on long, skinny skis, primarily on groomed tracks. Skate skis are somewhat shorter and wider; you travel at a much faster clip, pushing your skis outward on wide, groomed trails, in a motion that resembles in-line skating. Classic skiing feels like a more natural motion and, for a novice, is far less demanding, both physically and mentally, than skate skiing, a.k.a. "skating." A beginner can go out for a casual classic ski and have a fine time with minimal or no instruction. A first-time skater attempting to wing it, even one fit enough to win triathlons, may well collapse from a combination of exhaustion and frustration. Skate skiing is ultimately a blast and in many areas has overtaken classic skiing in popularity, but the learning curve is darned steep.

Contrast this to snowshoeing, also an excellent calorie burner but one that requires no skill and minimal fitness and carries a lower risk of injury than any other snow sport. The term *snowshoeing* may conjure up images of bearded Scandinavian trappers slogging across the tundra, their boots strapped to giant wooden tennis racquets, but today's snowshoes are compact, with frames made of lightweight aluminum. High-tech fabric stretches across the frame, preventing you from sinking into the snow.

Downhill skiing and snowboarding are also popular cold-weather workout options. Sure, you get a free ride up the mountain, but you more than make up for it on the way down. Just ask your hips, thighs, and buttocks after a long day on the hill. Beyond that, downhill skiing and snowboarding are terrific activities for working on balance, coordination, and agility. Because these activities can be particularly hard on your body, consider taking a "get in shape for ski season" class at the gym or spending four to six weeks strength training prior to your first day on the slopes.

Though these activities tend to be expensive, many mountains offer excellent beginner packages that come with lift tickets, rental equipment, and a half or full day of lessons. Many also offer couples and family packages, including some free meals. Shop around online and see what you can find.

» Checking out the benefits of stretching

» Knowing when to stretch

» Taking a look at various styles of stretching

» Going through a stretching routine

Chapter **3**

Strengthening and Lengthening Your Muscles

Maybe you've never considered yourself the weight-lifting type. Maybe you suspect that the size of one's muscles is inversely proportional to the size of one's brain. Maybe when you see a hulking guy on the street, you think, "He may be able to bench-press my minivan, but I can read a menu in French."

The truth is that weight lifting is an incredibly smart thing to do. It's not just a form of narcissism, and it's not just for bodybuilders. Heck, these days, even 80-year-olds are pumping iron. This chapter explains why you should, too.

This chapter also sets the record straight on what stretching can and can't do for you. (Hint: It can do a lot.) Fortunately, you needn't be able to do full splits to reap the benefits of stretching, and you can fit a stellar flexibility program into a few minutes a day. Whether you find stretching a relaxing pastime or a chore on par with cleaning your oven, this chapter shows you how to make the most of flexibility training.

Why You've Gotta Lift Weights

People who start lifting weights often tell you how much more fit, powerful, and energetic they feel . . . but enough about feelings. There's plenty of good, solid evidence that strength training does all that and more. At least one of the following reasons may get you to hoist some iron.

TIP

Throughout Book 4, the terms *weight lifting, weight training,* and *strength training* are used interchangeably, even though you don't necessarily need weight to build strength.

Staying strong for everyday life

If you don't use your muscles, they get smaller. This gradual slide toward wimpiness can begin as early as your mid-20s.

WARNING

People who don't exercise lose 30 to 40 percent of their strength by age 65. By age 74, more than one-fourth of American men and two-thirds of American women can't lift an object heavier than 10 pounds, such as a small dog or a loaded garbage bag. These changes aren't the normal consequences of aging. They're a result of neglect — of experiencing life from a recliner and the front seat of an RV.

Fortunately, strength is one of the easiest physical abilities to retain as you get older; certainly, you can do a lot more to halt strength loss than you can to prevent wrinkling skin, fading eyesight, or increasing affection for network television. One study, which included men up to age 96, found that by lifting weight, most seniors can at least double — if not triple — their muscle power.

So if you rarely lift anything heavier than a cellphone, it's time to build enough brawn to get along in the real world. Increased strength is what you need to unscrew the top off a stubborn jar of pickles, hoist your kid onto the mechanical horsy, and close a suitcase that's too full. Even if you have the stamina to sprint the full length of an airport to catch your plane, it's not going to do you much good if you can't lug along that overstuffed luggage.

Keeping your bones healthy

REMEMBER

Strong muscles and strong bones go hand in hand. The more weight you can lift, the more stress you can put on your bones; this stress is what stimulates them.

Most people start out with strong, dense bones — imagine them as poles of steel. But around age 35, most people — men included — begin to lose about 0.5 to 1 percent of their bone each year. For women, bone loss accelerates after menopause — 1 to 2 percent a year for the first five years and then about 1 percent annually until age 70. Then the loss slows back to 0.5 percent a year. In the five to seven years following menopause, women can lose up to 20 percent of their bone mass.

Ten million Americans are estimated to have *osteoporosis*, a disease of severe bone loss, and almost 34 million more are estimated to have low bone mass, placing them at increased risk for osteoporosis. When bones become extremely weak — picture them like chalk, porous and fragile — it doesn't even take a fall to break them. Someone with osteoporosis doesn't fall and break a hip; she breaks a hip and falls. An action as low-impact as a sneeze can cause a bone fracture in a person with osteoporosis.

Osteoporosis causes more than 2 million fractures a year, mostly of the back, hip, and wrist; by 2025, the toll is expected to be 3 million broken bones, according to the National Osteoporosis Foundation. About half of those who break their hips never regain full walking ability, and many of these fractures lead to fatal complications. Women account for about 80 percent of osteoporosis cases, but following a hip fracture, the one-year mortality rate is nearly twice as high for men as it is for women.

However, if you do everything right, you can decelerate this bone loss significantly — by about 50 percent. If you've already lost a lot of bone, you may even be able to build some of it back.

REMEMBER

Strength training alone can't stop bone loss, but it can play a big role. Also important are calcium, vitamin D, and aerobic exercise such as walking and jogging. (Swimming and cycling don't work as well because your body weight is supported, either by the water or the bike; when you have to support your own self, your bones respond by building themselves up.)

Preventing injuries

When your muscles are strong, you're less injury-prone. You're less likely to step off a curb and twist your ankle. Plus, you have a better sense of balance and sure-footedness, so you're less apt to take a tumble during a weekend game of touch football. Research shows that one out of every three people over age 65 falls at least once a year. Almost 10 percent of older people who fall are hospitalized for an injury, and about half of those cases involve broken bones.

Looking better

Now it's time to talk about pure, unadulterated vanity. Aerobic exercise burns lots of calories, but weight lifting firms, lifts, builds, and shapes your muscles. A marathon runner may be able to go the distance, but they won't turn any heads on the beach if they have a concave chest and string-bean arms. (They may also be a faster runner if they pumped up a bit.)

The fibers that make up muscle lose shape when they're inactive. As one researcher explained, "If you take a chunk of muscle from an active person and look at it under a microscope, the fibers hold together well. If the person is inactive, the fibers look like gelatin." Squishy muscles, as you can imagine, don't do much for your appearance. For example, if your abdominal muscle fibers get soft, they don't do as good a job holding in your internal organs, and your belly looks poochier.

There's no such thing as *spot reducing* — that is, selectively zapping fat off a particular part of your body. But you can pick certain areas, such as your butt or your arms, and reshape them through weight training. And if you have wide hips or a thick middle, you can bring your body more into proportion by doing exercises that broaden your shoulders and back.

Weight training also makes you look better by improving your posture. With strong abdominal and lower-back muscles, you stand up straighter and look more svelte, even if you haven't lost an ounce.

Speeding up your metabolism

Metabolism is one of those buzzwords that never fades from the news. At gyms, health-food stores, and juice bars, you can buy pills, powders, and "thermogenic herbs" touted to rev up your metabolism (and thereby help you burn extra calories without trying). All these claims are bogus. The best way to increase your metabolism is to build muscle, which you can accomplish by lifting weights.

How does this work? First, a couple of definitions: Your *metabolism* refers to the number of calories you're burning at any given moment, whether you're watching the weather forecast or riding a bike. But when most people use the term, they're referring to your resting metabolism, the number of calories your body needs to maintain its vital functions. Your brain, heart, kidneys, and other organs are cranking away 24 hours a day, and your muscle fibers are constantly undergoing repair. All these processes require energy in the form of calories simply to keep you alive.

REMEMBER

But here's the key: Your resting metabolic rate depends primarily on your amount of *fat-free mass* — everything in your body that's not fat, including muscle, bones, blood, organs, and tissue. The more fat-free mass you have, the more energy your body expends to keep going. Therefore, you want to build as much muscle as possible. You can't do anything to increase the size of your brain, but you certainly can make yourself more muscular, and lifting weights is the primary way to do just that.

Keep in mind, however, that packing on a few more pounds of muscle isn't going to turn your body into a calorie-burning inferno. For every 1 pound of muscle you gain, your body may burn an extra 10 to 15 calories per day. That's not a lot, especially if you compensate by eating one extra Hershey's Kiss (24 calories) per day. However, in the long run, even a small metabolic boost can be significant. If you burn an extra 25 calories per day, you can burn 9,125 calories in a year — enough to lose nearly 3 pounds, or at least prevent a 3-pound weight gain. Every little bit helps.

If that's not impressive, consider the flip side: If you don't lift weights, your metabolism will slow down every year, as your muscles slowly shrivel up. After age 40, metabolism typically slows by about 5 percent a decade. And with a more sluggish metabolic rate, you'll gain weight even if you eat the same amount of food. How's that for incentive to hit the weight room?

One final point: The metabolism-boosting benefits of weight lifting are particularly important if you're cutting calories to lose weight. Dieting alone tends to cause a loss in muscle as well as fat; if you lift weights while cutting back on your calorie intake, you can preserve muscle — and maintain your metabolism — while losing fat.

Flexibility Training: Getting the Scoop on Stretching

Stretching may be the most misunderstood aspect of fitness. You see people at the park bending over to touch their toes and think: *Hmm ... should I be doing that? How many seconds should I hold a stretch like that? Should I do it before I exercise or afterward?*

Truth is, even exercise scientists don't agree on all the ins and outs of stretching, also known as *flexibility training*. And finding the motivation to stretch can be tough. After all, getting your fingertips to touch behind your back is not exactly a process that puts a blowtorch to fat.

Understanding why you need to stretch

REMEMBER

Stretching is the key to maintaining your flexibility — in other words, how far and how easily you can move your joints. Here are some good reasons to make stretching part of your exercise routine:

>> **Maintaining good posture:** Flexibility is one of the keys to good posture, helping you look better and avoid muscle pain. When your front neck muscles are short and tight, your head angles forward. When your shoulders and chest are tight, your shoulders round inward. When your lower back, rear thigh, and hip muscles are tight, the curve of your back becomes exaggerated.

>> **Reducing back pain:** A regular stretching routine also can reduce pain and discomfort, particularly in your lower back. In fact, the pain often lessens when you begin doing simple stretches for your lower-back and rear-thigh muscles.

>> **Correcting muscle imbalances and improving coordination:** Say that your front-thigh muscles are strong but your rear thighs are tight and weak. (This is a common scenario.) As a result, you end up relying on your front thighs more than you should. Chances are you don't even notice this, but it throws off your movement in subtle ways — you may have a short walking stride or bounce too high off the ground. Muscle imbalances can eventually lead to injuries such as pulled muscles. They also contribute to clumsiness, which in itself can lead to injury.

>> **Keeping your range of motion later in life:** As you get older, your tendons (the tissues that connect muscle to bone) begin to shorten and tighten, restricting your flexibility. Scientists also suspect that collagen, one of the main materials in connective tissue, becomes denser with age, so your movements become less fluid. Studies show that by the time people are in their seventies, many people can move the majority of their joints only half as far as they could in their prime.

As you lose flexibility, you walk more stiffly and with a shorter stride and therefore have more difficulty stepping up to a curb or bending down to pick up trash. The danger is that you're at greater risk of falling, and this risk, combined with bone-density loss, can become a life-threatening situation. The good news: Stretching your rear-thigh, hip, and calf muscles can greatly reduce this risk, regardless of your age.

CAN STRETCHING PREVENT INJURY?

Can stretching prevent injury? The jury is still deliberating this one, and the body of evidence is contradictory. On the one hand, research shows that an active warm-up routine combined with preworkout stretching can significantly reduce the risk of injury to the muscles and their connective tissue while you're exercising. This is probably because the warm-up/stretch combinations heat up and elongate the muscles. However, this combo does not seem to diminish overuse injuries or injuries that happen when you aren't exercising.

Other studies show that stretching without a warm-up does not reduce injury rates at all, probably because it may actually make the joints less stable and less able to react quickly to sudden movements. Research does show that a warm-up without stretching can help prevent injury, so when it comes to injury prevention, it's unclear how important stretching is. But this much is clear: Preworkout stretching alone, without a warm-up, is not a good idea.

A few studies suggest that over the long term, postworkout stretches can improve strength and endurance performance and lower the risk injury. Just don't expect stretching to make your muscle less sore. For example, stretching right after running a marathon will not make you feel less stiff or achy the next day. It may even slightly increase your chances of getting hurt.

Nevertheless, runners continue to swing their legs up on the hood of a car to stretch their hamstrings before heading out for a run and walkers continue to hang their heels off the edge of a curb before they take a step. So ingrained is this preworkout stretch ritual that the message does not seem to be getting through to the average exerciser. Top athletes do seem to get it: When you watch any Olympic or professional competition, you see the athletes doing active warm-ups and using techniques known as PNF (proprioceptive neuromuscular facilitation) stretching or Active Isolated Stretching (AIS). Olympic swimmer Dara Torres actually hired two stretchers to travel with her to keep her muscles supple enough to continue swimming at the top of her game into her forties. Even yoga and Pilates, which are very flexibility-based disciplines, use active warm-up techniques before moving into static positions. (See Chapter 4 in Book 4 for more about yoga.)

Whether stretching reduces injury remains unclear, but regardless of whether you stretch before working out, continue to keep in mind the numerous other great reasons to take up flexibility training.

>> **Performing better in sports:** Flexibility is a key performance factor for many sports. Clearly, gymnasts, dancers, and skateboarders need a great deal of flexibility to excel. Swimmers need good shoulder flexibility. Runners, walkers, and cyclists require some flexibility but less than athletes in other sports (in fact, some studies have shown that having too much flexibility in certain sports, such as running and cycling, actually increases chances of injury). The point is that there seems to be an optimal amount of flexibility, depending on which activities you tend to pursue, but even the least athletic among us require a basic amount of stretching. (For more info on stretching and injury prevention, see the nearby sidebar "Can stretching prevent injury?")

Deciding when to stretch

Contrary to popular opinion, stretching is not the first thing you should do when you walk into the gym or arrive at the park for a jog. Don't stretch your muscles until you've at least warmed up thoroughly (see Chapter 1 in Book 4 for warm-up basics).

TIP

Before a workout, warm up and then stretch, or leave your stretching until after you're done exercising. Stretching at the end of your workout, after you've finished exercising but before you shower, may be the most convenient and beneficial time to stretch. A postworkout stretch is a great way to relax and ease back into the rest of your day.

WARNING

Be sure to stretch after — not before — you cool down (see Chapter 1 in Book 4 for more on cool-downs). Putting your head below your heart right after a workout can cause fainting and nausea. Before you lie down to stretch, make sure that you aren't feeling breathless and that your heart rate has dipped below 100 beats per minute and dropped at least 20 beats from when you stopped exercising.

Exploring Stretching Techniques

There are several different schools of thought on how to stretch. Here are four of the most common:

>> **Static stretching:** You move into a position and hold yourself in place for at least 15 seconds. The idea here is that you gradually stretch the muscle to the

point of its limitation. This is the most common type of stretching, and most experts consider it very safe.

>> **PNF stretching:** This technique has a name that sets a new standard for fitness jargon: *proprioceptive neuromuscular facilitation.* PNF involves tightening a muscle as hard as you can right before you stretch it. The theory behind PNF is that the act of tightening, or squeezing, causes the muscle to become relaxed and more "receptive" to the stretch. So after you tighten your hamstring for a few seconds, you're able to stretch it a little bit farther than usual immediately after you release the tension. PNF stretching is best done with a partner, and some gyms offer 45-minute private training sessions entirely devoted to this type of stretching.

>> **Active Isolated Stretching (AIS):** Using a rope, towel, belt, or band, you tighten the muscle opposite the muscle you're targeting for a stretch. Then you move the targeted muscle into a stretched position and hold it for about 2 seconds — that's right, 2 seconds — just long enough to elongate the muscle without triggering the rebound reflex. The *rebound reflex,* also known as the *stretch reflex,* is an automatic defense mechanism that causes muscles to tighten up and spring back to prevent tearing when they have been pulled too hard or too far or for too long.

The theory behind AIS is that when you *contract,* or shorten, a muscle, the opposite muscle has no recourse but to relax and lengthen. You repeat the process 8 to 12 times in each position before moving on to the next stretch.

So which type of stretching works best? There isn't a consensus among fitness professionals or exercise scientists. Static stretching seems to be the safest and easiest to learn though not necessarily the most effective. However, some exercise experts theorize that conventional stretching techniques can damage muscles by pulling on them too hard and triggering the rebound reflex.

PNF and AIS may well be the most effective, according to some studies, but these methods require more knowledge and skill and, in the case of PNF, the convenience of a partner.

TIP

You should start out with static stretching. As you gain some experience and your muscles begin to feel more well-oiled, doing some PNF or AIS is probably a good idea. The following section gives you a complete static routine.

LET'S ROLL! DOING A LITTLE MASSAGE

You may see people in the gym sitting or lying on a large foam tube, rolling it back and forth like they're rolling out cookie dough. In fact, they are doing a technique called *myo-fascial release,* a fancy name for self-massage. The theory is that the roller stretches muscles and tendons as it loosens up soft tissue and scar tissue and increases blood flow.

Rollers seem particularly effective for loosening the sides of the hips in an area known as the *iliotibial* (IT) band, for treating shin-splint pain, and for stretching any unusually tight muscle. You simply place your weight on the roller and roll it back and forth under the offending muscle. Or you move into a stretch and roll the device underneath the muscle while you remain in the stretch position.

There's little research here, but as with massage, many people feel that using rollers makes their muscles feel better. And there is research to show that any type of massage can be effective for increasing circulation and breaking up *muscle adhesions,* areas where muscle fibers are bunched together as if they are taped or glued together.

If your gym doesn't have a foam roller, you can pick one up on the cheap. A small one will run you about $15. You can get a similar effect from placing handballs in strategic places. For example, lie on your back and place the ball on the inside of your shoulder blade or gently sit on one and roll it back and forth.

Still Life: Doing Static Stretching

If you consider stretching too boring, too painful, or too complicated, you'll like this section. You find some guidelines for static stretching and get started with a thorough basic stretching routine.

Following a few rules of static stretching

Watch runners at the park or weight lifters at the gym. Chances are they have the wrong idea about stretching. Maybe they'll grab their heel for a split second to stretch their front thigh, or bend over for a moment to touch their toes. Entire classes of boot–campers start off by flopping over and grabbing their ankles with their knees locked tight in place. It's enough to make you cringe, and that sort of "stretching" isn't going to make you more flexible. It may even injure you.

Here are the basic rules for a useful and safe flexibility workout:

>> **Stretch as often as you can — daily, if possible.** Stretch after every workout, both cardiovascular and strength. If you stretch on days when you don't work out, warm up with a few minutes of easy movement like shoulder rolls, gentle waist twists, or light cardio activity. The American College of Sports Medicine (ACSM) recommends stretching at least three to five days a week, although stretching five to seven days is ideal for most people. Stretching three times a week seems to improve the bendiness of joints much more than stretching once a week, but stretching even more often seems to provide at least some additional benefits.

>> **Move into each stretching position slowly.** Never force yourself into a stretch by jerking or snapping into position. Blasting yourself into a stretch can sometimes be too much of a shock to a muscle and may cause an injury.

WARNING

Never bounce. After you find the most comfortable stretch position, stay there or gradually deepen the stretch. Bouncing only tightens your muscle — it doesn't loosen it. Forceful bouncing increases the risk of tearing a muscle.

>> **Notice how much tension you feel.** A stretch should rate anywhere on your pain meter from a feeling of mild tension to the edge of discomfort. It should never cause severe or sharp pain anywhere else in your body. Focus on the area you're stretching, and notice the stretch spread through these muscles.

TIP

>> **As you hold each position, take at least five deep breaths.** Deep breathing promotes relaxation. The consensus seems to be that holding a static stretch for 15 to 30 seconds is ideal. Get out a stopwatch and time your stretches until you get a sense of exactly how long 30 seconds really is.

>> **Perform each stretch two to four times.** Here again, studies compiled by the ACSM find this regimen to be the most effective.

>> **Stretch *all* your muscles.** Just because you stretch out your shoulders does not mean your hamstrings are any less tight. For stretching to be really effective, you have to take a full-body approach. Remember that old song "Dem Bones," which says "the thigh bone connected to the hip bone"? This is absolutely true of stretching. Any joint that is tight can throw off your posture or your stride or cause you discomfort.

Trying a simple static stretching routine

This section features a no-brainer stretching routine that won't pull your hamstrings like a rope in a tug of war. After you master these moves, the workout should take about five minutes.

This is just a starting point. It's a great idea to learn additional stretches; you can choose from literally hundreds, as you find out if you take up yoga, Pilates, or martial arts. Varying your flexibility routine allows you to stretch your muscles at a number of angles. Plus, you'll be able to give the necessary extra attention to the muscles you use most in your particular workout. For example, if you're a tennis player or rower, you may want to do a few extra upper-body stretches.

Neck Stretch

This stretch is designed to loosen and relax the muscles in your neck. To do the Neck Stretch, stand or sit comfortably. Drop your left ear toward your left shoulder, and gently stretch your right arm down and a few inches out to the side (see Figure 3-1), using your opposite hand to assist the stretch by gently pressing on the side of your head. Repeat the stretch on your right side.

As you perform the Neck Stretch, be sure to keep your shoulders down and relaxed.

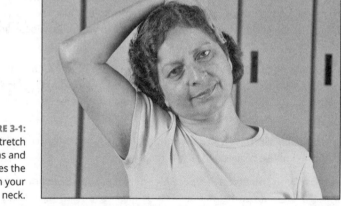

FIGURE 3-1:
The Neck Stretch loosens and relaxes the muscles in your neck.

© Matt Bowen

Chest Expansion

This stretch targets your shoulders, chest, and arms and helps promote good posture. Sit or stand up tall and bring your arms behind you, clasping one hand inside the other (see Figure 3-2). Lift your chest and raise your arms slightly. You should feel a mild stretch spread across your chest.

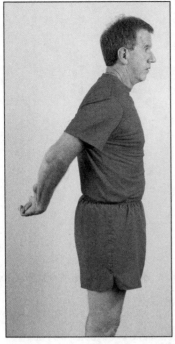

FIGURE 3-2:
The Chest
Expansion
promotes good
posture.

© Matt Bowen

TIP

Keep in mind the following tips as you perform the Chest Expansion:

>> Resist arching your lower back as you pull your arms upward.

>> Try to keep your shoulders relaxed and down.

>> Don't force your arms up higher than is comfortable.

Back Expansion

This move stretches and loosens your shoulders, arms, and upper- and lower-back muscles. Here's how to do it: Standing tall with your knees slightly bent and feet hip-width apart, lift your arms in front of you to shoulder height. Clasp one hand in the other. Drop your head toward your chest, pull your abdominals inward, round your lower back, and tuck your hips forward so that you create a C shape with your torso. Stretch your arms forward so that you feel your shoulder blades moving apart and you create an "opposition" to your rounded back. You should feel a mild stretch slowly spread through your back and shoulders. (See Figure 3-3.)

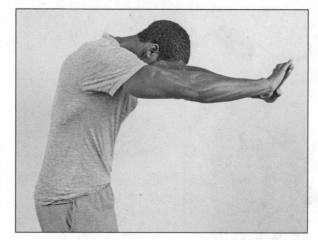

FIGURE 3-3:
The Back Expansion stretches your shoulders, arms, and back.

TIP

Keep in mind the following tips as you perform the Back Expansion:

>> Keep your abdominal muscles pulled inward to protect your lower back.

>> Lean only as far forward as you feel comfortable and balanced.

>> Keep your shoulders down and relaxed.

Standing Hamstring Stretch

This is a great stretch for your hamstrings (rear-thigh muscles) and your lower back. If you have lower-back problems, do the same exercise while lying on your back on the floor and extending your leg upward.

Stand tall with your left foot a few inches in front of your right foot and your left toes lifted. Bend your right knee slightly and pull your abdominals gently inward. Lean forward from your hips and press your buttocks backwards as if you're preparing to sit down, and rest both palms on top of your right thigh for balance and support (see Figure 3-4). Keep your shoulders down and relaxed; don't round your lower back. You should feel a mild pull gradually spread through the back of your leg. Repeat the stretch with your right leg forward.

TIP

Keep in mind the following tips as you perform the Standing Hamstring Stretch:

>> Keep your back straight and your abs pulled inward to make the stretch more effective and to protect your lower back.

>> Don't lean so far forward that you lose your balance or feel strain in your lower back.

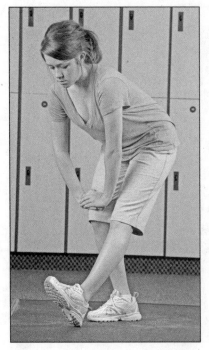

FIGURE 3-4:
The Standing
Hamstring
Stretch targets
your rear-thigh
muscles.

© Matt Bowen

Standing Quad Stretch

This stretch focuses on the quadriceps (front-thigh muscles). Be extra gentle with this stretch if you're prone to knee or lower-back pain. If back pain is an issue for you, you can do a similar stretch while lying on your side, bending your top knee and bringing your heel toward your buttocks.

Stand tall with your feet hip-width apart, pull your abdominals in, and relax your shoulders. Bend your left leg, bringing your heel toward your butt, and grasp your left foot with your right hand (see Figure 3-5). You should feel a mild pull gradually spread through the front of your left leg. Then switch legs.

Keep these tips in mind as you perform the Standing Quad Stretch:

TIP

>> Hold onto a chair or the wall if you have trouble balancing.

>> Don't lock the knee of your base leg.

>> If you're more comfortable, hold your foot with the hand on the same side.

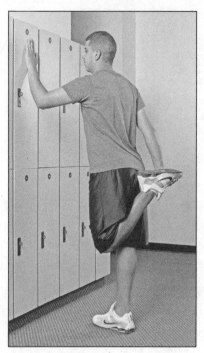

FIGURE 3-5:
The Standing
Quad Stretch
targets your
front-thigh
muscles.

Double Calf Stretch

This stretch offers some relief for the calf muscles, which tend to be tight and bunched up from daily activities such as walking and standing.

Stand with your feet together, toes facing forward, about 2 feet from a wall that you're facing. Pull your abdominals gently inward and don't round your lower back. With straight arms, press your palms into the wall and lean forward from your ankles, keeping your heels pressed as close to the floor as possible (see Figure 3-6). You should feel a mild stretch spread through your calf muscles.

TIP

Keep in mind the following tips as you perform the Double Calf Stretch:

>> Keep both heels flat on the floor or as close to the floor as your flexibility allows.

>> Keep your abs pulled in to prevent your lower back from sagging or arching.

>> To increase the stretch, bend your elbows, leaning your chest toward the wall.

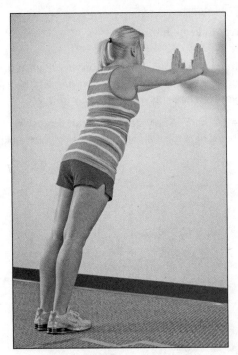

FIGURE 3-6:
The Double Calf
Stretch helps
relieve tightness
in your calf
muscles.

© Matt Bowen

Hip Stretch

This stretch is great for your outer hips and lower back. You can do this stretch while sitting or standing, but when you perform it from a lying position, it's easier to control the tension.

Lie on your back with your knees bent and feet flat on the floor. Lift your left leg up and place your ankle across your right thigh, a few inches below your knee so that your left knee is pointing out to the side as much as your flexibility allows; see Figure 3-7a. While keeping both knees bent, lift your right foot until your right thigh is perpendicular to the floor, and thread your hands through the center of your legs so that you can clasp your right leg. Gently pull your right leg toward your chest. (See Figure 3-7b.)

You'll feel this stretch in your outer thigh and buttocks and perhaps in your lower back. If you're very tight in your arms or shoulders, you may feel it there, too.

TIP

Here are a couple of tips to keep in mind:

>> To increase the stretch, keep your right hand on your thigh and, pulling it gently toward you, place your left palm gently on your left thigh just below your knee. Press your left knee outward and away from you.

>> If any of this is just too hard, simply stay in the start position with your left ankle perched on your right thigh and gently pressing your left knee outward.

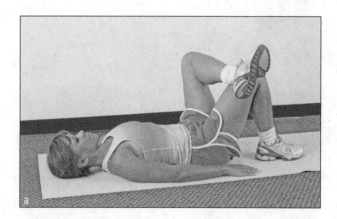

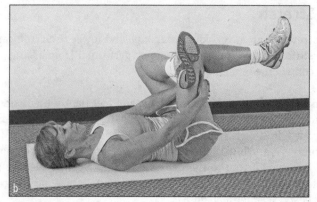

FIGURE 3-7:
The Hip Stretch increases hip and glute flexibility.

© Matt Bowen

Butterfly Stretch

This exercise stretches your inner thighs, groin, hips, and lower back. Take extra care to lean forward from your hips rather than rounding your lower back. This exercise may also cause some knee discomfort.

To do the Butterfly Stretch, sit up tall with the soles of your feet pressed together and your knees relaxed to the sides as far as they'll comfortably go as shown in Figure 3-8a. Pull your abdominals gently inward and lean forward from your hips. Grasp your feet with your hands and carefully pull yourself a small way farther forward (see Figure 3-8b). You should feel the stretch spread throughout your inner thighs, the outermost part of your hips, and lower back.

TIP

Keep in mind these tips as you perform the Butterfly:

>> Increase the stretch by carefully pressing your thighs toward the floor as you hold the position.

>> Don't hunch your shoulders up toward your ears or round your back.

>> To reduce stress on your knees, move your feet away from your body. To increase the stretch, move your feet toward your body.

FIGURE 3-8: The Butterfly Stretch targets your inner thighs, groin, hips, and lower back.

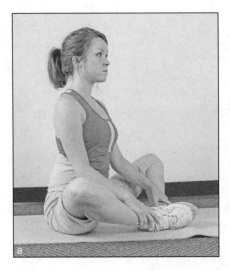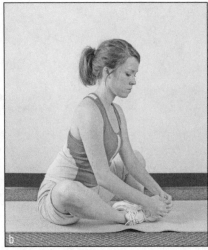

© Matt Bowen

Chapter **4**

All about Yoga

Here in the West, people tend to view exercise as a way to improve your body — to strengthen your heart, tone your muscles, and make your joints more flexible. Only in the past few decades has the mainstream fitness community come to accept what many other cultures have known for thousands of years: Exercise can also be good for your mind.

This realization has spawned a popular fitness catchphrase — *mind-body exercise* — and yoga is at the forefront. Everyone can benefit from adding yoga to their exercise repertoire. Yoga takes you away from the typical pump and grind and sweat and gets you to focus on how your body moves and feels. Some studies show that just eight weeks of yoga practice can change the brain so you are calmer and more focused, have a better memory, and can learn more easily. This chapter explains what yoga entails, helps you choose a style and a class that suits you, and shows you a few moves.

Looking at What Yoga Can Do for Your Body

Celebrity yoga disciples such as Jennifer Aniston, Madonna, and Gwyneth Paltrow wear their yoga bodies like badges of honor — as well they should. Clearly, yoga can shape your muscles; a yoga practice also helps you develop balance, strength, and coordination. Many athletes supplement their main sports or workout routines with yoga to balance out their fitness and help avoid injury.

TECHNICAL STUFF

And here's something interesting: Some studies suggest that yoga can be useful for weight loss, even though a typical yoga class burns only about 240 calories in 45 minutes, no more than a relatively slow walk. Because yoga enhances the skill of mindfulness — the ability to be present in the moment and consider what you're doing in a very thoughtful and nonjudgmental way — it appears that people who practice yoga tend to be more mindful about their food choices and portions.

REMEMBER

You can substitute yoga workouts for your regular program once or twice a week. For example, instead of lifting weights or doing a traditional stretching workout, do a session of yoga. Some mind-body classes are intensely demanding on the muscles, so make sure that you don't overload your workout schedule. For example, some yoga classes call for intense moves such as handstands and one-legged balance poses — great for the body but every bit as hard on you as doing squats with heavy weights or walking lunges. Resting your body between yoga workouts is important.

Finding a Yoga Style That's Right for You

There are many forms of yoga. Most include the same fundamental poses but differ in terms of how quickly you move, how long you hold each pose, how much breathing is emphasized, and how much of a spiritual aspect there is. Some styles offer more modifications to the really bendy and twisty moves, so they're more accessible to new exercisers and the flexibility challenged. Others are for people who can already touch their toes with their tongue. If you find that you dig yoga, experiment with some of the different styles. You may find you like one more than the others.

Here's a brief look at the main yoga options.

>> **Anusara:** Anusara, a relatively new form of yoga, has a deep spiritual element and a heavy focus on good posture and body alignment.

>> **Astanga:** Astanga, sometimes called Power Yoga, is one of the most physically demanding forms of yoga in terms of flexibility, strength, and stamina. You move from one posture to another without a break, so this style isn't recommended for beginners.

>> **Bikram:** Bikram, an intensely physical style of yoga, includes a lot of breathing exercises. The same 26 poses are performed in the same order during 90-minute classes that are usually conducted in a room heated to 100 degrees. (The heat is intended to make it easier to stretch.)

WARNING

If you have high blood pressure, are at high risk for developing heart disease, or already have heart disease, get your doctor's permission before taking a class conducted in a room at a high temperature.

>> **Hatha:** This is like a slow, easy, basic stretching class with an emphasis placed on breathing. The poses are basic, and sometimes the instructor includes a simple meditation. This is perhaps one of the most Westernized approaches to yoga.

>> **Integral:** Integral classes involve lots of meditation and chanting. However, integral yoga is one of the easier forms to learn because the postures are relatively simple with plenty of modifications offered for the flexibility-challenged.

>> **Iyengar:** Iyengar yoga instructors must complete a rigorous two- to five-year training program for certification, so the quality of teaching tends to be consistently good. Iyengar yoga involves props such as foam blocks and stretching belts. Instructors pay close attention to body alignment.

>> **Kripalu:** Kripalu, a less physical and more meditative style of yoga, emphasizes body alignment and breath and movement coordination. There are three stages in kripalu yoga. Stage One focuses on learning the postures and exploring your body's limits of strength and flexibility. Stage Two involves holding the postures for an extended time, developing concentration and inner awareness. Stage Three involves moving from one posture to another without rest.

>> **Kundalini:** Kundalini yoga was one of the first Westernized forms of yoga. Because it's designed to release energy in the body, it involves a lot of intense breathing exercises. Most of the poses are classic flexibility exercises.

>> **Sivananda:** This classic style of yoga is one of the most widely followed in the world and follows well-known poses, with an emphasis on relaxation and breathing.

>> **Vinyasa:** Often referred to as "vinyasa flow," vinyasa classes take you through numerous poses with little rest, though instructors tend to move at a manageable pace and encourage novices to try easier variations. Vinyasa is typically chant-free and excellent for developing flexibility and balance.

Getting Started

If you don't know downward-facing dog from walking your dog, taking your first yoga class can be daunting. Don't shy away! You'll quickly find that plenty of your classmates are new, too. To make your entry into the yoga world easier, following are tips on choosing a class, dressing like a yoga regular, and surviving your first session.

Taking yoga classes

Most health clubs offer yoga classes at no additional charge. You can find a wider variety of styles and techniques at yoga-only studios, which charge $10 to $25 per class. You can often opt for a series of classes for a reduced price per class. The same price structure holds for virtual classes you participate in via Zoom — an option that became quite popular during the COVID pandemic and continues to be an alternative. You'll likely also find classes aimed at different experience levels.

TIP

If you're a yoga novice, make sure you take a beginning class, and don't try to keep up with anyone else. Yoga can be extremely demanding, both in terms of flexibility and strength. Even if you can bench-press a heavy load in the gym, you may find yourself lacking the strength to hold a yoga pose for even 30 seconds. Yoga requires a different type of strength than weight-lifting does. For instance, many yoga poses require you to call upon the strength of your core and dozens of small spinal muscles that don't get much action in a weight-machine workout.

There's no national yoga certification, so this chapter can't list certain credentials to look for in a teacher. In the yoga world, it usually means a lot if you've studied with a certain yogi master, but most people have trouble evaluating this type of credential. Rely on your own judgment and word-of-mouth recommendations. A good yoga instructor wanders around the room, gently correcting class members' techniques and offering variations that allow less-flexible people to accomplish all the poses.

REMEMBER

Some yoga instructors don't take into account individual differences in fitness and flexibility, so it's up to you to know your own limits. Also, some classes may be too spiritual for you and that's your call.

TIP

Yoga offers an active timeout to energize your body and calm your mind. Most yoga classes end with several minutes of lying facedown on the floor. This come-down time, called shivasana, is low-key enough to make some people fall asleep, but after you get up, you feel recharged. Following shivasana, the instructor and class members typically sit with legs crossed and palms together at heart level.

The instructor bows her head and says, "Namaste" (pronounced na-mah-stay), a Sanskrit term meaning, "I bow to you," and the class bows and responds, "Namaste." This ritual is used as a sign of respect and mutual gratitude.

Looking at yoga equipment and clothing

Yoga doesn't require a large commitment of clothing and equipment. Just make sure you wear something comfortable that lets you move freely in all directions without riding up or falling down. You may be most comfortable in clothing that's close fitting (but not oppressively tight) so that it stays close to your body while you have your legs apart and torso inverted. You can spend plenty on stylish yoga outfits or just wear any old stretchy shirt and shorts or tights.

Unlike most other fitness activities that require a major investment in footwear, yoga is generally practiced barefoot.

The one piece of equipment you absolutely do need is a *yoga mat,* one that's sticky or tacky (that is, nonslip), as opposed to smooth or slippery. Look for a mat that's at least 68 inches long by 24 inches wide. Look for a yoga mat at your local sporting goods store, yoga specialty shop, gym, yoga studio, or at online shops (search for "yoga mat"). Many studios and gyms also have a variety of foam blocks, straps, and ropes to help you with your stretches, as well as blankets to use during meditations. You can also purchase these at the same place you buy mats.

Following yoga tips for beginners

TIP

Chapter 5 of Book 4 offers general advice for surviving a new exercise class with both your body and ego intact. Here are additional tips that pertain to yoga specifically:

>> **Watch the instructor, not other classmates.** Yes, this goes for all classes, but it's particularly important for yoga because yoga tends to include a lot of balance work. When you're standing on one foot with the other in the air and your arms intertwined like plant vines, it's better to keep your eye on the person most likely to stay upright.

>> **If a pose feels uncomfortable to you, skip it.** In a class coauthor Suzanne regularly takes, one pose makes her feel as if her lower legs are about to be twisted off at the knee. While the rest of the class does this pose, Suzanne kneels in child's pose (which is introduced later in this chapter) and contemplates how terrific her knees feel.

>> **Bail if the instructor confuses you.** Keep auditioning instructors, and you'll find one you click with. Some offer just the right amount of instruction about how to get into position and what it should feel like, and others stuff your brain with so much information that you start to feel that performing downward-facing dog is more complicated than flying a 747 jet. Some instructors do the workout with you, whereas others wander around the room and teach the entire class verbally.

>> **Bring a water bottle.** Many yoga classes are surprisingly demanding or lengthy, and a couple of sips mid-class may make the experience much more pleasant.

Trying a Yoga Routine

The following sections describe several basic yoga poses. Depending on the class, sometimes you simply move through them and sometimes you hold them for several seconds. These poses also allow for many modifications and adjustments, so you may want to peruse a website, pick up a book, watch a video or listen to a podcast, or take a class to get guidance on how these may best fit into your yoga practice.

Downward-Facing Dog

Downward-Facing Dog, also known as *Down Dog,* is the quintessential yoga move. In a typical yoga class, you may come back to down dog 50 times (or maybe it just seems like 50 times). Down Dog is an awesome stretch that spreads through the whole body but is especially effective for the lower legs, shoulders, arms, and lower back. Here's how to do it:

1. **Start on your hands and knees.**

   Sit or kneel on the floor on your hands and knees with your knees directly below your hips and your hands slightly in front of your shoulders. See Figure 4-1a.

2. **Exhale, and start to straighten your legs.**

   Lift your knees away from the floor, keeping your knees slightly bent and your heels lifted. Lengthen your tailbone upward so your body forms an upside-down V shape.

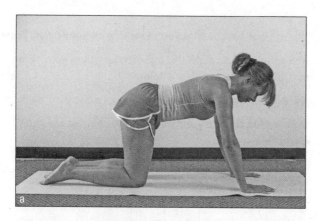

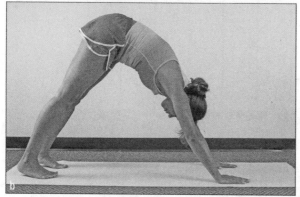

FIGURE 4-1:
Downward-
Facing Dog.

3. **Exhale, and push your top thighs back, stretching your heels onto or toward the floor — whatever your flexibility allows (see Figure 4-1b).**

   Straighten your knees but do not lock them. Firm your outer thighs and roll your upper thighs inward slightly.

4. **Firm your outer arms and shoulder blades. Hold the position before bending your knees and either returning to the start or moving into the next pose, or asana.**

Forward Bend

The Forward Bend can be extremely relaxing, because you stretch your back and legs. Here's how you do it:

1. **Start in a sitting position, with your legs out in front of you in a V (whatever width of V is comfortable for you), toes pointed up toward the ceiling.**

2. Pull up on your butt so that you're resting on your pelvic bone.

3. Stretch your arms straight up, trying to lengthen your spine as you stretch, and inhale (see Figure 4-2a).

4. As you exhale, lean your chest forward, keeping your back straight.

5. Point your chin toward your shins and your chest toward your thighs, as shown in Figure 4-2b.

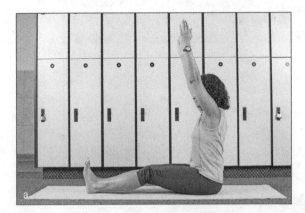

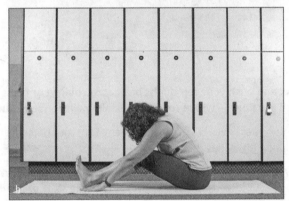

FIGURE 4-2: Forward Bend.

© Matt Bowen

Child's Pose

This move stretches your lower back and arms and relaxes your entire body. If you have knee problems, lower yourself into position with extra care. Here's what to do:

1. **Start in a kneeling position.**

2. **Drop your butt toward your heels as you stretch the rest of your body down and forward.**

3. **In the fully stretched position, rest your arms in a relaxed position along the floor, rest your stomach comfortably on top of your thighs, and rest your forehead on the mat (see Figure 4-3).**

   You should feel a mild stretch in your shoulders and buttocks and down the length of your spine and arms.

Ease into this stretch by keeping your shoulders and neck relaxed. Don't force your derriere to move any closer to your heels than is comfortable.

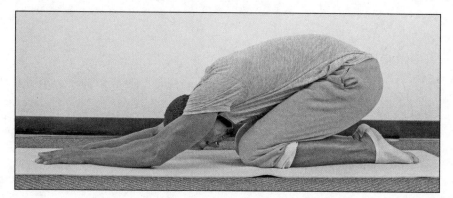

FIGURE 4-3:
Child's Pose.

© Matt Bowen

Modified Sage Twist

This unique pose rotates the spine from left to right, toning and relaxing as you go. Here's what to do:

1. **Start in a sitting position and extend both legs forward.**

2. **Bend your right knee and place your right foot on the floor, next to your inside left thigh.**

3. **Place your right hand on the floor behind you, palm down.**

4. **Take your left palm or fingertips and wrap around the outside of your right knee.**

5. **Inhale, extending and lifting your spine upward; exhale and twist your torso and head to your right side (see Figure 4-4).**

6. **Repeat with the left leg bent, twisting to the other side.**

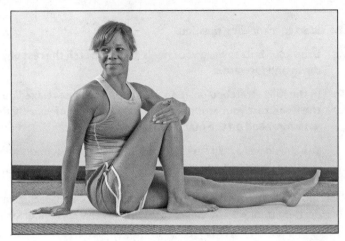

FIGURE 4-4:
Sage Twist
with a twist.

Cat Pose

The Cat Pose elongates your spine and eases tension in your back. Try it by following these steps:

1. **Rest on your hands and knees, with your belly facing the floor.**

2. **Inhale deeply.**

3. **Exhale and pull in your abdominal muscles, tailbone, and butt.**

4. **Pressing down on your hands, press your back toward the ceiling so your spine rounds, as in Figure 4-5.**

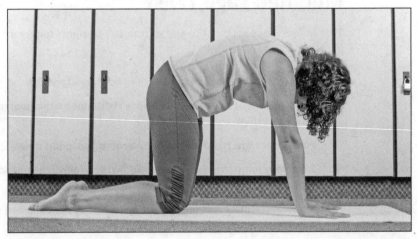

FIGURE 4-5:
Cat Pose.

Triangle Pose

Moving from a sitting or lying position to standing, the Triangle Pose stretches your spine and abdomen. Here's how you do it:

1. **Stand with your feet much wider than your shoulders, and place both arms straight out to the side, parallel to the floor, with palms facing up. See Figure 4-6a.**

   Both feet can be flat on the floor, or you can point your left foot, keeping your heel off the floor.

2. **Inhale deeply.**

3. **Exhale and bend to the left, as in Figure 4-6b.**

   Keep your knees straight and your hips facing forward. Don't twist your lower body; simply bend at your waist.

4. **Slide your left arm down your left leg as you bend, and then hold your leg or ankle.**

5. **Hold this position, slowly breathing in and out several times.**

   If you're able to, lift your right leg off the floor, anywhere from 3 to 18 inches, keeping your knee straight.

6. **Repeat, bending to the other side.**

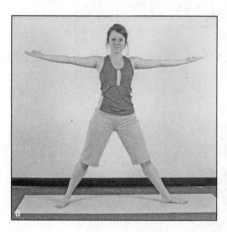 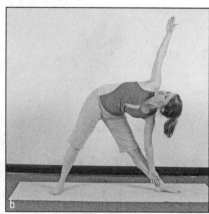

FIGURE 4-6: Triangle Pose.

© Matt Bowen

Sun Salutation

This move stretches your abdominal, lower-back, front-hip, and thigh muscles. If you're prone to lower-back pain, make a special point of tightening your core, and don't arch your lower back. Here's how to do the Sun Salutation:

1. **Kneel on the floor; then bring your left leg forward so that your foot is flat on the floor, your knee is bent, and your thigh is parallel to the floor.**

2. **Lift your arms straight up with your palms facing in.**

3. **Pull your abdominals gently inward, and keep your shoulders down and back.**

4. **Look to the ceiling, and as you stretch upward with your upper body, push your weight slightly forward from your hips into your front thigh (see Figure 4-7).**

   You should feel this stretch travel through your torso and upper body, including your arms. You should also feel it at the very top of your back thigh.

5. **Repeat with your right leg forward.**

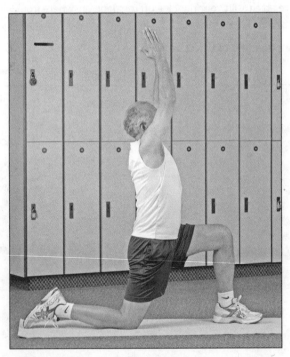

FIGURE 4-7:
Sun Salutation.

© Matt Bowen

TIP

Keep in mind the following tips as you perform the Sun Salutation:

» Hold on to something solid, such as a sturdy chair, with one hand if you have trouble maintaining balance.

» Don't lean so far forward that your front knee moves in front of your toes.

» Don't arch your lower back.

Chapter 5

Choosing an Exercise Class or Virtual Workout

I f you loved playing Simon Says as a kid, you'll love group workouts, whether in a class or on a screen. To burn fat, build muscles, and have fun, all you need to do is copy everything the instructor does (assuming you've chosen a good instructor).

Group exercise has experienced a creative explosion since the days of Richard Simmons. In addition to traditional classes like low-impact cardio, you can try Zumba, Pilates, and much more. Many classes use equipment, such as dumbbells, balls, jump ropes, and even treadmills.

To explore your options, you can start by downloading an app of an exercise style, and if it's appealing to you, find a gym that offers the class. Or start with a live class and if you prefer privacy, check out a streaming video. These days, geography doesn't hold you back.

This chapter covers some popular instructor-led offerings besides yoga and Pilates (see Chapter 4 in Book 4 for details on yoga). For each class described in this chapter, you find out how much you'll sweat, what you'll gain, and how you'll fare if you're a klutz.

Getting Through When You Haven't a Clue: Taking an Exercise Class

If you're new to exercise classes, you have plenty of company. Of all the latest creative offerings, group exercise is attracting many folks who traditionally have stayed away. Don't fret, either, about getting injured. Exercise classes are much safer than they were in the Jane Fonda era of ultra-deep knee bends, jerky moves, and high kicks now considered criminal today. Most health clubs and studios require the instructors to have experience and, in certain instances, certification. Many clubs audition teachers, do regular evaluations, and pay attention to participant feedback.

Signing up

TIP

To make life easier for yourself when you're just starting out, choose classes with the words *beginner, introductory,* or *basic* in the title. You'll get a much different impression of boot camp from a slower, simplified beginner class than if you accidentally wander into an advanced class and hear, "Okay, the name of today's circuit is Last Man Standing!"

Class fees vary widely. Some health-club memberships include unlimited classes, and others charge extra for specialty classes. Specialty studios charge $10 to $40 per class, and they may charge extra to rent the equipment. At many clubs and studios, you can save money by buying a package of classes — say, ten at once — but be sure to find out whether you must use the package by a certain date (some states have now made expiration dates illegal). Another option is to buy a month's worth of unlimited classes. Some clubs let you try out one or two classes for free. You also can seek classes in other places such as community centers and churches.

Knowing what to expect from a live instructor

REMEMBER

No matter what type of class you're taking, a teacher who is standing right in front of you should do the following:

>> **Ask questions at the beginning of the class.** Some examples include, "Any newcomers?" "Anyone with an injury I need to know about?" or "Is there anyone here who's never tried jump rope before?"

>> **Include a warm-up and a cool-down period.** The cool-down should be followed by stretching exercises.

>> **Give clear instructions so you always know where you are and what's coming next.** Your instructor may say, "Two steps right," and then point right with two fingers. They should cue the moves coming up next instead of springing a lunge on you at the last second.

>> **Speak in plain language.** The really obnoxious instructors say things such as "plantar flex at your ankle joint" rather than "point your foot." However, a good teacher should educate you. It's perfectly okay for an instructor to say, "Feel this move in your quadriceps — that is, your thigh."

>> **Watch the class rather than gaze at themselves in the mirror.** They should face the students at least some of the time and occasionally walk around adjusting everyone's form.

>> **Make the class entertaining.** You don't want your instructor to take your classes so seriously that they become a chore or a bore.

>> **Have an education.** It's a definite plus if your instructor is certified by one of the major national fitness organizations. However, some specialty fields, such as boxing and tai chi, don't have organized certifying bodies. Don't hold that against them, but do ask where your instructor was trained so you know that person does indeed have some training.

Getting the most out of your classes

TIP

Before the class starts, tell the teacher you're a novice. A good instructor will keep an eye on you and correct your mistakes without making you feel foolish. If you don't mind the spotlight, stand in the front — the instructor will be more likely to notice and correct you. If you're shy and prefer to make your mistakes more privately, stand in the back or get lost in the middle. Throughout the class, keep your eye on the teacher rather than a fellow student. And don't compete with anyone. This isn't the time to give your ego a workout.

If you get tired, just march in place or dial down your intensity. Don't stop cold and walk out in the middle of a class — you risk nausea or even fainting. But don't be afraid to bail if the instructor isn't a good fit for you.

If the class is good, even if it leaves you feeling like a clod, come back for more. Skills and fitness take time to develop. You'll feel pretty darn good when you master a class that used to wipe you out.

Considering popular classes

Two classes that have the same name may be completely different. One body-sculpting class may use dumbbells; another may use rubber exercise tubes. And of course, no two teachers have the exact same style. Still, all body-sculpting classes, like other types of classes, have common characteristics. Here's a rundown of the most common classes around.

TIP

A recent trend is quick fitness classes — 15- to 30-minute classes that help people sneak in a workout in the busiest of days. Some gyms tack these on the end of longer classes so you have the option of supplementing your first class or running into the classroom just to work your abs or your thighs.

HIIT (high-intensity interval training)

Short bursts of very intense effort followed by recovery periods are the basis of high-intensity interval training. The bursts of effort can range from 20 seconds to a minute or so and the less-intense periods last 10 seconds to several minutes — the energy bursts may be longer or shorter than the recovery periods. A whole session is generally no longer than half an hour.

HIIT is a good cross-training regimen. For example, if your workout of choice is running, you can benefit by substituting a HIIT session on your non-running days.

What it does for you: The intense energy expenditure raises your metabolic rate even post-workout, burns calories, promotes fat loss and muscle gain. HIIT improves your oxygen consumption, reduces your heart rate and your blood sugar.

The difficulty factor: The exercises themselves are generally familiar — running, cycling, doing squats, and so on – but you do them at a very high level of intensity, often to the point of exhaustion.

Signs of a sharp instructor: You want an instructor who is a very good timekeeper — someone who lets you know how much more time you need to expend maximum energy and when the recovery period is over.

TIP

Tips for first-timers: HIIT is an exercise for healthy hearts, so check with your medical professional before embarking on a session.

High- and low-impact classes

High- and low-impact classes are the original Jane Fonda–Richard Simmons–style classes that ushered in the era of group classes. Don't know who these people are? Doesn't matter. You still see these classes form the core of many large gyms' group fitness schedule. Fads and trends may come and go, but high- and low-impact classes remain like barnacles on the sides of a ship, albeit with name changes like Cardio Push, Let It Go Low, Get High, or Eighties Flashback.

What it does for you: You get in shape and burn calories.

The difficulty factor: Difficulty depends on the class. With *low-impact,* you always have one foot on the floor; you don't do any jumping or hopping. *High-impact* moves at a slower pace, but you jump around a lot. High/low combines the two types of routines.

Signs of a sharp instructor: Instructors should spell out the terminology, rather than just say, "grapevine left, grapevine right."

TIP

Tips for first-timers: Shop around for a teacher you like who plays music that inspires you; there's nothing like a little "Eye of the Tiger" to get you going in the morning.

Body sculpting or kettlebells

Body sculpting is a nonaerobic, muscle-toning class. Look for names like Total-Body Power or Hot Body Blast. Most sculpting classes use weight bars, exercise bands, dumbbells, or a combination of these gadgets. You perform traditional weight-training moves in a class setting. Some focus on one specific body part; core conditioning classes have become especially popular. Kettlebell classes, in which you swing ball-shaped weights with handles on them, also are common.

What it does for you: Body sculpting gives you strength and muscle tone and lowers your risk of bone loss but only if you lift heavy enough weights. Sculpting classes are ideal if you're interested in the fundamentals of weight training but don't have the bucks to throw down for a personal trainer, you're too shy to enter the weight room, or you're unmotivated to lift on your own.

The difficulty factor: Prepare to be sore if you're a novice or if you usually do different exercises. Almost anyone can do body-sculpting classes the first time out if they're taught well. Kettlebells are a little harder to get in the swing of (we couldn't resist the pun!), because you have to figure out how to control the weights and not send them flying through a window or into your neighbor.

Signs of a sharp instructor: Instructors should tell you to use moderately heavy weights so that you don't do more than 15 reps per set. You don't develop much strength or tone if you do dozens of reps with very light weights. The instructor should correct your form and remind you where you should feel the exercise. Watch for a warm-up and cool-down, too.

Tips for first-timers: Prepare yourself for muscle soreness the day or two after your workout. First-time Kettlebellers should take a class designed for novices. A bit of technique is involved in the stance, swing, and selection of the correct weight for each exercise.

Circuit training and boot camp

Circuit training or boot camp is a fast-paced class in which you do a series of exercises, usually alternating sustained cardio exercise with weight training, boxing, or athletic movements. *Circuit training* is like a game of musical chairs: Everyone begins at a *station* (that is, a place where an exercise is done), and when the instructor yells "Time!" or some such phrase, everyone moves to the next free station. Some classes alternate an aerobic activity (such as stepping or stationary cycling) with a muscle-strengthening activity (such as using weight machines). *Boot-camp classes* are like circuit training classes on steroids; they're far more intense, and the exercises are typically more complex and challenging.

What it does for you: Both type of classes increase strength and cardio fitness and burn lots of calories. However, you don't get the same level of conditioning as you would from doing your cardio and strength training separately. If you take circuit classes, aim to get in an additional 20 minutes of straight aerobic exercise at least three days a week.

The difficulty factor: Moderate. Circuit training can be intense, but it's quite adaptable to the individual and requires minimal coordination. If your instructor is more interested in letting spit fly in your face than giving technique pointers, participant injury rates are likely to be high. Depending on the circuit and the moves, you may be stumbling over your feet or punching air when you should be smacking the punching bag. Stick with it, though, and you'll get the hang of it. If you have a short attention span and an adrenaline rush, this is the workout for you.

Signs of a sharp instructor: If an instructor swaggers in with a *Full Metal Jacket* attitude, get out quick! Good instructors are aware of each class member's level and modify the moves accordingly. They recognize that operating at a fast pace does not mean throwing caution and good technique to the wind.

Tips for first-timers: Pay attention to how you feel. Many people are surprised by how challenging this type of workout can be.

Boxing and martial-arts-inspired classes

A boxing or martial-arts-inspired class usually takes the training moves of a boxer, kickboxer, or martial artist and choreographs them to music. However, some instructors don't use music and instead choose to count or call out commands. You do some or all of the following: jump rope, shadow-box, do forward kicks, punch, and do the fancy footwork that boxers do in the ring and martial artists do in the movies.

What it does for you: This class develops power and endurance. These workouts also improve your coordination, strength, agility, and balance.

The difficulty factor: After one of these classes, you'll know why boxing athletes and martial artists are renowned for their fitness. Most classes are geared toward advanced exercisers, although some clubs offer beginner and multilevel classes, too. Many of the classes require decent coordination to master the footwork and handwork, but if you like to sweat and think at the same time, sign up.

What to wear: You can buy specialty boxing and martial-arts shoes, although medium-to-high-top cross-trainers are fine. Most gyms supply boxing gloves and other additional equipment needed.

Signs of a sharp instructor: Go for classes taught by someone with good boxing and/or martial arts skills, rather than, say, a yoga instructor who's just futzing around with a jump rope. Most teachers don't have these certifications, because there really isn't any formal organizing body in these specialties, but some instructors do have degrees of belt or rankings of some sort. If they don't, it's best if they've at least attended some instructional seminars.

TIP

Tips for first-timers: Pay attention to how you feel, and skip or modify moves that feel too difficult or uncomfortable. Don't give up; boxing gets easier.

Dance-based workouts

A dance-based workout is a cardio routine with choreography borrowed from dance moves. Classes range from simple moves with a little attitude thrown in to what seems like a tryout for a dance competition. At many urban clubs, you find funk aerobics, hip-hop, and even *salsa hip-hop,* a funky class spiced up with salsa dance moves. Look for names like Cardio Jam and Zumba (a fusion of Latin and international music). Taking an actual dance class in, say, ballet, tap, or modern can also give you a mighty good workout, so don't overlook that option.

What it does for you: These classes develop heart and lung power and really improve your posture, body awareness, flexibility, coordination, and agility. You teach your body to move in complex ways and use muscles you didn't know you had.

The difficulty factor: Difficulty depends on the level of the class. Dance classes are so popular now, perhaps because of the popularity of reality-TV dance contests, so a class is out there for every level and every style. Even if you have two or even three left feet, you can find a class you can get through without feeling your joints were carved from wood. And secretly, who hasn't always wanted to feel light on their feet?

What to wear: You can wear your typical tights and T-shirt, but don't be surprised if you're the only one. Some classes tend to have their own style of dressing: high-top sneakers, off-the-shoulder tops, baggy shorts, sexy bras, oversized socks. In many classes, you slip your shoes off and leave them at the door.

Signs of a sharp instructor: Good instructors break down complicated moves into a series of smaller ones before putting them all together. They repeat, repeat, and repeat sequences until they're drilled into your brain.

TIP

Tips for first-timers: If your parents didn't pass down the dancing gene in your DNA, start with a beginner class or something super basic like Zumba. Dance, more than any other style of class, can leave unprepared novices in the dust.

Cardio-machine classes

Cardio-machine classes are group classes taught on stationary bicycles, rowers, treadmills, or just about any other cardio machinery. These classes follow the same basic pattern: You pedal, walk, run, step, or row while the instructor talks you through a visualization of an outdoor workout. ("You're going up a long hill now — you can't see the top yet . . ."). During the class, you vary your pace and intensity, sometimes pushing yourself as fast as you can, other times cranking up the intensity and going slowly, and other times breezing in recovery mode.

What it does for you: A cardio-machine class burns lots of calories, ratchets up your cardio fitness, strengthens your thigh and calf muscles, and — if you so desire — prepares you for the real outdoor deal.

The difficulty factor: Most equipment classes last 30 to 90 minutes and are geared toward all levels of exercisers, depending on which class you take. However, even beginner classes are a bit more challenging than novice classes of other breeds. You don't need much coordination, but you do need the wherewithal to push through even when you feel tired.

What to wear: For non-cycling machine classes, wear what you'd typically wear to exercise on that piece of equipment. For cycling classes, most studio-cycling bikes have the same hard, narrow seats as outdoor racing bikes, so a pair of padded bike shorts or a gel seat can help keep your fanny happy. Most bikes have water-bottle cages so you can stash your water within easy reach. Some studios such as SoulCycle (in major cities like New York and Los Angeles) provide shoes, but if your club doesn't, wear stiff-soled shoes; walking and running shoes are too soft. Many bikes have clipless pedals so you can wear outdoor cycling shoes with cleats that click into the pedals.

Signs of a sharp instructor: Good instructors know all the nuances of the equipment and share all this insider info with the class. Rather than stay parked on their piece of machinery, they walk around and make technique adjustments.

TIP

Tips for first-timers: Show up early to your first class so you have plenty of time to make your equipment adjustments and familiarize yourself with all the buttons and knobs.

Specialty classes

Specialty classes are your flavor-of-the-month classes, though some have more staying power than others. Health clubs and studios dream up exotic routines such as pole dancing, trapeze school, and stiletto strength (which prepares your body for walking in high heels) in an effort to attract people into the exercise studio. Often these classes are gone in three months, but if they've served their purpose, which is to get your butt off the couch and bouncing on a trampoline, they've done their job.

The difficulty factor: The skills required are all over the map, as is the quality of instruction and effectiveness of these workouts. But give 'em a try. Exercise in any way, shape, or form beats eating chips and channel-surfing any day of the week.

Signs of a sharp instructor: Often the instructor is the mad-genius inventor of the class or a loyal disciple. To this we say either "Great!" or "Good luck with that."

Tips for first-timers: Usually everyone's a first-timer, so you're in good company.

Working Out with an Onscreen Instructor

You may feel silly prancing around your living room in front of your screen or mirror, but if you're short on time, avoiding potentially crowded places, feel self-conscious about your body, or are taking care of kids at home, a virtual workout may be a better option for you than a live class.

With the advent of the COVID pandemic, in-person classes of every description quickly became virtual classes, and workout classes were no exception. You can find any type of workout you want virtually via online live or recorded classes, DVDs or other media, Zoom classes, and interactive subscription services.

REMEMBER

Safety is an important consideration, especially if you don't have much exercise experience and you're working out in an unsupervised setting. Follow these safety tips:

>> **Clear adequate space in front of your screen.** You don't want to bang your shins on anything or knock over a lamp.

>> **Gather all the equipment you need before your workout.** This way, you don't have to stop mid-workout and rummage through the closet for your jump rope or hand weights. Place your mat or chair or bench at a 45-degree angle to the screen so you get a good view of the instructor without having to crane your neck or compromise your technique.

>> **For cardio and strength-training workouts, wear proper shoes instead of working out in bare feet or socks.** In any case, don't jump around on concrete or tile floors. You may want to buy a board made of springy wood similar to what you find in good aerobics studios. These boards help absorb impact.

>> **Even if the instructor doesn't do it on the screen, gauge your intensity by checking your heart rate or taking the talk test during or immediately following an intense portion of the workout.** Chapter 1 in Book 4 explains these methods.

REMEMBER

Taking a class through a Zoom connection or through your on-demand fitness app means you're in control of who sees and hears you during your workout. You don't have to feel pressure to keep up with anyone else. You can turn off video and/or mute yourself at any time, so if you need to wipe sweat from your brow or blow your nose, you can do that in private (and with the nose-blowing, your classmates will thank you). At the same time, you can develop camaraderie through a virtual connection, virtually sweating with the same people class after class.

You can build an extensive workout library through online classes for less than one month's worth of gym membership dues. If you're really creative, you can probably do it for close to free. You may even get more imaginative routines than many health-club instructors can drum up.

You have a range of options for joining a virtual workout:

>> **Streaming and downloads:** Many services, such as Amazon Prime and iTunes, feature video workouts (either for free or at a low cost). If you don't mind exercising in front of your computer or TV, you can be waving your arms

and lifting your knees in no time. (For a low-tech freebie, head to the local library and rent DVD exercise titles.)

You can find free workouts at various levels including low-impact routines from AARP.org to make-your-muscles-sing workouts from PopSugar.com.

>> **Online workout subscriptions:** With an online workout subscription (think Peloton and similar platforms), you can fire up a workout any time, day or night. Most are excellent. There are a lot of categories to choose from, such as 10-minute workouts, cardio, toning, yoga, HIIT (high intensity interval training), and so on. Most subscription services offer both a workout library and live, interactive classes. Prices vary, but many programs offer trial subscriptions.

>> **Apps and YouTube:** Here's a freebie tip: Flip to the App Store on your smartphone. Here you can find tons of free workout apps. Others cost just a few bucks.

As for YouTube, you can also find some good workouts there, although you need more patience and persistence than with apps. YouTube searches can yield surprising and frustrating results. You may search for abdominal exercises and wind up looking at ads for laundry detergent — presumably because of the washboard reference — but you may also stumble upon the most amazing Pilates class.

REMEMBER

If you're exercising to a recorded class, make use of these tips:

>> **Don't try to keep up with the instructors.** They practiced the routine for weeks before it was recorded. Look for someone in the video who goes at your pace. Many good videos feature demonstrators who exercise at different levels. At the start of the workout, the lead instructor should say something like, "If you're a beginner, keep your eye on Valerie." If you get winded, keep moving by marching in place or walking in a circle.

>> **If you're just starting out, follow a workout that includes several short sessions rather than one long one.** The shorter workouts last 5 to 25 minutes as opposed to 30 to 90 minutes. They're usually programmed to include a warm-up and cool-down.

>> **Remember the pause button.** Use it if you need to get water or you just need to catch your breath. Take advantage of all the extra features the workout has to offer, such as the ability to customize the music, the workout intensity, and the length of the workout.

5

Providing Your Body with Top-Notch Nutrition

Contents at a Glance

CHAPTER 1: **Eating Clean for a Healthier Body, Mind, and Soul**..317

What Clean Eating Really Is 318

Considering the Dangers in Processed Foods.................322

Surveying the Benefits of Eating Clean.....................326

CHAPTER 2: **Applying Eating Clean Principles to Daily Living**..331

The Principles of Clean Eating 332

Managing Cravings and Feelings of Deprivation 339

CHAPTER 3: **Nutrition Basics: You Really Are What You Eat**..345

Figuring Out What Your Body Needs (And What It Doesn't Need)...346

Considering the Roles of Proteins, Carbs, and Fats 356

Getting the Vitamins and Minerals You Need to Stay Healthy . . . 362

Protecting Your Health with Fiber..........................371

Water: The Essential Nutrient 373

CHAPTER 4: **Eat More, Eat Often** 375

Listening to Your Body 376

Getting Started with Good Food Choices....................381

Chapter **1**

Eating Clean for a Healthier Body, Mind, and Soul

E ating clean has been getting a lot of press lately — in books, websites, seminars, and various other media outlets. But what exactly is eating clean? Is it a diet? If so, what kinds of foods can you eat (and not eat) on the plan? And what is "clean" food, anyway?

Perhaps you've tried just about every other diet on the planet and you're tired of counting calories, carbs, and fat grams. If that's the case, you've come to the right place! One of the best things about the eating clean plan is that after you get the basics down pat, you don't have to keep track of your fat or protein intake or add up any points. After all, the plan's main focus is eating whole foods, which are naturally nutrient dense and low in calories.

Like most other diets, the eating clean plan offers several guidelines for following it, but another one of the great things about this plan is that you get to decide how much of your diet will be clean (and how much won't). You're in control, so if you decide that 90 percent of your diet is going to be clean, you can still fit some processed foods into your diet. If you decide to start out with a 50–50 mix, half of your diet will consist of clean foods while the other half includes the foods you already eat and enjoy.

This chapter defines clean eating and looks at the differences between whole foods and processed foods. You discover some of the dangers of processed and refined foods and find the benefits of eating clean. Finally, you understand food's effect on your body, mind, and soul and see how following the eating clean lifestyle can improve all three.

What Clean Eating Really Is

Clean eating is the act of basing your diet on whole, unprocessed, and preferably organic foods. In other words, when you eat clean, you try to eat as low on the food chain as possible; choose foods that are not processed, but just as they are harvested. By focusing on whole foods, your diet automatically becomes higher in vitamins, minerals, and phytochemicals and lower in refined sugar, bad fats, and food additives.

The following sections take a closer look at what *clean* really means and cover the difference between whole and processed foods. Then you discover the six degrees of clean eating so that you can decide what's right for you.

Eating clean doesn't mean cleaning your food before eating it

Eating clean doesn't mean washing all your food, although you certainly do need to rinse produce before adding it to a recipe or eating it raw. The basic principle of this plan is eating whole foods, which include unprocessed fruits and vegetables, lean meats, nuts, seeds, legumes, and whole grains. The *clean* part simply means that the food is unprocessed. In other words, clean, whole foods don't have ingredient labels because they consist of only one ingredient!

TIP

Think of eating clean as cleaning up your life. Just as you'd like to live life in a house free of clutter, you need to remove the clutter from your diet. What makes up the clutter in your diet? Junk foods, refined sugar, additives, preservatives, trans fats, white flour, artificial flavors, and toxins — just to name a few! (Check out Chapter 2 in Book 5 for more details on how to apply eating clean principles to your daily life.)

But following the eating clean plan is more than just choosing to eat whole foods. You get to eat more often, too! Because people will eat anything within reach when they're so hungry it hurts, the eating clean plan involves eating smaller meals plus at least two snacks throughout the day. Spreading out your food intake helps keep your blood sugar stable, which evens out your mood, improves your concentration on tasks during the day, and can even help reduce the risk of some diseases.

REMEMBER

Essentially, the eating clean plan calls you to do the following:

>> Eat the foods made by nature, not man.

>> Plan to eat five or six meals and snacks throughout the day.

>> Avoid processed foods (in other words, anything in a box with a label).

>> Use healthy cooking methods.

>> Eat before you become super hungry.

>> Stop eating when you're satisfied, not stuffed.

>> Don't count your calories, fat grams, or points.

>> Enjoy your food and appreciate its flavor.

The difference between the eating clean plan and other diets is that this plan is a lifestyle, not a complicated regimen that restricts entire categories of food. With fewer chemicals to deal with, your body becomes better able to concentrate on keeping you healthy.

Chapter 3 in Book 5 explains how eating clean can improve your body on the cellular level. Don't be scared; you don't need a science degree to eat clean. But you do need to understand that you literally are what you eat. Your cells, tissues, organs, and entire body will be happier when you eat a great diet.

Comparing whole versus processed foods

To really get a feel for the difference between whole and processed foods, take a look at the following ingredient list. Can you guess what this product is just by reading the ingredients in it?

Water, xylitol, modified food starch, cocoa processed with alkali, milk protein concentrate, hydrogenated vegetable oil, salt, sodium alginate, sucralose, acesulfame potassium, artificial flavor, artificial color

We don't blame you if you have no clue what this food is. It's full of ingredients you don't recognize and can't pronounce, and it's a perfect example of why the eating clean diet is so good for you. After all, why eat this sugar-free instant chocolate pudding mix when you could make your own chocolate pudding with chemical-free, whole ingredients, like milk, eggs, and bittersweet chocolate?

Whole foods are foods that grow in the garden, roam freely on farms, or swim in the sea. Think about the food chain you learned about in science class. Single-celled animals, plants, and plankton are at the bottom. Small fish and other tiny animals eat the single-celled animals, and bigger animals eat the small fish and other tiny animals, and so on up the chain. People (and sharks) are at the top, so everything eaten by the creatures lower on the chain becomes part of the creatures at the top.

To understand all the health benefits of eating clean, you need to consider another food chain: the processed food chain. A plain apple, a handful of chickpeas, or an organic egg are at the bottom. As you move further up the chain, manufacturers manipulate the food until it becomes more artificial ingredients than real food. The foods at the top of this chain include traditional snack foods, fast food, and foods packed with additives, preservatives, and artificial flavors.

Manufacturers end up stripping processed foods of many of their nutrients either to make them easier to combine with other ingredients or to change their characteristics. In contrast, whole foods come to you just as nature intended — bursting with flavor, color, texture, and nutrients.

The foods that are part of the eating clean plan are at the bottom of the processed food chain. They don't have labels, they don't carry preparation instructions, and they certainly don't have ingredient lists. These foods should fill your shopping basket each time you go to the supermarket.

TIP

Of course, some processed foods are perfectly acceptable on the eating clean plan. Whole-grain pasta is obviously processed, but it's minimally processed. Read the label; if it lists whole grains, water, and perhaps salt, it's a pretty clean food. Cheese is another processed food, but if you choose a natural cheese that doesn't come loaded with additives and artificial colors, it still fits into the eating clean plan.

Gaining control with six degrees of clean eating

One of the best things about the eating clean plan is that you're in control. In other words, you get to choose how much of the eating clean plan you implement. You can go all out and make 100 percent of your diet clean. Or you can choose to eat an occasional fast-food meal or include some processed foods in your diet. The choice is yours!

Table 1-1 shows the six degrees of clean eating. Take a look at what each degree entails, and think about which one best fits your life.

TABLE 1-1 ## The Six Degrees of Clean Eating

Degree	What You Eat When Following This Degree
20%	At the beginning of your eating clean adventure — or if you're trying to wean kids (or a reluctant spouse) off a junk food diet — start by changing one meal in a five-day week into a clean meal.
40%	Add another clean meal a week to your plan to continue the eating clean journey. You can also start at this level.
50%	If you want to live an eating clean lifestyle, 50% is really the minimum degree to shoot for. At this level, you get some of the benefits of the eating clean diet plan but can still eat a few fast-food meals and the occasional junk food. Just try to make the nonclean 50% of your diet a bit healthier! Make homemade potato chips instead of eating processed, flavored chips; use multigrain pasta in place of white; and enjoy just one brownie rather than five.
60%	Now you're getting more serious! At this level, most of your foods are clean and unprocessed, but you still eat processed foods two or three days a week. You have to do more cooking, but you're also saving money because you're eating out less and buying fewer processed (and expensive) foods.
80%	Many people stop at this level of clean eating. The vast majority of your meals are clean, using whole, unprocessed foods, but you can still include some bottled pasta sauce and bakery bread in your diet.
100%	Not many people can follow a true clean eating plan all the time, but if you can, bravo! If you've been diagnosed with a serious illness, this level may be the best option for you. Or if you're sick and tired of feeling sick and tired, the pure eating clean plan may help you feel better.

REMEMBER

Of course, you can set your target somewhere in between these six degrees. Heck, your plan may vary between 100 percent clean and 60 percent clean within the same day! If you're serious about living the eating clean lifestyle, though, aim for making whole foods the basis for at least 50 percent of your diet. Don't worry about backsliding or falling off the eating clean wagon; just focus on the big picture and enjoy your food and your life. (See Chapter 2 in Book 5 for tips on how to deal with backsliding and get back on the eating clean wagon.)

Considering the Dangers in Processed Foods

Are processed foods really as bad as some people think? In a word, yes. Consider just one example: trans fats. Manufacturers make these fake fats by bubbling hydrogen through liquid oils. Although this process (called *hydrogenation*) sounds like something out of a Frankenstein movie, it's not that complicated. The hydrogen simply transforms the oil into a solid substance. Hydrogenation is a very inexpensive way to make solid fats, which is why food processors love it.

For years, doctors (yes, doctors!) recommended that people eat margarine made with this method rather than butter or simple oils. Now, of course, researchers know that trans fats may be one of the culprits behind America's skyrocketing heart disease rates. The fake fats literally become part of your cell walls, making them flabby and changing their ability to interact with other parts of your body. Nobody wants flabby arms, let alone flabby cell walls!

The following sections look at some of the preservatives and additives packed into processed foods and explain why you should avoid them. These sections also consider whether fortified foods are really any better than unfortified foods and explain why breaking the junk food habit is so important to your health.

Preservatives and additives

Surprisingly enough, the U.S. Food and Drug Administration (FDA) and U.S. Department of Agriculture (USDA) haven't tested many of the preservatives and additives used in processed foods because they're on the Generally Recognized as Safe (GRAS) list. A chemical's presence on this list means that it has been used for so long (since before 1958) — with no known harmful side effects attached to it — that the FDA allows manufacturers to use it in food without any required testing.

The FDA defines *safe* as "a reasonable certainty in the minds of competent scientists that the substance is not harmful under its intended conditions of use." That's not exactly a ringing endorsement! And the phrase *intended conditions of use* needs some further explanation; see the nearby sidebar "How many chemicals do you consume?" for details.

The FDA has developed four different classifications of chemicals that manufacturers add to processed food:

- **Food additives:** This category includes preservatives, flavor enhancers, emulsifiers (calcium stearoyl di laciate, polyglycerol ester, and monoglycerides, among others), vitamins and minerals, and chemicals that control the pH of a product.

- **GRAS substances:** These products are the ones that have "existing evidence of long and safe use." These substances have not been tested by the FDA or USDA.

- **Prior-sanctioned substances:** The FDA or USDA tested and approved these products before the government developed the GRAS list.

- **Color additives:** This category includes color enhancers and additives.

The FDA doesn't guarantee that the chemicals included in the GRAS list and the prior-sanctioned substances list are safe, but it doesn't test them unless some new evidence shows that they may be unsafe. You may have heard of the artificial sweetener cyclamate. It was in the GRAS list until testing found that it caused cancer in animals; then the FDA removed it from the list.

WARNING

The FDA has removed some chemicals from the market. Red Dye #2 and Violet #1, for example, were removed from the market after Congress passed the 1960 Color Additive Amendment. Before the amendment passed, manufacturers used 200 food dyes; less than 35 of those dyes passed the testing process and were declared safe. So how much damage was done by the 165 unsafe food dyes? Think of it this way: Some manufacturers used to put lead in butter to give it that beautiful yellow color or chalk in milk to make it look thick and creamy!

Many people, especially those who eat clean, don't want to wait for some food additive, pesticide, or preservative to be declared dangerous retroactively. They'd rather take control of what they put into their bodies and consume as few of these chemicals as possible — through the eating clean diet, of course. (Find out more about these chemicals in Chapter 2 of Book 5.)

Of course, a few preservatives and additives may be perfectly safe if consumed in small amounts. But many people really don't like the phrase *may be.* Do you really want to be a guinea pig in a huge experiment conducted on the population? If you want to gain more confidence about the safety of the foods you eat, give the eating clean plan a try and avoid processed, refined, and packaged foods as much as you can.

HOW MANY CHEMICALS DO YOU CONSUME?

One of the problems connected with the chemicals in your food is how much of each particular food you consume. If your diet consists mainly of fast food and the amount of hormones in that beef burger you love is considered "safe in a reasonable diet" but you eat 400 hamburgers a year, you're going to ingest more than the amount of hormones the FDA approved. Similarly, if you love asparagus, eat it three times a week, and can't afford to buy organically grown produce, you'll be getting more than the studied dose of pesticides used to grow that particular product.

To reduce your exposure to preservatives, additives, and other chemicals added to food, vary what you eat. Don't subsist on fried chicken and roasted potatoes. Add different types of fresh fruits and vegetables, even if they aren't grown organically, and you can reduce your exposure to many chemicals.

Label claims (also known as marketing hype)

Many processed foods have lots of claims plastered all over their labels. "Fortified with calcium!" "Strengthens your immune system!" and "Made with real fruit!" are just some of the banners you see on packaged foods these days. But what, if anything, do these claims mean?

Many fortified foods have only some (key word *some*) of the nutrients that manufacturers removed during processing added back in. For instance, a cereal made from white flour may have vitamins and fiber added back in. But the amounts added back in aren't even close to 100 percent of what was removed in the first place. The process to turn the wheat grain into white flour permanently strips out many of those nutrients.

Although eating fortified foods is better than eating unfortified foods, it's not as good as eating the whole foods in the first place. Unfortunately, many people blissfully put these fortified products in their shopping baskets, unaware that many of the claims on the packages have no real meaning.

The FDA does regulate some label claims, but many companies change a word or two to get around these regulations. Then the claim becomes misleading. For example, most flavored strawberry juices don't actually contain strawberries. The "real fruit" you see on the label claim is actually pear concentrate, and the "strawberry" is present only in the form of artificial flavoring.

The following list presents some common label claims and explains what they actually mean:

>> **Made with organic ingredients:** Only 70 percent of the ingredients in the food must be grown organically.

>> **High or rich in . . . :** These food products must have 20 percent of the Recommended Dietary Allowance (RDA) of the nutrient in question per serving.

>> **Zero trans fats:** The product can contain up to 0.5 grams of artificial trans fats per serving. But be aware that if you eat more than one serving, those partial grams can add up fast.

>> **More, fortified, enriched:** For this designation, the product must contain 10 percent of the RDA of the nutrient in question per serving or more than a similar product contains.

>> **Natural:** This claim means the product can't contain anything synthetic. But it can still be high in sodium, fats, and sugars.

>> **Made with whole wheat:** This claim doesn't mean that the food contains no refined grain products. In fact, the food has to contain only a tiny amount of whole wheat to legally use this label.

Understandably, these claims can confuse consumers. The claims don't tell you about substances that you may need or want to avoid; you have to read the ingredient list for that information. Funny how these claims, when clearly explained, don't seem as wonderful as you'd think! If a food has "more vitamin A" but the "more" is only 10 percent of your RDA and the food has enough sodium to put you over your limit for the day, is it really a healthy choice?

REMEMBER

Overall, eating foods without labels is less complicated and better for you. When you buy whole, unlabeled foods, you can be pretty sure that what you see is what you get.

Junk food addiction

The term *junk food junkie* used to be pretty popular in the American lexicon. People used it as a joke, but unfortunately, that term is very accurate because junk food is actually quite addictive.

Consider this: A study published in *Nature Neuroscience* found that your brain reacts to junk food just like it does to addictive drugs such as heroin. Kind of scary, right? You've likely seen pictures of heroin addicts, who will do anything for that next hit.

One of the most dangerous things about addiction is that over time, the addict has to consume more and more of the addictive substance to create the same amount of pleasure in the addict's brain. That fact is what causes the death of many drug addicts; eventually they overdose.

That fact is also what can cause the illness and death of junk food junkies; eventually the ever-increasing consumption of empty calories, lots of sugar, refined ingredients, sodium, and artificial additives wear out the body. With little or no vitamins, minerals, and phytochemicals to help the body repair itself, junk food junkies eventually come to the end of the line and develop a disease. To think that manufacturers actually develop junk foods to be as addictively appealing as possible!

REMEMBER

The eating clean plan helps remove your addiction to junk food simply by substituting whole foods that are healthy and nutritious for the unhealthy, addictive junk foods. This process takes time, though, so don't think you'll find an easy way out of the junk food maze. But you can get out of it, and with some thought and effort, you can get your family off the junk food treadmill, too. One of the best things about the eating clean lifestyle is that the more you follow it, the better you feel, so you get on an upward spiral toward good health rather than a downward spiral into sickness.

Surveying the Benefits of Eating Clean

So other than containing clean, natural ingredients rather than artificial chemicals, what can clean, whole foods do for you? Eating a clean diet can help you live longer, make you stronger, prevent disease, and maybe even treat some diseases. These claims may sound like one of those late-night infomercials, but they're all true — backed up with scientific research conducted by real doctors wearing lab coats!

The following sections look at how you can use the eating clean lifestyle to obtain and maintain good health. They discuss how to eat clean to lose weight, to prevent disease, and to lead the longest, most active life you can.

Overall good health

WARNING

If you've been blessed with good health, you're lucky. After all, your genes do play a part in whether you develop disease. But scientists estimate that 310,000 to 580,000 deaths in the United States every year are caused by an unhealthy diet and lack of physical exercise. After all, your diet has a very real effect on your health:

JUNK FOODS: FAKE EVERYTHING

You know that junk foods contain artificial colors and flavors, along with sugar and salt to increase their addictive qualities. But do you know that junk food manufacturers also manipulate texture? Texture and flavor are the two big players in food's appeal. Emulsifiers, thickeners, fats, and stabilizers increase the *mouthfeel*, or texture, of processed foods. In other words, manufacturers artificially manipulate their foods to make them more pleasing to your mouth. This artificial mouthfeel gives junk food an advantage over regular food, so you tend to crave it more than whole foods. After you realize that the whole mouthfeel is just as artificial as the ingredients, you may be able to say no the next time you crave a triple-fried cheese doodle. Try a crisp apple or some cauliflower instead.

>> Diet causes up to one-third of all cancers.

>> Poor diet causes most cases of obesity.

>> A diet based on processed foods, junk foods, and refined foods is a major risk factor for developing heart disease.

>> Not getting enough vitamins, minerals, and phytochemicals in your diet puts you at greater risk for catching infectious diseases.

>> Eating too much sugar, alcohol, and bad fat can reduce the efficiency of your immune system.

The eating clean plan can help you stay as healthy as you can be by putting your dietary focus on whole foods that pack a nutritional punch. No matter what the current state of your health is, you can feel better and get healthier if you ditch the refined, overly processed foods and start concentrating on eating healthy foods.

The characteristics of overall good health are

>> Stamina

>> Normal body weight

>> Normal blood pressure

>> Good blood cholesterol counts and other normal blood parameters

>> A healthy heart

>> Good digestion

>> Clear skin

>> Mental acuity

Overall good health has many more markers, of course, but the point is that good health isn't perfection. It isn't about achieving a model's body or looking like your favorite movie star. Good health means that your body is able to do what you want it to do, whether that's to hike Mount Annapurna or take a walk around the block.

Weight loss and disease prevention

More than 60 percent of all Americans are overweight. Even with messages about nutrition being blasted all day long, through every form of media, Americans are getting more and more overweight. What's going on?

Many nutritionists think the problem is what's in the food most people eat. Your body wasn't made to use all the chemicals and artificial ingredients packed into much of the American diet. And it certainly wasn't made to consume as much sodium, fake fat, and sugar as many people do today. Plus, your body was made to efficiently process food and store fat since your ancestors couldn't guarantee that they'd get three square meals a day. When Americans are faced with unlimited quantities of food available 24 hours a day, something has to give. Often, that something is their waistbands.

REMEMBER

The key to healthy, sustained weight loss is to gradually lose weight by eating a nutrient-dense diet of filling foods, which is exactly what the eating clean plan is all about. On the plan, you eat more often and you eat foods that are satisfying and very nutritious. After you get into the clean eating plan, you really won't have any more room in your life (or your stomach) for the junk food that made you overweight in the first place!

Remember the thousands of deaths caused every year by poor diet and lack of exercise discussed in the preceding section? Well, people don't die because of a poor diet; they die because of the diseases caused (or exacerbated) by that poor diet. Those diseases include

>> Heart disease

>> Cancer

>> Diabetes

>> Hypertension

>> Stroke

>> Autoimmune diseases

>> Osteoporosis

Disease occurs when something goes wrong in your body. Cells grow too fast, and your body is so busy filtering toxins that it takes longer to respond to infection. Over time, these factors can lead to a serious disease.

REMEMBER

The eating clean diet really is the model for eating to prevent disease. One of its main focuses is on getting plenty of phytochemicals, which help prevent inflammation, keep your immune system strong, and keep your cardiovascular system running smoothly. The only way to get your phytochemicals is to eat lots of whole fruits, vegetables, nuts, seeds, and grains.

A longer, more active life

A good motto for the eating clean life is "It's not only the years in your life, but the life in your years!" Everyone wants to live a long life, of course, but if that life is full of preventable pain, disease, and suffering, all bets are off. Living a long life should mean being able to easily walk up stairs, walk around the block, and participate in active hobbies well into your 80s and 90s.

REMEMBER

Fortunately, the eating clean diet can help you do just that. If you're blessed with basically good health, eating whole foods prepared in a clean way is one of the best ways to keep yourself healthy. Of course, no diet can guarantee good health or a long life. But you can tip the odds in your favor with the eating clean plan.

Chapter **2**

Applying Eating Clean Principles to Daily Living

E ating clean isn't just about the food you put in your mouth; it's a total lifestyle. By buying, preparing, and eating whole foods, you're affecting far more than your waistline and your health. You're making a positive impact on the world around you.

The eating clean lifestyle doesn't restrict you from eating any foods except processed foods. So you don't have to become a vegan or vegetarian (although you can if you want to!), and you don't have to count carbs, fat grams, or calories. By eating lower on the food chain, you save money and improve your health while making the world a better place to live.

One of the main benefits of this lifestyle is its simplicity. Because you don't have to keep track of calories, fat grams, or carbohydrates, planning meals is a lot less complicated than it is for other diets. Plus, the eating clean diet includes every food group, so you don't have to feel deprived. You don't have to worry about going hungry, either, because you get to eat satisfying meals and snacks throughout the day.

This chapter looks at the principles of clean eating, including eating for your health, consuming whole foods, avoiding processed foods, and figuring out how to enjoy healthy foods. We also show you how to handle feelings of deprivation and cravings that may undermine your clean eating efforts.

The Principles of Clean Eating

Depending on who you talk to, different clean eating plans have different principles. This flexibility is another reason why so many people find this lifestyle rewarding and doable. As long as you eat whole foods and avoid processed foods, you can create the clean eating lifestyle that works best for you.

The following sections look at the overall eating clean platform. You can pick and choose which facets appeal to you and your family. Then you find out how to make clean changes in your diet. Finally, you look at the real flavor of real food and understand how to appreciate it.

REMEMBER

The reason this chapter stresses *lifestyle* rather than *diet* is that most diets fail. Only 5 percent of all dieters stay on their diets and keep the weight off for more than a few years. Because clean eating is a lifestyle choice, the benefits you reap from it last a lifetime.

Getting your footing on the eating clean platform

The eating clean movement really started in the 1960s thanks to the efforts of Adele Davis and other health food authors. At that time, health food stores started springing up around the country, and people told jokes about tofu eaters who dressed in natural fibers and sandals and ate nuts and berries. In 1987, Ralph Nader wrote the book *Eating Clean: Overcoming Food Hazards,* which focused on the hazards of processed foods. But then Corporate America started pushing convenience foods and time-saving products above everything else. Mixes, frozen dinners, and junk foods started crowding whole foods off grocery store shelves.

After decades of Americans' eating processed foods and, not coincidentally, watching their population become more obese, fad diets became more and more popular. But they weren't successful, because following a really restrictive diet for long periods of time is nearly impossible. Everyone falls off the wagon, and many people have a hard time getting back on — which is why, after losing weight, more than 90 percent of overweight people eventually put the weight back on. On the other hand, the clean eating lifestyle has become more popular as more people realize how simple it really is. It's a lifestyle you can live with for the rest of your life.

REMEMBER

The basic planks of the eating clean platform are as follows:

>> **Eat whole, unrefined, and unprocessed foods that are low on the food chain.** Buy bunches of broccoli, whole heads of lettuce, corn on the cob, cantaloupe, whole chickens, and unrefined grains rather than processed foods, such as broccoli in sauce, packaged salads, canned corn, and lunch meat.

>> **Eat a wide variety of unprocessed foods.** Today's markets and grocery stores offer many more fruits and vegetables today than they did a few years ago. Try unusual foods such as passion fruit, salsify, or broccoli rabe. Experiment with unfamiliar foods to help make mealtime more interesting.

>> **Avoid artificial substances, including artificial flavors and colors, preservatives, and artificial sweeteners.** These items can harm your health by literally becoming part of your body's cell structure and changing some basic biological mechanisms. These changes weaken your body's ability to stay healthy.

>> **Cut back on sugars, especially processed sugars such as high fructose corn syrup and artificial sweeteners.** That means no more soda pop or other sugary drinks. Your body processes these ingredients differently, and they provide nothing but empty calories.

>> **Avoid trans fats and artificial fat substitutes.** The trans fatty acids found in shortening, lots of baked products, and snack foods may be behind the skyrocketing heart disease rates in this country, so don't eat them. Two more reasons why you should avoid artificial fats are that they cause unpleasant side effects and no one really knows about their long-term safety.

>> **Choose low-fat, not nonfat, dairy products.** Nonfat products use processed and artificial substances, such as additives and starches, to mimic the texture and flavor of fat.

>> **Choose foods that are nutrient dense.** In other words, for every calorie a food provides, it should also provide vitamins, minerals, protein, carbs, fiber, and good fats. Good fats include the fats found in nuts, olive oil, and lean meats, especially seafood. On the other hand, you find empty calories, which are calories with little or no nutritional value, in snack foods, cookies, candies, and soda.

>> **Combine protein, complex carbohydrates, and healthy fats at every meal for the most satisfaction.** This combination helps stave off hunger and

gives you more energy than you get from consuming something that's sugary or salty.

>> **Drink lots of water.** Try to drink several glasses of water a day. If you don't enjoy the taste of plain water, you can also drink unsweetened tea. Drinking plenty of water helps keep your digestive system running smoothly. Avoid drinking fruit juices, because they can be high in sugar and calories.

>> **Eat five or six minimeals a day rather than three large meals.** Make breakfast your largest meal, with whole-grain cereal or toast with butter or peanut butter and some form of protein, such as a hard-boiled egg. Your other meals need to include protein, carbs, and fat, such as celery sticks with nut butters and dried fruits or sandwiches made with sliced chicken and vegetables such as avocado and tomatoes.

>> **Practice portion control, especially when you eat more than three meals a day.** Each meal should be about 300 to 400 nutritious calories. Figure out what ½ cup of brown rice or other whole grain or fruits and vegetables looks like, because that's how big a typical serving is. A serving of bread is one slice; a serving of meat is 3 ounces, or about the size of a deck of cards. With time, eating proper portions will become second nature. Depending on which meal schedule works best for your day, you can adjust the amounts accordingly. For more information about portion sizes, see www.niddk.nih.gov/health-information/weight-management/just-enough-food-portions.

Making clean changes in your life

Clean changes in your life aren't difficult to make, but they do take some gumption, perseverance, and practice. When you make a concentrated effort to eat lower on the food chain, notice how this decision affects other areas of your life. To be successful, you have to think about food and eat differently, which will no doubt prompt changes in other areas of your life.

REMEMBER

As you adopt an eating clean lifestyle, you may also

>> **Lose weight and gain more energy.** Eating healthy foods with lots of vitamins, minerals, fiber, protein, complex carbohydrates, and good fats automatically makes you healthier. Of course, adding exercise to your new lifestyle is also important. As you feel stronger and gain more energy from the foods you eat, exercising will be much easier.

>> **Add fun exercise to your life.** Go for a walk with your kids, play on a jungle gym, take up a new sport, or invest in a gym membership. The combination of healthy eating with regular exercise can improve all parts of your life. With more confidence in how you look and feel, who knows what you can achieve?

>> **Improve your skin condition and overall appearance.** People who eat clean food also enjoy clear and smooth skin, thick and shiny hair, and bright eyes. The saying "you are what you eat" is absolutely true. Do you really want to be a nacho cheese chip?

>> **Spend more time cooking at first.** Before you can eat whole, unprocessed foods, you need to, well, process them. Don't panic. Cooking whole foods doesn't have to be difficult. After all, making simple meals, such as baked chicken with a chopped salad, isn't time-consuming. Plus, you're learning a valuable skill.

>> **Spend more time planning meals at first, now that you aren't relying on fast food or convenience foods to feed your family.** As you get into the eating clean lifestyle, you accumulate more recipes and ideas for clean foods, so the planning gets easier.

>> **Spend more time shopping for food and reading labels.** Especially at first, allow more time for shopping. Picking out the ingredients for a chopped salad takes longer than buying a frozen dinner. Keep reminding yourself that the health and life benefits are well worth the extra time and effort.

>> **Shop more often.** Because the foods you're buying aren't laced with preservatives, their shelf life is shorter. So shop more often and buy a bit less each time you shop.

>> **Produce less waste.** You can compost most food waste (except meats). Plus, you no longer buy foods that are wrapped and sealed in many layers, so you use less packaging. That's good for the earth and your garbage bill.

>> **Make preparing and eating food an event.** Use the time to talk to your family and teach them skills. Let each family member plan a meal or two in a week or a month, and take the time to find out more about the food and the cuisine behind each meal.

Discovering real flavor

Flavor in food is what makes eating enjoyable. But flavor doesn't come only from the reaction between foods and the taste buds on your tongue. Taste is only a small part of the flavor equation. The other important characteristics of flavor include aroma, color, temperature, and something called *mouthfeel*, which is the texture of food.

Processed foods are infamous for including artificial flavors and colors, along with tons of added sugar and salt. These ingredients interfere with your body's natural appetite centers, spurring you to eat more and crave more of these unhealthy foods. When you embark on your clean eating lifestyle, you'll notice some changes in how food tastes.

Your tongue has five different types of taste receptors that are bundled into buds and that react with the ions and molecules in food and then send messages to your brain through chemical reactions. Sour and salty taste receptors detect ions, while the others detect molecules. The five types of taste receptors are

>> **Sour:** The acid in foods stimulates these taste receptors, which have channels that pick up the hydronium ions found in foods such as lemon juice and balsamic vinegar.

>> **Salty:** The sodium ions in food stimulate these taste receptors.

>> **Bitter:** G-protein receptors on specialized taste buds perceive alkaloids (certain amino acids or proteins) in food, which cause bitter flavors, and directly activate neurons in the brain. Human bodies are hard-wired to detect bitter taste because many poisonous plants are bitter.

>> **Sweet:** Hydroxyl groups on sugar molecules stimulate your sweet taste receptors by using a protein called *gustducin,* which prompts reactions on the tongue that the brain recognizes as sweet.

>> **Umami or meaty:** The glutamic acid salts, which are part of the amino acids found in meats, cheeses, and some vegetables, stimulate these taste receptors.

Spicy or hot flavors don't stimulate any of the taste receptors. The so-called spicy flavor is actually the perception of pain, which the nerve endings just below the taste buds detect. That's why your tongue takes a few seconds to register the spiciness and heat when you bite into a jalapeño pepper.

A single taste bud has dozens of taste-receptor cells that include all five of the basic taste sensations. (Contrary to popular belief, they aren't grouped around the tongue in separate sections.) With the addition of salt, sugar, and flavor enhancers, processed foods are formulated to stimulate salty, sweet, and umami taste receptors, which are collectively called *appetitive tastes.* The threshold for tasting these substances is very low.

Clean foods activate your taste receptors without any help from artificial ingredients. Their flavors are much more pure. After just a short period of time on the eating clean diet, you'll start to recognize the clean taste of natural foods. Table 2-1 lists some clean foods with the five basic taste attributes plus spicy.

Combining the foods in Table 2-1 and choosing foods that incorporate more than one flavor can enhance your eating experience. (Now, that sounds like a restaurant commercial, doesn't it?) Think about an apple: It's both sour and sweet. The sweetness makes the sour flavor more pronounced, and vice versa. Plan your meals using this concept. Include some clean foods that have several flavors to enhance every meal.

TABLE 2-1   **Flavorful Clean Foods**

Food	Sweet	Sour	Salty	Bitter	Umami	Spicy
Bananas, mangos, melons, honey, agave nectar	X					
Yogurt, pomegranates, tamarind		X				
Kelp, pickled foods			X			
Spinach and dark greens, broccoli, Brussels sprouts, celery, eggplant, grapefruit				X		
Mushrooms					X	
Peppers, herbs, spices, ginger, radishes, raw onions and garlic, horseradish						X
Apples, oranges, strawberries	X	X				
Cooked onions and garlic, carrots, tomatoes	X				X	
Lemons, limes		X	X			
Tea, vinegar		X		X		
Mint		X				X
Kale, asparagus			X	X		
Meat stocks, lean meats, soy products, nuts, shellfish			X		X	
Kohlrabi				X		X
Miso					X	X
Natural cheeses		X	X		X	

Even though junk foods are designed to hit all the right taste buds, you can use a biological advantage to appreciate clean and healthy whole foods: More than 80 percent of what you perceive as flavor is actually aroma. Processed foods include artificial ingredients that mimic aromas of clean foods. But clean foods are full of natural aromas that make their flavors much more complex and satisfying than their artificial counterparts.

TIP

Don't forget the important impact that color, texture, and temperature have on the flavor experience. To use your natural flavor-detecting abilities to fully appreciate clean foods, pay attention to these three flavor factors and try out the following tips:

>> **Eat more slowly.** When you chew your food slowly, you give your taste buds time to detect the different flavors and aromas being released. Not only is

gulping down food bad for your digestion, but it also keeps you from experiencing all the flavors natural foods have to offer. Chewing also releases vapors into the back of your mouth, which stimulate your sense of smell. Chewing food for a longer period of time releases more flavor.

>> **Put away the salt shaker.** Many people have become used to the flavor of salt. As a result, they need more and more salt to satisfy the salty appetite center of the brain. Foods may taste bland at first on the eating clean plan, but your taste buds will gradually adjust to less sodium and the natural flavors of the foods will become more prominent.

WARNING

There is an exception to this rule: If your blood pressure is low (100/60 or less on either reading), you may have weak adrenal function and need salt. These people feel better and are healthier with more added salt, not less. If that's you, check with a physician skilled and knowledgeable in natural, nutritional medicine before making a decision to cut back on salt.

>> **Smell your food before you taste it.** You shouldn't sniff each bite before you put it in your mouth, a practice that can be construed as rude in some cultures. But breathe in over your plate before you start eating. Notice the rich smell of meats, the clean spiciness of a vegetable salad, and the sweet, complex aroma of herbs and spices.

>> **Plan meals with different textures.** Texture is an important part of flavor assessment. For example, if you make a whole meal of foods with soft textures, it will seem less interesting and more bland. Try to incorporate crisp, chewy, smooth, soft, and hard textures in your meals.

>> **Incorporate as many colors as possible on your plate.** You eat with your eyes before you eat with your mouth! No wonder your meal seems more appetizing when it contains reds, greens, browns, and yellows than when it's all beige or brown. Biting into a deep-red strawberry is more satisfying than biting into one that's pale and anemic-looking. As an added bonus, eating more colorful foods means giving your body more nutrients.

>> **Plan meals with different temperatures.** The contrast between hot and cold enhances the eating experience. Think about eating some warm grilled bread topped with a cold tomato salsa.

REMEMBER

Appreciating your food's natural flavors is easy to do on a clean diet because clean, whole foods hit all the flavor points that are built right into your anatomy. Foods that are less processed take more time to eat, forcing you to slow down and really notice the flavor and aroma of your food. The natural flavors of clean foods are more pleasing than artificially flavored and colored foods, especially when you get used to eating foods without so much added salt and sugar. Whole foods offer different textures and colors, making the meal much more appetizing. And you can serve clean, whole foods at any temperature or mix of temperatures, which adds interest to meals.

Managing Cravings and Feelings of Deprivation

For many people, just the thought of switching to a healthy eating plan is depressing. After all, life without chocolate chip cookies or nacho cheese chips seems pretty sad to a lot of people. To deal with these types of thoughts, you need to unleash your natural taste sensors and reprogram your brain so you start craving good foods.

The following sections look at the biological factors behind cravings and feelings of deprivation, and you discover what you can do to rewire your brain so that you enjoy eating (and even crave) healthy foods.

Understanding cravings

Did you know that the cravings you feel are real and not the result of low willpower and that they may actually be food addictions? Food companies understand the relationship between cravings and addiction, which is why they load processed food with salt, sugar, unhealthy fats, food colorings, and additives.

Food cravings and hunger have both psychological and physical facets. True hunger is a physical response to low blood sugar. But stress, boredom, aromas wafting through the air, and tempting television commercials can trigger food cravings. Unlike the actual need for food, however, a craving diminishes over time. If you give yourself some time and space to process what you're actually feeling, the craving will probably subside. Plus, the only way to satisfy cravings is by eating one particular food; you can satisfy true hunger with any nutritious food.

In a 2010 study published in *Nature Neuroscience,* scientists at the Scripps Research Institute showed that you can activate the same biological mechanisms that drive addiction to tobacco, cocaine, or heroin to create food addictions. A constant diet of foods such as cheeseburgers, chips, and candy can turn into a vicious cycle of addiction and cravings. As the body becomes obese, reward and pleasure centers in the brain deteriorate, requiring more and more processed junk foods to satisfy them. This phenomenon is called *sensory overload,* and it creates a vicious cycle of cravings for junk food that result in more weight gain, which increases cravings, which result in more weight gain . . . you get the picture. If you don't break this cycle — by changing your eating habits — you'll likely end up suffering from obesity, type-2 diabetes, and other diseases.

Refined carbohydrates like those found in cakes, cookies, and white bread cause insulin levels to spike. The rapid rise in blood glucose levels causes the release of insulin, which plays an important role in cravings by

>> Storing refined carbs by converting them to fat

>> Slowing down production of fat-burning hormones

>> Telling your body to hold on to its stored fat

>> Making you hungry more quickly

Eating a lot of junk food, or foods high in sugar and refined carbohydrates, may literally rewire your brain, creating a chemical imbalance. This imbalance occurs in the area of the brain that creates feelings of reward and satiety. When this change occurs, compulsive eating habits and addiction usually follow.

The main problem with food addiction is that people need to eat to live. While cocaine addicts can change their lives to avoid the addictive substance, people can't avoid food. But you can take control of this cycle by applying the clean eating principles discussed in the earlier section "The Principles of Clean Eating."

Your brain also associates many of the foods you crave with pleasurable events. For example, if your mother always made chocolate cake on cold, snowy days or baked some fabulous chocolate chip cookies when you had a bad day at school, you may have come to associate those foods with comfort and warmth. So you're probably not craving the food; you're craving the feelings the food engenders! To overcome these types of psychological cravings, look for other ways to create the feelings you long for: Snuggle up next to a fire in the fireplace, wrap yourself in a blanket with a good book, or play a quiet board game with your family.

Although fighting cravings and food addiction takes a lot of effort and hard work, you can be successful by following these tips:

>> **Keep food that tempts you out of the house.** If that candy bar isn't readily available but some sweet grapes or crunchy baby carrots are, you'll be much more inclined to reach for healthy snacks when you're hungry.

>> **Go for a walk or get some exercise.** These activities stimulate the production of feel-good chemicals in your brain, which give you feelings of wellbeing and satisfaction.

>> **Delay satisfying your cravings for 20 minutes.** Research shows that if you can wait 20 minutes to eat what you crave, the feeling will usually subside. If you're still hungry after that period of time, have a clean and healthy snack.

>> **Take chromium supplements to help you get rid of the sugar and carb cravings.** This crave-control process can take months, but a controlled study found that chromium supplementation can significantly reduce carbohydrate craving and improve depression in women. However, many individuals need as many as 1,000 micrograms of supplemental chromium daily to achieve this effect. Fortunately, chromium supplementation is very safe; the Environmental Protection Agency (EPA) says that 70,000 micrograms daily is the upper limit.

>> **Have a small portion of the food you're craving, especially when you're just starting your new lifestyle.** Have a few spoonfuls of that ice cream you love rather than a bowlful and then distract yourself by partaking in a pleasant activity, such as a walk or a game. By satisfying the craving in small ways, you can head off a larger binge later.

>> **Stick with your eating clean plan and feel your cravings diminish.** When you eat clean, whole foods, you feel better and stronger and have more energy. Compare these feelings to the feelings you have after bingeing on chocolate candy or a fat-laden, heavy fast-food meal. You don't need much more motivation to stay the course!

>> **Cravings intensify when you think you're hungry, but you may just be thirsty or tired.** Have a drink of water, brush your teeth, and go to bed!

Dealing with deprivation

Human beings are complex creatures who are trained to respond to emotions by eating. When babies get hungry, they feel uncomfortable and cry; the parent responds with food and cuddles. You don't have to be a rocket scientist to see the connection that can build up between love, comfort, and food.

When you eliminate the foods you've relied on for comfort throughout your life, you're naturally going to feel deprived at first. Several factors cause feelings of deprivation, and, fortunately, you can address all of them with a clean eating plan. Chapter 4 of Book 5 discusses emotional eating and eating because of cues other than hunger, but you can feel deprived for other reasons, too.

The following list describes some of the reasons why you may feel deprived when you first start your eating clean plan and offers some tips for how to deal with those feelings:

>> **You don't consume enough calories.** Because you're eating more whole foods, more foods with fewer calories, and more fiber, you may not be getting enough calories, especially if you live a very active lifestyle. Unless you're

obese and continue to gain weight, consider adding more high-calorie foods to your diet, especially foods high in protein and good fats, such as lean meats, cheeses, and nuts.

>> **You eat a bland diet.** Make sure to season your food well (but not with salt!) and use condiments, herbs, and spices to keep the food interesting. Experiment with recipes from different ethnic cuisines and don't be afraid to try new foods to spice up your plate.

>> **You miss foods you're used to eating.** If you're used to eating lots of chips and dip, you don't have to eliminate those types of foods completely. Think of ways to incorporate the same flavors and textures by using clean foods. Instead of eating processed chips with a luridly orange artificially flavored cheese dip, make some kale chips and eat them with a spiced edamame dip. Instead of eating chocolate chip cookies, have a small bar of dark chocolate, maybe chopped and sprinkled over yogurt flavored with fresh fruit.

>> **You focus too much on food.** Food is only part of your life. Yes, you do need to eat to stay alive. But if food occupies most of your consciousness, think of ways to make it a smaller part of your life. Try to add more interest and stimulation to your daily routine. Take up a hobby. Learn something new. Make new friends and interact with other people in your life.

REMEMBER

Don't forget to be kind to yourself! You're attempting a complete life makeover, which is an honorable and responsible thing to do. Just trying something new can be very rewarding. Think about how you're really feeling and try to address emotional issues honestly without burying them in food.

Understand that you're not going to stick perfectly to this plan and resolve to enjoy the process. If you can involve your family in this new lifestyle, all the better. By getting your family and friends involved, you create a built-in support system with people who will support you in your journey to improve your life.

REMEMBER

Learn to trust your body's signals. A feeling of deprivation means your brain is trying to tell you that something isn't right. Whether you're dealing with stress or you have unresolved emotional issues, numbing yourself with food isn't the answer. Listen to your body and try different ways to soothe and tame bad feelings. Food is only the solution to hunger — nothing else.

Living with lapses and backsliding

One guarantee in any diet or lifestyle change is that you will fall off the wagon. No one can eat a perfect diet forever. Life is full of too many temptations. So accept that you won't eat clean 100 percent of the rest of your life and figure out how to deal with your lapses.

DO CRAVINGS SIGNAL NUTRIENT DEFICIENCIES?

Some people think that cravings are a sign that you're deficient in the nutrient that the food you crave provides. This theory may have some truth to it, but the types of foods that people crave usually aren't nutrient dense; they're full of sugar, fat, and salt. And you likely aren't deficient in any of those food components. Rather, if you crave sweets or chocolate, you may be deficient in nutrients like the vitamin B complex, chromium, zinc, and magnesium. But eating a chocolate bar isn't a good way to satisfy this deficiency because it contains only about 50 mg of magnesium; the recommended daily allowance (RDA) for that mineral is at least 300 mg per day. Snacking on foods like nuts, seeds, and legumes provides more of the needed minerals and other nutrients along with fiber and protein.

One real biological craving, called *pica,* is when people who are deficient in iron or other minerals crave nonnutritive things like soil, flour, raw rice, and chalk. After they fix their iron deficiency, those cravings subside. So you can't blame your craving for double chocolate chip ice cream on a calcium deficiency!

TIP

To deal with lapses and missteps, try these ideas:

>> **Build lapses and breaks into your eating plan.** Aim to eat clean 50 to 70 percent of the time, especially when you're first getting started. In other words, let yourself have a few potato chips or a reasonable serving of ice cream occasionally. By doing so, you curb feelings of deprivation, which can cause backsliding. Plus, if you know that you can have a treat later in the day, you'll be more likely to pass up that tray of baked goodies at lunch.

>> **Set aside some fairly clean foods that are better for you than the typical junk food.** For instance, if you really enjoy a creamy, cold, sweet bowl of ice cream, sweeten some yogurt with agave nectar and fruit and freeze it for a clean treat. You have infinite possibilities for creatively satisfying cravings without reverting to old bad habits.

>> **Recognize that you strayed from your clean eating plan and get back on track.** Many people simply give up when they give in to the cravings for junk food or sweets. Don't give up! Just resume your clean eating plan. Try to recognize what event or emotion triggered your lapse and write about it in a food journal (see Chapter 4 in Book 5 for details). Then think of ways to deal with that issue instead of turning to junk food.

REMEMBER

After you've been on the clean eating plan for a month or two, you'll find that eating a clean diet is actually more satisfying than eating your old diet ever was. You'll feel better and have more energy. Just as you can get stuck in a vicious downward spiral of eating and craving junk, you can achieve a healthy upward spiral of eating and craving clean!

Chapter **3**

Nutrition Basics: You Really Are What You Eat

Everyone has heard the phrase "you are what you eat," but did you know that it's literally true? Your body uses everything you put into it for some particular purpose: It uses proteins to build muscles and repair injuries; carbohydrates to create energy; fats to make cell membranes supple and to lubricate joints; and vitamins and minerals to keep your cells alive and healthy.

Getting the right amounts and combinations of these nutrients isn't easy. But the eating clean diet is one of the best ways to achieve the perfect balance of nutrients, calories, and taste. After all, whole foods automatically provide more nutrients, especially micronutrients, than any supplemented or enhanced processed food. This chapter looks at what your body needs to perform at its peak capacity. You find out how your body uses food, and you look at what your body doesn't need. This chapter also breaks down the roles of proteins, carbohydrates, fats, vitamins, and minerals, and explains how your body uses them. Finally, you get the low-down on your body's fiber and water needs.

Figuring Out What Your Body Needs (And What It Doesn't Need)

Without food, you would die. How long you could survive depends on your fat stores and overall health, but most people can only survive for a few months without food.

Consider this: Your body is an amazing machine. It efficiently extracts nutrients from the food you eat, processes that food, storing essential nutrients to ensure survival over a long period of time, and heals itself by using the nutrients it gets from food. The following sections look at how your body uses food, what happens when you take in more calories than you need, and what happens when you don't get the nutrients essential to good health.

How your body uses food

Your body's digestive system breaks down everything you put into your mouth and then uses what the body needs for basic functions.

Your digestive tract includes your mouth, esophagus, stomach, intestines, rectum, and anus. Your mouth starts breaking down food, and your esophagus takes the food to your stomach, which breaks it down further. The intestines further digest and absorb nutrients, and the rectum and anus dispose of the solid material you don't need.

Other organs in the digestive tract include the liver, gallbladder, and pancreas. The liver produces bile (which is stored in the gallbladder) to aid in your body's digestion, particularly of fats and oils. The liver itself starts the process of "reassembling" fully digested food into a form useful to the human system, and it processes toxins for disposal. The pancreas produces digestive enzymes that work on fats and carbohydrates, as well as on the proteins that the stomach hasn't completely digested. A complex system of nerves, blood vessels, enzymes, and hormones keeps everything working smoothly.

From one end to the other

Here's a step-by-step look at how your body uses food:

>> **Your mouth starts the digestive process.** Your teeth break down the food you eat, and digestive enzymes from your salivary glands start to break down starch. You swallow, thus moving the food through the esophagus. Although the action of swallowing is voluntary and you control it, you give up control as

the food starts moving down the esophagus. From that point on, nerves and muscles control the food's path.

>> **Your stomach is the food's next stop.** A normal stomach, when empty, has a very acidic pH of 1.5 to 3.5, which makes sense because it produces hydrochloric acid (HCl) to digest your food. Depending on its dilution, hydrochloric acid can have a pH from 0 or below to 3.0. (At those concentrations, it can burn through your clothes in seconds!) With the aid of *pepsin,* a protein-digesting enzyme produced almost exclusively in the stomach, your stomach starts processing protein and, to some extent, fats, carbohydrates, and fiber. Your stomach contracts to mechanically break down the food and mix it with pepsin. The stomach's muscle movements also move the food into the small intestine.

>> **Your small intestine continues the digestive process.** Enzymes from the pancreas and bile from the liver and gallbladder enter the small intestine to digest the food as it leaves the stomach.

The small intestine absorbs many nutrients through small fingerlike projections called *villi* and even smaller projections called *microvilli.* These projections increase the surface area of the intestine so that your body can quickly and efficiently absorb nutrients into the bloodstream. Any food that your body can't digest in the small intestine goes onto the large intestine.

>> **The blood that has absorbed nutrients from your small intestine goes to the liver.** The liver acts as a processing plant by filtering out harmful toxins. It then reassembles some of the digested nutrients and passes them on to the rest of your body, where your cells use them for energy and tissue repair and replacement.

>> **Your large intestine is the final step on the digestive journey.** Fiber, water, bacteria, and other foods your body can't or won't digest travel through the large intestine, which is your body's last chance to retrieve nutrients from the food you ate. Your body expels whatever's left.

The macronutrients of food

REMEMBER

The three main components, or *macronutrients,* that make up food are carbohydrates, proteins, and fats (including oils). Your body uses each component in different ways. (For more about these nutrients, see the later section "Considering the Roles of Proteins, Carbs, and Fats.")

>> **Carbohydrates:** Your body uses carbohydrates for energy. It breaks them down into individual sugars, which your cells then transform into energy. A very small proportion of the carbohydrates you consume aren't used for energy.

>> **Proteins:** Your body uses proteins for repair and muscle function. It breaks them down into amino acids, which the body then uses to repair cells, improve muscle function, and make certain hormones that originate from cholesterol, neurotransmitters, and enzymes.

>> **Fats:** Fats are an essential component in every diet because they provide your body with energy, heat, and essential fatty acids. Plus, your body stores fat to fight against future starvation.

Your body uses vitamins and minerals to process macronutrients and to regulate growth and metabolism. These substances promote health by increasing efficiency of cell repair and production. They also prevent illness and keep your body running at maximum efficiency. (See the later section "Getting the Vitamins and Minerals You Need to Stay Healthy" for more details.)

What happens to additives and chemicals

Eating processed foods means consuming preservatives, additives, and artificial ingredients. What happens to these chemicals? How does your body process them?

WARNING

Put bluntly, your body isn't designed to process and incorporate preservatives, additives, stabilizers, and other artificial ingredients. Because many of these ingredients are fat–soluble, your body stores them in its fat instead of using them for energy or cell repair. Unfortunately, however, they don't just sit benignly in your body's fat. They can change cell structure and metabolize. Some even become carcinogens, which can, over time, cause cancer.

Here are just some of the artificial ingredients used in processed foods, along with a quick summary of what happens to them after they enter the body:

>> **Antibiotics:** Farmers feed many animals, particularly poultry and pigs, antibiotics to reduce the death rate from infection, which occurs in very crowded conditions, and to enhance growth and weight gain. The residues of these chemicals remain in the processed meat that humans eat. Overuse of antibiotics creates super bacteria that evolve to resist every antibiotic, which, as you can imagine, isn't good for the human population. Unfortunately, consuming small amounts of antibiotics in food is the best way to help these superbugs evolve. Antibiotic-resistant bacteria are becoming a huge problem in the medical field. There may come a day when a simple cut or scrape could lead to a life-threatening infection that is no longer treatable.

>> **Aspartame:** This artificial sweetener becomes a neurotransmitter during digestion, meaning that it can cross the blood-brain barrier. After it crosses that barrier, it can damage and kill brain cells. The body quickly processes

aspartame and breaks it down into methanol, which the body can then convert into formaldehyde. This particular conversion can cause changes in cell structure, leading to disease and chronic health conditions.

TECHNICAL STUFF

Anecdotal evidence has revealed that aspartame is a good ant poison. When this product is damp, often — but not always — ants will carry it back to the nest, and within a few days, all the ants disappear.

Aspartame accounts for more than 75 percent of the adverse reactions to food additives reported to the FDA. Many of these reactions are very serious, including seizures and death. A few of the 90 documented symptoms listed in the FDA adverse reaction reports include

- Breathing difficulties
- Depression, anxiety attacks, fatigue, and irritability
- Dizziness
- Headaches/migraines
- Hearing loss
- Heart palpitations
- Insomnia
- Joint pain
- Memory loss
- Muscle spasms
- Nausea
- Rashes
- Seizures
- Tachycardia
- Vision problems
- Weight gain

» **Caffeine:** Caffeine is a quickly processed and relatively safe psycho-active stimulant, which is why so many people consume it in the morning. It raises your blood pressure and blocks adenosine receptors in your brain, thus reducing drowsiness. It also increases dopamine production, stimulating your brain's pleasure centers and reinforcing feelings of addiction. Caffeine is a *diuretic,* which means it removes water (as well as minerals such as calcium, zinc, and magnesium) from your blood and cells. But with long-term caffeine use, this diuretic effect lessens or disappears completely.

>> **High-fructose corn syrup (HFCS):** The body partially processes this chemically concentrated sugar and stores it as fat. In fact, the body metabolizes it into fat very quickly. High-fructose corn syrup doesn't suppress the body's production of *ghrelin,* a molecule that stimulates the appetite, so your brain doesn't get the message that you've eaten enough food. Plus, the liver converts high-fructose corn syrup into triglycerides, which, when present in excess, can increase the risk of heart disease.

>> **Hormones:** Most factory farms feed hormones and *pseudo-hormones* (unnatural molecules that imperfectly mimic real human hormones) to the animals they raise for meat so that they grow bigger faster. The animals store the chemicals in their fat, which humans then eat. These hormones and pseudo-hormones can affect human growth and development. For example, too much estrogen and pseudo-estrogen increases breast and prostate cancer risk.

>> **Monosodium glutamate (MSG):** This ubiquitous additive, which is also known as *free glutamic acid,* is present in many processed foods and affects the body in many ways, including the following:

- MSG is an *excitotoxin,* which means it overstimulates and damages brain cells.

- MSG may be addictive, so you may crave foods that have MSG and eat more of them, creating a vicious cycle.

- MSG stimulates the umami taste bud, fooling your body into thinking that the food you're eating is nutritious.

- MSG changes the diameter of your blood vessels, which is why some people feel warm and develop headaches after ingesting it.

- MSG stimulates the pancreas, causing it to produce more insulin, so blood sugar levels drop and you get hungry sooner.

- MSG intake has been implicated in the development and exacerbation of diseases such as Parkinson's, multiple sclerosis, stroke, obesity, and depression.

MSG does occur naturally in meats and other foods, but it's bound up in the protein complexes of those foods and has less of an effect than the added MSG.

>> **Nitrates and nitrites:** These chemicals are used in processed meats such as hot dogs and bacon. They can bind with *hemoglobin,* the molecule in your blood that carries oxygen throughout your body, thus causing dizziness, headaches, and rapid heartbeat. Your liver converts nitrates into *nitrosamines,* which are carcinogenic in animals and probably humans, too. Nitrites are carcinogenic in humans.

» **Olestra:** You find this artificial fat in snack foods. At first, snack-food manufacturers touted olestra as a simple way to lose weight because the body doesn't digest it, meaning that it travels right through the body. Unfortunately, this indigestible property causes some severe and unpleasant physical reactions, which can keep you chained to the bathroom. Plus, the fake fat binds to fat-soluble vitamins your body needs and takes them right out of your body.

» **Trans fats:** These fake fats, made by hydrogenating polyunsaturated fats such as corn oil, are one of the most dangerous artificial ingredients. They raise your risk of heart attack, stroke, diabetes, high blood pressure, and cancer.

WARNING

Because your body doesn't recognize that trans fats are artificial, they become part of your cell membranes, making the cells weaker. Consuming trans fats increases the level of LDL cholesterol (the bad stuff) in your blood. Your body easily stores trans fats but can't easily retrieve them for fuel, so they cause weight gain.

Keep in mind that the FDA says most of these ingredients are safe for human consumption, at least in tiny amounts. (A big change on the regulation of trans fats happened in 2015.) After all, some of them do help preserve food, keeping it safe for long storage periods and long transit times from the factory to the grocery store. But knowing what you know now, you can be the judge of what you want to ingest. Just remember that whole foods don't need artificial chemicals to stay safe, look better, or taste better.

REMEMBER

One of the best things about the eating clean plan is that you avoid processed foods, chemicals, and additives that can harm your body, and you eat whole foods, which contain all the protein, fat, carbohydrates, vitamins, and minerals that your body needs, in the correct amounts and proportions.

What happens to excess macronutrients and calories

It's too bad your body doesn't discard the excess carbs, protein, fat, and calories you consume like it discards waste, fiber, and too much liquid. Human bodies evolved to hang on to fuel simply because starvation was part of life for early humans. If you eat only once a week or once a month, your body will hold on to all the calories it can as a hedge against starvation. Of course, now that you have 24-hour supermarkets and pizza delivery, starvation is the least of your worries.

Your body is extremely efficient. It extracts and uses the energy it needs from the food you eat and converts the excess into fat, which it then stores in your body. Too many calories equal excess fat. But all calories are not equal (the laws of thermodynamics aside). After all, human bodies aren't machines made out of metal and moving parts; every body is different. For example, simple carbs and sugars trigger insulin responses in the body, which tell it to store fat. In some people, this response is very easy to trigger; as a result, a high-carbohydrate diet makes them put on weight. On the other hand, for most people, the body has to work harder to digest proteins than it does to digest carbs, which means they gain less weight on a high-protein diet.

Understanding how your body processes excess nutrients

When you consume too many carbohydrates, proteins, and fats, your body processes the excess nutrients in different ways:

>> **Carbohydrates:** The body breaks down carbohydrates into glucose, which it then uses for fuel. The body converts excess glucose into glycogen and sends it to muscles and the liver. If your body has too much glycogen, your liver converts it into fat and stores it in fat cells.

>> **Proteins:** The body processes proteins into individual amino acids and peptides, which your liver sends into your bloodstream to maintain and repair cells, and make some hormones, neurotransmitters, and enzymes. The body converts excess proteins into fat and stores it in fat cells.

>> **Fats:** The body breaks down fats into fatty acids, cholesterol, glycerol, and triglycerides in a process called *lipolysis*. Because fats are a rich source of energy, the body uses them in cell production. Oils are also fats; they contain fatty acids that the body uses in the metabolism process to keep your cells healthy and strong and to help move oxygen through your bloodstream. Some fatty acids (omega-3 and omega-6) are essential nutrients. The body stores excess fat and oil as fat (go figure!).

WARNING

You can eat too much of each of these macronutrients. For example:

>> If you consume too much protein and not enough carbohydrates, you put stress on your kidneys and throw your body into *ketosis* — when your body burns fat rather than carbs for energy. The strain on your kidneys can lead to kidney disease, kidney stones, osteoporosis, and eventually ketoacidosis, a condition that's dangerous for diabetics. In addition, too much protein can cause gout in some people. Consuming high-fructose corn syrup can induce higher levels of uric acid, which also leads to gout. Researchers are finding that higher levels of uric acid are particularly damaging to the kidneys.

>> Eating too many carbohydrates can be problematic for most people. Compared with individuals who do *not* have a genetic predisposition to type-2 diabetes (approximately two-thirds of all Americans), individuals with this genetic predisposition (the other one-third) have considerably more insulin secretion after eating the very same amount of carbohydrates. This "over-the-top" insulin secretion leads to insulin resistance. To overcome this resistance, even more insulin is secreted, which leads to even more insulin resistance. This never ending loop ultimately "crosses over" to type-2 diabetes, with its higher risk of further complications including heart disease, kidney failure, and many others.

People *without* the genetic predisposition to type-2 diabetes will still gain excess weight when they consume too many carbohydrates, but have much less chance of actually developing type-2 diabetes with all its possible complications.

>> Eating too much fat can lead to obesity, which puts strain on your organs and bones and can lead to diseases like heart disease, cancer, diabetes, and arthritis. Some people, however, can eat as much fat as they want on the Paleo diet and still lose weight, if they have a certain metabolism that predisposes them to type-2 diabetes.

REMEMBER

When you eat clean, you eat whole foods that contain good proportions of fat, carbs, protein, vitamins, minerals, and fiber. Whole foods take longer to eat and digest, which means you feel satisfied longer. As a result, you're less likely to overeat and your body's energy input and output stay in balance, keeping you at a healthy weight.

SO WHAT'S A CALORIE?

So what is this ubiquitous calorie? Here's the scientific definition: A *calorie* is the energy needed to raise the temperature of 1 cm^3 of water by 1 degree Celsius. In other words, a calorie is stored energy. Your body stores energy in the form of fat, which your body keeps in fat cells for quick access if needed. Your body converts the fat to glucose, which your cells use to create energy.

The macronutrients you consume have different numbers of calories per gram:

- Proteins have four calories per gram.
- Carbohydrates have four calories per gram.
- Fats have nine calories per gram.

Examining the connection between excess calories and weight gain

If you eat the same number of calories that you burn, your weight stays the same. If you don't take in enough calories, you lose weight. And if you eat more calories than your body burns, you gain weight. Seems pretty straightforward, right?

As with many so-called rules, you need to consider some exceptions. For instance, for people with type-2 diabetes and people whose families have a history of this disease (about 36 percent of the population), eating large amounts of proteins, fats, and oils and very few, if any, calories from carbohydrates can lead to weight loss — which is why high-protein/low-carb diets are so popular, and why those 36 percent should follow this diet for better health.

WARNING

But these diets are very acid-forming, causing your blood pH to lower and forcing your body to take calcium from bones and teeth, thus leading to the development of gout or osteoporosis. For these reasons, be sure to work with a physician who is knowledgeable in nutritional and natural medicine before you try a low-carb diet.

Each pound of fat contains 3,500 calories. To lose a pound of fat a week, you need to burn 500 more calories a day or eat 500 fewer calories a day. The number of calories you need in a day depends on your sex, age, weight, and activity level. Younger people, men, and more active people need more calories. Older people, women, and people who lead more sedentary lifestyles need fewer calories.

Your body uses calories (or energy) to

>> **Keep you alive:** Respiration, brain function, and muscle activity all require energy. Just being alive burns up a certain number of calories every day. The specific number of calories burned varies from person to person and is called your *basic metabolic rate,* or BMR. People with so-called high metabolisms usually have less efficient bodies that burn up more calories than most just to stay alive.

>> **Repair damage:** Cells in your body die every day, and your body must replace them. You need energy to make new cells. You also need energy to repair or discard cells that free radicals and oxidation damage.

>> **Keep you active:** Even sleeping and resting require energy. But if you move around, run, or exercise, your body uses more energy. You burn calories through metabolism to provide energy to your cells so you can move your muscles.

What happens if you don't get the micronutrients you need

Did you know that you can be overweight and malnourished at the same time? Overweight people don't lack access to macronutrients (proteins, carbs, and fats); they lack access to micronutrients — vitamins and minerals. A serious deficiency in some micronutrients can lead directly to disease. For example, beriberi develops when you don't get enough vitamin B1 in your diet, and scurvy can develop when you don't get enough vitamin C. A minor deficiency in micronutrients can lead to conditions such as high blood pressure, depression, and a weakened immune system.

Here are just a few things micronutrients (vitamins and minerals) do for your body:

» Help maintain a proper oxygen level in your brain

» Fight *free radicals,* which are unstable forms of oxygen that damage cells

» Keep your red blood cells healthy so that they can transport oxygen to your body's cells

» Keep your nerve cells healthy so that your body can react to stimuli and stay healthy and so that you can maintain a regular heartbeat and calm mood

» Regulate your hormone balance so that diseases such as diabetes don't develop

» Keep bones and teeth healthy by regulating calcium and phosphorus balance

» Create and maintain enzymes so that your body can digest food and transform it into energy and cell components

REMEMBER

By eating whole foods, especially fruits and vegetables, you can provide your body with the micronutrients it needs, including the micronutrients no one knows about! Scientists don't know every single micronutrient your body needs. But whole foods contain them, in just the right proportions. And organically grown foods contain even more of these nutrients.

Missing out on micronutrients hurts your body. Diseases may not develop for months or years, but they will develop. Providing your body with a constant supply of vital micronutrients is one of the best ways to get healthy and stay healthy.

Considering the Roles of Proteins, Carbs, and Fats

All food is made up of proteins, carbohydrates, and fats. These macronutrients provide energy for your body, building blocks for cell maintenance and repair, and compounds such as hormones and enzymes that help your cells function properly.

The following sections look at the composition of proteins, carbs, and fats and explain why you need all of them in your diet. You also look at what roles the macronutrients play in your body's function and find out how to find the best clean sources for each one.

Clean proteins: Amino acids, the building blocks of life

Proteins should comprise about 30 percent of your diet. (But if you have type-2 diabetes or you're overweight and type-2 diabetes runs in your family, you may need to eat more protein in a diet such as the Paleolithic diet; talk to your doctor for details.)

Proteins are made up of *amino acids*, which are individual molecules that are literally the building blocks of your body. Amino acids come in dozens of varieties. Nine of them are called *essential amino acids*, meaning that you must get them from a food source because your body can't make them — not even from other amino acids. The Protein Digestibility Corrected Amino Acid Score (PDCAAS) evaluates the quality of protein sources and the body's ability to digest them. Eggs have a score of 100 on this scale, which means they're a perfect source of protein.

As your body breaks down food, the proteins travel to the liver, which converts them into amino acids. The body uses these amino acids to build and repair tissue, provide energy, and produce enzymes, neurotransmitters, and certain hormones. If you don't eat enough protein, your body will start to break down the protein in your muscles to use for cell repair and other functions. You don't need to combine proteins at every meal, but you should try to combine proteins over a week.

Most Americans get more than enough protein. Unless you're an elderly person who doesn't eat enough or you have a special dietary need, or you have significant low stomach acid and don't digest enough protein into enough amino acids, you don't need protein supplements or shakes to get the protein your body requires. And people with hidden gluten sensitivity don't absorb enough amino acids for good health. Clean protein comes from meats, dairy, eggs, and whole foods such as whole grains, legumes, nuts, seeds, and beans. On the clean eating plan, you consume the right amount of good-quality protein.

Complete proteins: Everything you need

Some foods contain *complete proteins*, which are proteins that contain all nine essential amino acids. These foods include

» Meat, such as beef, chicken, fish, lamb, pork, and shellfish

» Dairy products, such as cheese, milk, and yogurt

» Quinoa, soybeans, and amaranth, which are complete proteins that may have a score of less than 100 on the PDCAAS

» Eggs, which are an excellent source of protein, in terms of both value and digestibility

TIP

If you eat these protein sources, you don't have to worry about whether you're getting enough protein because you definitely are. But if you eat a vegetarian or vegan diet, eating the right kind of protein is something you need to think about. This is easy to remember: Just eat all the plant foods available to you, including vegetables, fruits, nuts, seeds, and legumes.

Incomplete proteins: Combining to get what you need

Foods that don't contain all nine essential proteins are called *incomplete proteins*. If you don't eat enough complete proteins, you need to combine different incomplete proteins (making them *complementary proteins*) to get the essential amino acids your body needs. Here are the incomplete proteins you need to eat:

» **Grains and legumes:** Eat a meal of vegetarian lentil soup with whole-grain bread or a meal of beans with rice.

» **Grains and nuts or seeds:** Consume whole-grain breads with almond or peanut butter.

» **Legumes and nuts or seeds:** Eat chickpeas with walnuts, blended together into hummus.

Carbohydrates: Energy for your body

You hear a lot of buzz about carbohydrates (or *carbs*, as they're often called) in the media these days. Proponents of high-protein diets claim that carbs are bad for you. Well, eating too much of any one food component is bad for you, but carbohydrates in and of themselves aren't bad. In fact, carbohydrates should comprise about 40 to 50 percent of your diet (less if you're concerned about type-2 diabetes and should follow the Paleo diet plan).

Carbohydrates come in two types: complex and simple. *Complex carbohydrates* are the kind you want to include in your diet. They're long chains made up of *simple carbohydrates* (or sugars), such as glucose, sucrose, lactose, and fructose.

You find complex carbohydrates in the following foods:

» Whole grains, such as wheat, barley, buckwheat, oats, quinoa, brown rice, wild rice, and amaranth

» Vegetables, such as carrots, potatoes, corn, cabbage, asparagus, cauliflower, dark greens, zucchini, broccoli, celery, cucumbers, garlic, and onions

» Fruits, such as apples, grapefruit, pears, strawberries, plums, oranges, berries, and dried fruits

» Legumes, such as pinto beans, chickpeas, lentils, kidney beans, and split peas

Focus on these foods when you're planning the carbohydrate part of your diet. Because they've been minimally processed (and fit into the eating clean lifestyle!), they offer more to your body than simple carbohydrates. For example, complex carbohydrates provide fiber, vitamin B, and minerals, such as iron, magnesium, and selenium. Plus, your body digests them slowly, which can help stabilize your blood sugar levels. Fortunately, whole foods included in the clean eating plan contain lots of complex carbohydrates.

Unlike complex carbohydrates, simple carbohydrates raise blood sugar quickly and provide instant energy, especially in those genetically pre-disposed to type-2 diabetes. However, the quick spike of energy you get from foods with simple carbs soon leads to a slump in blood glucose, which means you get hungry quickly, your mood drops, and your energy lags. Foods that contain simple carbohydrates include the following:

» Table sugar

» Corn syrup and other syrups

» Fruit juices

» Candy

» Sweetened beverages such as pop and soda

» White rice and pasta

» Baked goods made with white sugar and white flour

» Sweetened processed cereals

REMEMBER

Always read the labels on food packages! Foods high in simple carbs are usually also highly processed and contain additives and preservatives (which means you need to avoid them if you're eating clean). Be sure to avoid any product that contains added simple carb ingredients such as glucose, fructose, dextrin, maltodextrin, galactose, maltose, or anything with the suffix *-ose*.

Although complex carbohydrates are made up of chains of simple carbohydrates, the foods that contain complex carbohydrates also have fiber and lots of vitamins and minerals. You don't find fiber, B vitamins, and potassium in a lemon drop! But you do find those nutrients in a slice of whole-wheat bread.

Essential and clean fats

Fats are the third macronutrient in food. Despite the popularity of low-fat diets, you need to incorporate essential fats (omega-3 and omega-6 fatty acids) into your daily diet. In fact, fat should comprise about 30 percent of your diet. Many nutritionists recommend eating a diet higher in protein, higher in fat, and lower in carbs.

Fats provide the following benefits to your body:

>> Provide insulation and padding for your organs and skeletal system

>> Aid in metabolism and become part of your cellular structures

>> Aid in growth and reproduction

>> Allow the fat-soluble vitamins (A, D, E, and K) to travel through your body

But the type of fat you eat is important. You need to avoid trans fats and restrict the amount of saturated fats you eat (the following section explains why). To get the most benefits from the fats you eat, stick with the clean fats you find in foods such as nuts, avocados, olive oil, fatty seafood, and seeds.

Taking a look at what fats are made of

Fats consist of chains of fatty acids and glycerol. The fatty acids have long chains of carbon atoms bound to hydrogen atoms. They're classified according to the number of hydrogen atoms attached to the carbon atoms. If a fat is missing a hydrogen atom, it uses a double bond to join two carbon atoms and to replace the hydrogen atom.

The three kinds of fats are

>> **Saturated fats:** When all the carbon atoms in the fatty acid chain are paired with hydrogen atoms, the fat is *saturated*. Saturated fats are solid at room temperature. They include butter, hydrogenated shortening (note the name — hydrogen is added to oil to make it solid), and animal fats.

>> **Monounsaturated fats:** These fats have one double bond in their fatty acid chain. They're liquid at room temperature. Monounsaturated fats occur in avocados, olives, coconuts, and nuts, especially macadamia nuts. These stable fats are the best for your health.

>> **Polyunsaturated fats:** These fats have two or more double bonds in their fatty acid structures. They're liquid at room temperature. Polyunsaturated fats come from vegetable sources and include sunflower, safflower, and corn oil. (Canola oil is also polyunsaturated, but you should avoid eating it because it comes from a genetically modified, or GMO, plant.) The problem with polyunsaturated fats is that they're unstable and can easily oxidize, causing inflammation in the body.

Getting more omega-3s and fewer omega-6s

Like the essential amino acids that are so important to your body's health, essential fatty acids play an important role in your body. Essential fatty acids consist of a straight chain of hydrocarbons with a carboxyl group on one end. They're classified by their length and by where the double bond, which is a bond between carbon atoms in molecules, exists in their chain:

>> *Omega-3 fatty acids* have the double bond in the number 3 position and include alpha-linolenic acid (ALA), eicosapentaenoic acid (EPA), and docosahexaenoic acid (DHA).

>> *Omega-6 fatty acids* have the double bond in the number 6 position and include linolenic acid (LA) and gamma-linolenic acid (GLA).

You must consume these nutrients in the food you eat because your body can't make them on its own. Your body can manufacture omega-9 (with the double bond in the number 9 position) as long as you consume enough omega-3 and omega-6 fatty acids. You need to keep these different fatty acids straight because the ratio of fatty acids in your diet is crucial to good health. Fatty acids play a role in the following bodily processes:

>> Functioning of the central nervous system — brain, nerve endings, and spinal column — which can help prevent depression and other mental problems

>> Production of hormones called *eicosanoids,* which monitor and regulate the activity of your cells

>> Regulation of insulin sensitivity, which can help prevent diabetes

>> Production of prostaglandins, which regulate your heart beat, blood pressure, clotting, and immune system

>> Increasing HDL cholesterol (the good stuff) and reducing LDL cholesterol (the bad stuff) in your blood

REMEMBER

The tricky part about fatty acids is that the ratio of omega-3s to omega-6s in your diet plays a critical role in your health. Nutritionists say that you should consume these two fatty acids in a ratio from 1:1 to 1:4 (omega-3s:omega-6s). But most American diets consist of foods that place the omega-3s:omega-6s ratio at 1:25. This unbalanced ratio may be a prime cause of many of the diseases that affect today's population.

In ancient times, the Paleolithic men and women ate a diet that included meats and fish, both of which are high in omega-3 fatty acids. Even though their lifespans were shorter (roaming wild animals and no antibiotics certainly played a part in this fact), they had fewer diseases like heart disease and cancer.

As civilization developed, grains, such as corn and wheat, became the basis of much of the human diet. Even the animals humans use for meat today are fed corn and wheat rather than the grasses they eat naturally. And guess what? Those foods are higher in omega-6 fatty acids. The modern diet of processed foods, especially highly refined carbohydrates, is messing with the essential fatty acid ratio necessary for good health.

WARNING

If you consume too many omega-6s in relation to omega-3s, your body develops inflammation much more quickly and easily. When you consume too many omega-6s, your body breaks them down into compounds that destroy proteins and promote inflammation.

The foods that are higher in omega-3 fatty acids include

>> Fatty fish, including salmon, tuna, krill, and mackerel

>> Seeds, such as flaxseed and sesame seeds

>> Nuts, such as walnuts, Brazil nuts, and pistachios

>> Dark-green vegetables, including broccoli, collard greens, and spinach

>> Legumes, such as kidney beans and navy beans

The foods that are higher in omega-6 fatty acids include

>> Refined vegetable oils, including corn, soybean, and cottonseed oil

>> Meats from animals fed a diet high in corn and wheat

>> Foods cooked in vegetable oils

>> Processed foods, including commercially fried foods and frozen foods

>> Fast foods

TIP

When choosing the types of fats you consume, try to include more foods rich in omega-3 fatty acids. (The American diet is rich in omega-6 fatty acids, so you don't have to worry about not getting enough of that particular type of fat.) To get enough omega-3 fatty acids, many people consume fish oil supplements. But if you follow the eating clean diet plan, you'll automatically reduce your intake of many of the foods high in omega-6 fatty acids and increase your intake of omega-3s. As a side note, older men should avoid consuming too much flaxseed because excess omega-3 fatty acids from plant sources (not from fish) can increase the risk of prostate cancer.

Getting the Vitamins and Minerals You Need to Stay Healthy

The right amount of carbohydrates, fats, and proteins keeps your body running and helps it repair cells. But how exactly do they do so? The answer is vitamins and minerals. Where macronutrients are the fuel your body needs to work properly, micronutrients (that is, vitamins and minerals) are the workers that help your metabolism go.

Your body can't manufacture vitamins or minerals, so you need to get them in the foods you consume. Eating whole foods is the perfect way to get just the right amount of these valuable micronutrients.

The following sections look at what role vitamins and minerals play in your body, which are important to good health, the recommended daily allowance (RDA) for each, and which foods are the richest in these micronutrients.

Recommended daily allowances and reference intakes

The government has set minimum amounts of nutrients you need every day to prevent disease; these amounts are called *recommended daily allowances* (RDAs). The government established these numbers during World War II when the government found that many recruits for the army and navy were malnourished. You see RDA numbers on the labels of supplements and on many foods.

Another important nutrient-related number, or set of numbers, is the *DRI*, which stands for *dietary reference intakes.* The National Academy of Sciences developed the DRI in 1997 to address some nutritional concerns, such as the amount of non-essential nutrients everyone needs to consume and the safe upper limits of supplements. The Department of Agriculture is currently reviewing the DRI to see whether it should replace the RDA. The DRI includes the following four numbers:

>> **Recommended daily allowance (RDA):** The amount of nutrients that 98 percent of healthy adults need to meet their dietary needs

>> **Adequate intake (AI):** The recommended daily amount of nutrients that have no established RDA

>> **Tolerable upper levels (UL):** The maximum amount of nutrients (such as fat-soluble vitamins) that can be harmful when taken in large doses

>> **Estimated average requirement (EAR):** The amount of nutrients that meets the needs of 50 percent of a population

Don't worry if you're not much for numbers. Unless you're a dietician, you really don't need to know any of these terms except the RDA. Just remember that the RDA values are set at a minimum value necessary to prevent diseases, including scurvy and rickets. For optimum health, you probably need more than the RDA in many circumstances. Check with a physician skilled and knowledgeable in natural medicine if you're uncertain. Also, the RDA values are set for healthy adults. If you're ill, you need more vitamins.

REMEMBER The best way to get plenty of nutrients is, of course, to eat whole foods in a good variety. But you may want to supplement your diet with vitamins and minerals. In that case, you also need to know the UL values so that you don't get sick from vitamin or mineral overdose.

The role of vitamins

Vitamins play a key role in metabolism: They assist the enzymes that break down the macronutrients you eat so that your body can use them. They also assist in building new molecules in our bodies. Without vitamins, you would die. And although a lack of vitamins can cause disease, too many of some types of vitamins can also be harmful to your health.

The two kinds of vitamins are water-soluble and fat-soluble. Each type plays a different role in metabolism, growth, and repair. The following sections explain these two types of vitamins in more detail.

REMEMBER

Regardless of which type of vitamins you consume, try to get as many of them as you can through whole foods because they're the most *bioavailable* (or most easily absorbed) in that form. Supplements can be a good idea, but look for natural, not synthetic, supplements to avoid chemicals, colorings, and preservatives.

Note: Vitamins are present in whole foods and vegetables in very small amounts, but these small amounts are crucial to good health. They're measured in milligrams (mg; 1/1,000 of a gram), micrograms (mcg; 1/1,000,000 of a gram), or International Units (IU). An IU is the amount of a vitamin that produces a biological effect.

Water-soluble vitamins

You find *water-soluble vitamins* in plants and animals. Your body doesn't store them, so you must consume them in one form or another every day. They include

>> **Vitamin C:** You find this vitamin, which is also called *ascorbic acid,* in citrus fruits and other fresh fruits and vegetables. You should consume a minimum of 45 mg of vitamin C every day to prevent *scurvy,* a vitamin-deficiency disease that results in weakness, rough skin, paleness, and bleeding gums. Your body uses vitamin C to produce *collagen,* a connective tissue that's found throughout your body in skin, bones, muscles, tendons, and blood vessels. Vitamin C helps speed up wound healing and acts as an antioxidant against free radicals that can cause cancer, stroke, and heart disease. It also helps detoxify.

REMEMBER

Textbooks of genetics and pediatrics often point out that the human need for vitamin C results from a genetic defect we all share. Check with a doctor skilled and knowledgeable in natural medicine for a recommendation about what amount of vitamin C is best for optimal health for you.

>> **B-complex vitamins:** This collection of vitamins includes B1, B2, B3, B5, B6, B12, folate, and biotin. You find these vitamins in fish, meat, poultry, fresh vegetables, and whole grains — just the foods you eat on the clean eating plan! Your body uses B-complex vitamins to metabolize carbohydrates, proteins, and

fats so that your organs can run properly. These vitamins are particularly important to the health of your brain, heart, liver, and kidneys. They also help form healthy blood cells, minimize the risk of depression, and prevent birth defects. The amount of B vitamins you need varies throughout life.

Your body uses B-complex vitamins quickly when you're ill or under stress, so you need to make sure you get enough of them on a daily basis. Deficiency in vitamin B3 (niacin) causes *pellagra,* which manifests as skin lesions, weakness, confusion, and sensitivity to sunlight. Deficiency in vitamin B1 (thiamine) contributes to *beriberi,* which can cause heart failure.

TIP

Water-soluble vitamins are sensitive to light and heat. So look for vitamin containers that are dark colored and store your vitamins in a cool, dark place. Also try to consume uncooked foods that are high in these vitamins.

Fat-soluble vitamins

You find *fat-soluble vitamins* in fruits and vegetables, dairy products, nuts, and meats. Your body can store these vitamins in your fat cells and your liver, and they need fat to carry them to your intestine, where they're absorbed. You can skip a day or two with these vitamins, but for the best health, try to consume some fat-soluble vitamins every day. The fat-soluble vitamins include

>> **Vitamin A:** You find a precursor to this vitamin in brightly colored fruits and vegetables, such as sweet potatoes, cantaloupe, and carrots. But you find actual vitamin A in beef liver, fortified dairy products, cheese, and eggs. Vitamin A helps protect your eyesight and keeps your gastrointestinal tract running smoothly. It also aids in bone and tooth strength and growth, and promotes estrogen production in women and testosterone in men. You need a minimum of 4,000 to 5,000 IU of vitamin A every day. More than this amount is often useful to reduce the chances of catching a cold or the flu. Check with a physician skilled and knowledgeable in nutritional medicine about what might be good for you.

>> **Vitamin D:** This vitamin is often added to dairy products, and you find it in oily fish and eggs (though the amount in eggs is very small). It's also called the *sunshine vitamin* because your body produces a vitamin D precursor in your skin when it's exposed to sunlight (without sunscreen). Vitamin D helps keep your bones and teeth strong and helps your body absorb calcium and phosphorus, two essential minerals. If you don't get enough vitamin D, you can develop *rickets,* a disease in which your bones become fragile and bend. Research in the last two decades has found that vitamin D also reduces risk of breast, prostate, and colon cancers. Research has also found that higher levels of vitamin D are associated with lower risks of dying of anything (technically called *all-cause mortality*) with the exception of trauma.

The best way to get vitamin D is to get some sun exposure every day. In climates where getting plenty of sun exposure isn't possible, take a supplement every day. For the best health, children need a minimum of 800 to 1,000 IU daily, and adults need a minimum of 2,000 to 3,000 IU daily. Check with a physician skilled and knowledgeable in natural medicine to determine what amount is best for you.

>> **Vitamin E:** You find this vitamin in dark leafy greens and vegetables, nuts, whole grains, butter, eggs, and beef liver. Vitamin E helps protect the other vitamins and fatty acids from oxidation and free radicals. As an antioxidant, it's important to cell health. You need a minimum of 10 to 15 IU of vitamin E every day, but in many cases, 100 IU or more is best for optimal health. In fact, many physicians skilled in natural and nutritional medicine recommend 300 to 400 IU daily. Talk to your doctor about how much vitamin E is right for you.

TIP

Vitamin E is actually four very similar molecules, termed alpha-, beta-, delta-, and gamma-tocopherols. When together in a supplement (as they are in nature), they're collectively called *mixed tocopherols* and should always be taken together. Research shows that taking alpha-tocopherol alone can actually increase certain health risks.

>> **Vitamin K:** Vitamin K has two natural types: K1 and K2. K2 has several subtypes, the best known at present being MK4 and MK7. You get all the natural types of vitamin K by eating leafy dark-green vegetables, and you find both vitamins K1 and K2 in beef liver. Friendly bacteria in your intestine makes one type of vitamin K2, and you find another form of vitamin K2 in meat and animal protein. Vitamin K is essential to efficient blood clotting and strong bones. Without enough vitamin K, you'll bruise easily and bleed profusely when your skin is cut, and in extreme cases, you can hemorrhage to death. You need a minimum of 80 mcg of vitamin K every day.

The role of minerals

When nutritionists talk about *minerals*, they don't mean chunks of iron or rock salt. They mean the chemical elements, or micronutrients, that are necessary to support a healthy body. Minerals support the biochemical processes of life: metabolism, enzymatic and hormone activity, and cell production.

The following sections look at which minerals you need to incorporate into your daily diet, what each one does, and what can happen if you don't get enough of them.

Identifying the minerals your body needs

The amount of most minerals you need every day is very small. Even so, getting minerals in proper amounts is essential for good health. And just like with vitamins, clean, whole foods are the best way to get the right amount and proportion of the essential minerals.

The government has established an RDA for 14 essential minerals, which include calcium, phosphorus, and magnesium. Here's what you need to know about these key essential minerals (*mg* stands for milligrams):

>> **Calcium:** You find calcium in dairy products, canned fish with bones, nuts, seeds, and leafy green vegetables. Some processed foods (such as orange juice) are fortified with calcium. You need about 1,000 to 1,300 mg of this mineral every day. Children, nursing mothers, and pregnant women need more. Calcium deficiency can be serious, leading to heart arrhythmia, bones more likely to fracture, and muscle spasms.

>> **Phosphorus:** Phosphorus plays a critical part in life because it's a component of your DNA. You find phosphorus in most foods simply because it's so essential, but dairy products, fish, and meats are especially good sources. This mineral helps build and maintain strong bones and teeth and is essential for a strong metabolism. The molecule your cells use to get energy is called adenosine triphosphate (ATP), and your body uses phosphorus to make it. The RDA for phosphorus ranges from 700 mg for most adults to 1,200 mg for children and teenagers.

WARNING

One troubling source of phosphorus is soft drinks. Phosphoric acid in those sweet beverages can reduce calcium levels in your blood, leading to weakened bones and teeth. So don't get most of your liquid intake from soft drinks!

>> **Magnesium:** You find magnesium in green vegetables (because magnesium is present in chlorophyll, which makes plants green) and in nuts, cocoa, and soybeans. Magnesium plays a part in the production of ATP (the energy molecule described in the preceding bullet) and many aspects of metabolism. It also helps keep your bones strong, dilates blood vessels, helps prevent muscle spasms, and has many other functions. You need about 400 mg of magnesium a day.

>> **Potassium and sodium:** These electrolytes are closely linked. In fact, many Americans get too much sodium and not enough potassium because of a diet high in processed foods. Nutritionists think that the main problem with sodium intake isn't that people consume too much; it's that they don't get enough potassium. Eating whole foods is the best way to achieve a good sodium/potassium balance.

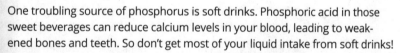

Nutrition Basics: You Really Are What You Eat

Potassium helps the muscles contract and plays a major role in nerve transmission. It also helps maintain the body's pH balance and controls blood pressure. Consuming more potassium can help counteract the effects of too much sodium. You find potassium in fresh vegetables and fruits (particularly in their skins). Especially good sources of potassium include raisins and dates, bananas, sweet and russet potatoes, and white beans.

Sodium also plays a part in muscle contraction and nerve transmission, and it keeps your body's fluid level constant and helps your body absorb nutrients. Too much sodium can increase the amount of fluid in your body, which puts strain on your heart muscle and blood vessels. Some people are more sensitive to sodium consumption than others.

>> **Chloride:** Your body uses this mineral to produce the hydrochloric acid your stomach needs to digest food. Cells also use chloride to obtain energy from the macronutrients you consume. You need about 2,300 mg of chloride daily. Table salts (sodium and potassium chlorides) are the main source of this mineral. Potassium chloride is definitely preferable for those with high blood pressure. Research has shown that potassium chloride can lower blood pressure.

>> **Iron:** Iron has two sources: heme and non-heme. Good sources for heme iron include red meats, poultry, and fish. Your body absorbs heme iron more easily than it does non-heme iron, which you find in leafy green vegetables, cocoa, and dried fruits. Non-heme iron is less likely to oxidize, and because it's paired with phytochemicals in plants, the risk of free radicals is even lower. But if you get much of your iron from non-heme sources, you need to get 1.7 times more iron than if you get most of your iron from heme sources. Iron deficiencies can cause anemia, fatigue, and increased risk of infection.

Children, younger men, and menstruating women need about 15 mg of heme iron per day. Older women and men need about 10 mg of heme iron, and pregnant women need about 30 mg of heme iron every day. Your body can store iron, so overdoses of this mineral are possible, especially because iron can oxidize easily and create those nasty free radicals. The tolerable upper limit (UL) for iron is about 40 mg.

>> **Zinc:** Zinc is important for prevention of macular degeneration (the gradual loss of vision) and is essential to the production of testosterone and growth hormones. Your body also uses zinc to make enzymes that help it process and digest carbohydrates and alcohol. Low levels of zinc are often responsible for poor wound healing. The RDA for zinc is about 8 to 11 mg per day. Most foods that are high in protein are high in zinc as well: beef, poultry, and seafood. Oysters have the highest zinc content. But you also find this mineral in dairy products, beans, whole grains, and some vegetables, such as potatoes and pumpkins.

» **Chromium:** If you've seen the movie *Erin Brockovich,* you've heard of this mineral in its unhealthy form. There are two types of chromium: chromium 3, or trivalent chromium, and chromium 6, or hexavalent chromium (the bad, unhealthy stuff). Trivalent chromium is the one your body needs, and it's found in many foods. Chromium is used for metabolism of carbs, fat, and protein. It's also critical to the function and action of insulin. Adults need about 25 to 35 micrograms per day; research shows that individuals with type-2 diabetes themselves or in their families may need considerably more. Chromium is found in mushrooms, brewer's yeast, broccoli, whole grains, grapes and grape juice, beef, and garlic.

» **Copper:** Copper is used to make red blood cells, collagen, elastic tissue, adrenalin, and nerve fibers. This trace mineral regulates blood pressure and heart rhythm and acts as an antioxidant. It's also used in enzyme manufacture and function. The RDA for copper is 2 milligrams per day. Consuming more than 10 mg a day can cause serious side effects, including liver damage, nausea, and muscle pain. Copper is found in fish, legumes, nuts, lentils, soybeans, spinach, and seeds.

» **Iodine:** Iodine and iodide are both necessary for optimal body function. Iodine's best known use is in the thyroid gland for the synthesis of its many hormones. Low iodine often causes *goiter,* a term for an enlarged thyroid. Our bodies also use iodide to kill germs. Iodine is "preferred" by breast tissue, where it joins with a fat normally present there to actually kill many types of breast cancer cells. Iodine and iodide both help women maintain healthy levels of estriol, an important anticarcinogenic estrogen.

Lack of maternal iodine can lead to diminished mental capacity in infants and children. Low iodine levels can also contribute to diminished mental capacity in children and adults. Although our thyroid glands contain the most iodine, our breasts, ovaries, pituitary glands, salivary glands, and bile made by the liver contain more iodine and iodide than the rest of our bodies. Most adults need a minimum of 120 to 150 micrograms of iodine and iodide per day; pregnant and lactating women need up to 290 micrograms per day. Japan and Iceland — where considerable seaweed and fish are eaten — have the highest iodine intakes and the lowest rates of breast cancer in the world. This mineral is found in powdered kelp, which is available as a mild spice, other seaweed products, fish and other seafood, iodized salt, chard, lima beans, sesame seeds, mushrooms, garlic, and dairy products.

» **Manganese:** This trace mineral is used to form and create bone and cartilage. It's also a key element in metabolism and helps synthesize amino acids. Manganese is sometimes called the "brain mineral" because it's important for memory and brain function. You need about 3 to 5 milligrams of manganese per day. Good food sources include nuts, seeds, legumes, whole grains, bananas, oranges, and strawberries.

Low levels of manganese can lead to infertility, because our brains need it to stimulate the "releasing hormones" that ultimately lead to adequate progesterone and testosterone synthesis.

>> **Molybdenum:** Molybdenum is key to sulfur metabolism and detoxification. Because all proteins contain sulfur, that makes molybdenum very important in protein metabolism. If you have a bad reaction after eating at a salad bar or drinking certain wines, it's usually due to sulfites used as preservatives. Sometimes taking additional molybdenum can improve your sulfite metabolism enough that the reaction no longer occurs. Molybdenum also helps produce uric acid, a normal component of blood. Adults need a minimum of 45 to 50 micrograms of molybdenum every day. You can find molybdenum in whole grains, nuts, legumes, and dark leafy greens.

>> **Selenium:** Selenium acts as an antioxidant in the body and may help prevent cancer, particularly prostate cancer. Areas in the United States that have higher levels of this mineral in soil have lower cancer rates. It works with vitamin E to help prevent free radical damage to your cells and helps detoxify the body. Adults need about 55 to 60 micrograms of selenium per day. It's found in whole grains, seafood, meats, and nuts, especially Brazil nuts.

Putting clean minerals to work

Like vitamins, minerals assist your body in retrieving energy from macronutrients so that your cells can work, grow, repair themselves, and replace themselves. The minerals in plants, dairy products, and meat all come from the soil. Some nutritionists are concerned that as more and more farmers deplete their soil, the amount of minerals naturally present in these foods also decreases. After all, soil does wear out over time; unless farmers replenish it with decaying plant matter, nutrients disappear from the soil.

Artificial fertilizers, pesticides, and herbicides also take their toll on the soil. Naturally occurring bacteria in the soil convert minerals into the form that plants can use, and those bacteria don't take kindly to poisons such as pesticides. Herbicides, especially fungicides, can negatively affect the mineral content in soils. Some plants have a symbiotic relationship with fungi that helps them pull more minerals and nutrients out of the soil. When farmers use fungicides on their crops, those plants have a reduced mineral content. In fact, studies published by Dr. Linus Pauling have found that the mineral content of fruits and vegetables, from the time frame of 1940 to 1991, has decreased from 20 to 70 percent!

If you're concerned about this trend, consider taking a good multivitamin and mineral supplement, or try to buy organic foods from farms that practice sustainability. Or do both! Sustainable farms practice organic farming techniques and rely on letting fields lie fallow to keep the soil healthy. They also plant *cover crops*, such as clover, which return nutrients to the soil.

Protecting Your Health with Fiber

What is *fiber*? It's a complex carbohydrate and the part of fruits, vegetables, nuts, seeds, and whole grains that your body can't absorb or digest. If it doesn't provide any nutrients and your body can't digest it, why is fiber so important? It helps keep your digestive system running smoothly, adds bulk to stools, helps lower cholesterol levels, helps with satiety, and may help prevent against some types of cancer.

Two types of fiber exist: soluble and insoluble. Both are important to good health. The best sources of fiber are the whole foods that are central to the clean eating plan. The following sections look at the different types of clean fiber, discuss where to find them, and explain what fiber does for your body as it travels through your gastrointestinal (GI) tract.

Surveying the different types of clean fiber

The two types of fiber, which perform different functions in your body, are classified by whether they dissolve in water. Insoluble fiber doesn't dissolve in water, and soluble fiber does. Fiber is partially fermented by bacteria in your intestines, which helps maintain a good balance of healthy bacteria. It also performs other functions in the trip through your GI tract. Here's the lowdown on what the two types of fiber do:

>> **Insoluble fiber:** This type of fiber helps food and other materials move through your gastrointestinal system. It also makes going to the bathroom a bit easier. In other words, if you eat a lot of clean, fiber-rich, whole foods, you won't have a problem with constipation.

Insoluble fiber helps prevent the development of *diverticulitis* (inflammation of the small pouches in the colon that develop as you age; when these pouches become inflamed, they can harbor bacteria). It also slows the absorption of sugar into your bloodstream and helps control the acidity in your intestines. The bulk provided by insoluble fiber keeps things moving in your intestines, which may help prevent cancer.

You find this type of fiber in the bran of wheat and corn, in seeds and nuts, in other whole-grain products, and in fruit and vegetable skins. Leafy vegetables and fibrous vegetables such as green beans are also good sources of insoluble fiber.

>> **Soluble fiber:** This type of fiber dissolves in water and forms a gel material. Nutritionists now know that this type of fiber is critical to good health. It can lower blood cholesterol levels and stabilize glucose levels, which may help prevent type-2 diabetes. Soluble fiber binds with bile acids in the intestines,

removing them from your body. Your liver then makes more bile acids from the cholesterol in your blood, which reduces overall cholesterol levels. This type of fiber can also reduce inflammation and blood pressure.

Soluble fiber keeps you feeling fuller longer after a meal by slowing down the rate at which your stomach empties so that you don't want to eat again too soon. Good sources of soluble fiber include nuts, barley, fruits, vegetables, oat bran, dried legumes, and psyllium husks.

Bulking up your fiber intake

The average American consumes only about 12 grams of fiber per day. But nutritionists recommend that women eat 20 to 38 grams of fiber per day and that men eat 30 to 38 grams per day. The more calories you consume, the more fiber you should include in your diet. If you eat the recommended five servings of fruits and vegetables and six servings of whole-grain products every day, you can easily meet those fiber requirements.

Getting your fiber from processed foods is okay (check the labels to see how many grams are in a product), but eating whole grains, fruits, vegetables, legumes, nuts, and seeds is the best way to get enough fiber in your diet. In contrast, many processed foods that claim to be enriched with fiber are also high in sugar and trans fats (think those huge bran muffins sold in coffee shops). So depend on whole produce as your main fiber source.

TIP

When you increase your fiber intake be sure to also increase your water intake. Fiber works best when paired with water; water helps it move smoothly and easily through your GI tract. Find out more about the importance of water later in this chapter.

WARNING

It's possible to eat too much fiber! So take heed if you're eating whole foods on the eating clean plan and taking fiber supplements. Too much fiber can stop the absorption of minerals because the food speeds through your intestine too quickly. More than 45 to 50 grams of fiber a day is too much.

Chew on this: Connecting fiber and weight loss

Fiber plays an important role in maintaining a healthy weight. Most importantly, you feel more satisfied when you eat high-fiber foods. They add bulk to your stomach so you feel full longer.

Also, high-fiber foods take more time to eat because you have to chew them more before swallowing. (Think about it; you can't just gulp down a couple of apples like you can a handful of chocolate candies.) That extra time spent chewing helps give your stomach time to signal to your brain that you're full.

WARNING

Just because fiber is a good thing and it can help you lose weight doesn't mean you should go on a fiber binge to lose 15 pounds in a week. If your diet hasn't been high in fiber and you want to increase your intake, you have to do so slowly. If you add too much fiber to your diet too quickly, your body will rebel. You'll develop gas, bloating, and cramping as the bacteria in your intestines suddenly start to work overtime on the added fiber. So add fiber gradually to allow your system to adjust.

Water: The Essential Nutrient

You would die without water — and quickly. Your body is made up of about 65 percent water. You can survive for months without food, but you can survive only a few days without water. Every function in your body needs water. You need it for nerves to process signals in your brain; for blood flow; for cell function, repair, and reproduction; for nutrient absorption and waste elimination; for normal metabolism; and for respiration.

Most nutritionists say that you should consume 8 to 12 glasses of water a day. That sounds like a lot, but if you drink a glass of water with or before each meal, you'll consume six glasses a day on the clean eating plan without even trying. (The clean eating plan recommends that you eat six times a day. See Chapter 2 in Book 5 for details.) You also get water from the food you eat, especially foods like watermelon, peaches, and berries. Think juicy fruits!

TIP

To make sure you get enough water every day, do the following:

>> Bring a water bottle with you whenever there may not be a clean and easily available source.

>> Drink a glass of water when you wake up and another before you go to sleep.

>> Eat more of the foods, such as fruits and vegetables, which can be good sources of water.

Chapter **4**

Eat More, Eat Often

How many times have you looked at the plate of food you allow yourself and wished it contained more? Do you feel deprived when you go "on a diet" and wish you didn't feel so hungry? If you follow the eating clean lifestyle, those days are gone for good. When you eat clean, you get to enjoy many wonderful benefits, including better health and more energy. But best of all, you get to eat more food more often.

The key, of course, is that the types of foods you eat must be nutrient dense. In other words, for each calorie, the food must supply a reasonable amount of vitamins, minerals, fiber, and other nutrients. Empty calories, which are usually found in junk foods and processed foods, just aren't worth the costs to your health and your pocketbook and have no place in the eating clean lifestyle.

This chapter explains how to listen to your body and let it tell you when it's hungry or thirsty and when you just want to eat for emotional reasons. You find out what real hunger cues are and what satiety really means. You also discover what you should eat and when you should eat it, how to develop and enjoy mini-meals, how to work the eating clean lifestyle into your daily routine, and ways to enjoy your clean food with natural flavor enhancers.

Listening to Your Body

Do you know what being hungry really feels like? Of course, you've felt hunger pangs, especially on days that are so busy you can't find time to eat. But many people have lost the connection between their body's hunger signals and true hunger.

The following sections look at how your body tells you that you need more food, what forms your body's signals take, and how you can sometimes mistake other emotions or triggers for real hunger. You also find out what satiety means and how to determine when your stomach is really (and comfortably) full.

REMEMBER

The trick to eating clean is knowing how to recognize healthy hunger cues and how to defuse unhealthy cues. When you understand how your stomach and your brain work together and can identify the triggers that prompt overeating and craving, you can do something to stop the cycle of bad food choices.

Decoding hunger cues

Scientist Ivan Pavlov proved that you can prompt hunger in many different ways. Through his experiments, he demonstrated that his dogs would start drooling when they heard a dinner bell. They learned to associate the sound of the bell with food appearing, and their bodies responded. Human beings aren't much different!

Hunger is one of life's biological drives. You have to eat to stay alive, and your body tells you when you need food. But in this modern world, images of food — reminders of everything from chocolate doughnuts to french fries — constantly bombard you. After all, Madison Avenue's efforts to make you crave different kinds of food have been very successful over the years! But with the eating clean lifestyle, you have to figure out what real hunger feels like.

REMEMBER

You can separate hunger into two basic categories. One is the normal hunger that comes when your body needs food to repair and maintain itself. The other is the hunger that occurs when you respond to external cues, such as a picture of food, or internal cues, such as stress or sadness. Within these two hunger categories, you experience several different types of hunger, including

>> **True physiological hunger:** A type of hunger caused by a drop in blood sugar, changes in hormone levels, and an empty stomach and intestine. The brain decodes these signals and sends messages to the rest of your body, making your stomach growl and ache and sometimes causing a headache or feeling of weakness. You must recognize these hunger signals to keep your body properly fueled and healthy.

>> **Psychological hunger:** A type of hunger triggered by thoughts and emotions, such as worry, anxiety, or anger, or by the sight or smell of food. Eating junk food, binge eating, and eating out of habit rather than a physical need for nourishment feed this type of hunger.

>> **Appetite:** An interest in or craving for food. Appetite is linked to the physical need for food, but it can override the body's signals that you have eaten enough and can spur you on to eat more than you need — sometimes much more.

Tracking hunger in your household

The biggest challenges to eating well and maintaining a healthy body are understanding and untangling psychological hunger and appetite from physical hunger.

To help you understand the differences between the main hunger types, conduct a little experiment in your household over the next few days. Explain that physical hunger is going to be the standard that prompts eating in your household. Tell your family that they have to pay attention to their own hunger cues. Proposing a hunger rating system, where 1 is "extraordinarily hungry" and 10 is "extraordinarily full," may help. The goal is to stay within the range of about 3 to 7; that is, eat when you feel hunger pangs but aren't uncomfortably hungry and stop when you feel satisfyingly full. Meeting this goal takes some practice, but eventually everyone will become familiar with this natural way to control food intake.

TIP

If you discover that you eat for emotional reasons and have a hard time controlling such impulses, stock your house with healthy foods rather than cupcakes and potato chips. If the tempting, unhealthy foods aren't within easy reach but good snacks such as apples with cheese are, your diet will automatically improve.

Ignoring external cues

When everyone in your household understands the difference between physical hunger and psychological cravings, start tackling the external cues that drive you to eat even when you're not really hungry. After all, before you can succeed with the eating clean lifestyle, you must change your bad eating habits.

TIP

To get your body used to eating for health and hunger (rather than for psychological reasons), do the following:

>> **Turn off the television and computer during meal times.** Meal-time distractions turn your attention away from the food in front of you and your body's physical feelings and usually lead to overeating. The goal is to avoid mindless eating, which results when you don't concentrate on your plate.

>> **Slow down meal times.** Take time to talk to your fellow eaters, put down your fork and knife occasionally during a meal, and wait for your stomach to tell your brain it's full. That message takes 20 minutes to travel from your stomach to your brain. And you can eat a lot of food in those last few minutes before the signal arrives!

>> **Understand portion control and proper serving sizes.** Most people are used to the supersized portions restaurants serve. But did you know that a healthy serving of meat is only about the size of a deck of cards and that a serving of ice cream is only ½ cup? Practice measuring food to get used to correct serving sizes until dishing out proper portions becomes second nature to you.

>> **Try to separate emotions from eating.** Stress can prompt overeating or craving unhealthy foods. If you're stressed or angry and want to eat, wait 10 to 15 minutes. If, after that time, you're still hungry — according to physical, not emotional, cues — go ahead and choose something healthy to eat. If you aren't hungry, you know the trigger was emotional or external and not a genuine need for food.

Identifying thirst cues

Water is a basic element of life. In fact, human bodies are about 65 percent water. When your body needs more water, it lets you know through thirst cues. But did you know that people often mistake thirst for hunger?

If your stomach starts rumbling and you want to eat, get a drink of water. Not soda, not coffee or tea — just plain water. Then wait a few minutes. If you were thirsty, not hungry, your craving for food will abate. Drinking water to see whether you're thirsty rather than hungry is especially important if you had something to eat less than three hours ago or if you haven't had any water in the last hour.

Drinking lots of water helps your body do the following:

>> Keep your metabolism at the proper level

>> Decrease food cravings

>> Burn stored fat

>> Maintain muscle tone

>> Increase energy levels

In fact, drinking water or eating a clear soup before a meal is a great way to help fill up your stomach and control hunger pangs. Keeping your body properly hydrated can help you recognize the true feelings of hunger.

Understanding satiety

Satiety (pronounced say-*tie*-uh-tee) is the feeling of satisfaction you have after eating. It doesn't mean that you're full or that you've eaten so much you're uncomfortable. Figuring out what satiety means to you is important to your eating clean lifestyle.

To help you better understand what satiety means, consider the satiety index that Dr. Susanna Holt developed to rank foods according to how satisfying they are to eat, how much of those foods you must eat to feel full, and how soon you feel hunger pangs after eating them. The index uses an ordinary piece of white bread as the baseline score of 100. Foods that stave off hunger longer receive higher scores, while foods that prompt feelings of hunger more quickly rank lower. Not surprisingly, foods with more fiber, complex carbohydrates, and protein fill your stomach faster, are more satisfying to eat, and keep your blood sugar levels stable longer. Foods high in protein are the best at staving off hunger, while whole grains and fruits and vegetables that are high in fiber are better at helping you feel satisfied longer.

The following foods rank lower on the satiety index:

>> **Candy bar:** Score 70

>> **Doughnut:** Score 68

>> **Potato chips:** Score 91

>> **Cake:** Score 65

The following foods rank higher on the satiety index:

>> **Cheese:** Score 157

>> **Fish:** Score 225

>> **Apples:** Score 197

>> **Baked potato:** Score 322

>> **Oatmeal:** Score 209

The fact that the higher-ranking foods are clean while the lower-ranking foods are highly processed is no surprise. Not only does your eating clean lifestyle improve your health and wellbeing, but it also helps you feel more satisfied after each meal. Now that's a healthy reward you can build on and learn to enjoy!

The following sections describe two more factors that play a role in satiety — food flavors and stomach processes.

Factoring flavors into the satiety equation

Satiety is more than just a lack of hunger. Your appetite is a complex biological mechanism that engages many parts of the brain. When you eat a meal that contains a lot of different flavors, you activate more appetite centers in your brain. For example, a meal with sweet, salty, sour, and meaty (also called *umami*) flavors turns on many appetite centers in your brain, and you have to eat until all those centers signal that they're satisfied to feel full.

The problem with processed foods is that many of them are high in sugar and salt. As a result, processed foods prompt a lot of appetite centers in your brain, causing you to have to eat more to satisfy them. But you don't really taste all the flavors in processed foods. For example, you know that processed cereals are high in sugar, but did you know that many are also high in salt? The sugar wakes up the sweet appetite center of your brain, and the salt prompts the salty appetite center, urging you to eat more.

This concept plays into what Dr. David Kessler, a former U.S. Federal Drug Administration (FDA) commissioner, calls *hypereating* (an obsessive need to consume processed foods that change brain chemistry). Combinations of sugar, salt, and fat trigger appetite centers in your brain that release feel-good hormones called *endorphins*. In other words, processed foods literally give you feelings of happiness, comfort, and euphoria, very similar to what a drug addict feels after a hit. Food companies understand this fact very well, which is why so many processed foods contain exactly those ingredients in very specific combinations.

Nobody wants to eat a bland diet. Lucky for you, you don't have to. By eating whole foods, you get the best of both worlds — healthy nutrients and flavor! The key is to choose flavorful, high-volume, and nutritious foods with low density. For example, foods that are high in water and fiber, such as grapes or oranges, are more satisfying to eat than fruit juice. Although eating processed foods is often easier because they're usually low volume, eating clean foods is the healthier, more satisfying way to go. Almost anyone can quickly eat an entire package of potato chips, which weighs about 12 ounces, but eating an entire baked potato, which weighs about the same amount, takes more time and is more satisfying and nutritious.

Keeping your stomach busy longer

The rate of *gastric emptying* (how long your stomach takes to process food and empty into the small intestine) also plays a role in satiety. How long your stomach takes to process the food you eat depends on how much fiber, protein, carbohydrates, and fat the food contains. Fruit juices, for example, travel through your stomach quickly because they contain only simple carbs, which break down very quickly; the stomach doesn't have to process any solids.

But a meal full of grains, vegetables, and lean meats takes longer to process. The food stays in your stomach longer, which means you feel more satisfied for a longer period of time. Again, whole foods — the critical part of the eating clean lifestyle — have slower gastric-emptying rates, while highly processed foods have faster gastric-emptying rates.

REMEMBER

Sheer bulk of the food counts, too. The later section "Knowing what (and what not) to eat" compares the calories and nutrients in a clean meal to those in a processed meal. Not surprisingly, the clean meal has fewer calories and more nutrients, but if you look at the plates of food side by side, you notice something else. The clean plate also has much more volume.

Because you eat with your eyes as well as your mouth, just looking at a plate full of food can help you feel more satisfied. For example, a big salad, full of nuts and vegetables, such as mushrooms, avocado, and tomatoes, is more satisfying to eat than a small fried burrito from a fast-food joint.

Getting Started with Good Food Choices

Most Americans suffer from too much choice. Grocery stores are packed full of foods that, unfortunately, aren't very good for you. Although packaged foods taste good and are convenient, the toll they take on your health and your body is very high.

Making good food choices is a basic step toward the eating clean lifestyle. The following sections look at what the eating clean diet means and what kinds of food you should put in your shopping basket. They compare the calories and nutrition of a typical American fast-food meal with those in a clean meal, and they look at the best times to eat to keep your body properly fueled.

Knowing what (and what not) to eat

Did you know that the average American consumes enough extra calories every seven days to gain more than 50 pounds a year? This alarming statistic corresponds to the explosion of processed food and fast-food availability in modern culture.

The visual and emotional cues you face on a daily basis, along with the chemical makeup of processed foods and your body's natural responses to these cues, make eating a healthy diet very difficult. But you can change course with a little bit of effort, some simple rules, and a better understanding of what your body really needs. Read on to find out what you need to know.

Choosing the right packaged foods (if you must)

You've heard of the food chain that has algae and amoeba at the bottom and lions and tigers at the top, but you may not know about the other food chain — that is, the processed food chain. In this food chain, foods in their natural state, such as apples, greens, berries, and whole grains, are at the bottom, and processed foods, such as sugary snack cakes and fast-food burgers, are at the top. If you eat low on the food chain, you'll automatically eat a clean diet. So think about food in its natural state before you buy it. A gelatin fruit salad packed in a little plastic cup with chunks of peaches floating in it is very different from a fresh peach picked right off the tree.

REMEMBER

If you're still buying foods with a label, use the following rules to help guide your choices:

» **Read the labels.** If a product like whole-wheat bread contains more than five or seven ingredients, put it back on the shelf. You don't have to stick to a certain ingredient count; just make sure that the number of ingredients is about what you would use if you made the food from scratch.

» **If you can't pronounce, spell, or understand ingredients on the food label, don't buy that particular product.** Your body doesn't need artificial flavors or chemicals made in the lab. Even chemicals the FDA regards as safe may be problematic in the future.

» **Avoid foods that have sugars, processed ingredients, or fat as the first or second ingredient on the label.** These foods are made up of empty calories that don't provide much nutrition.

» **Choose foods that are low on the food chain.** In other words, choose foods that are as close as possible to their natural state. Pick up a head of cabbage rather than a bag of coleslaw. Choose a bag of apples rather than a bottle of sweetened applesauce. If you do so consistently, you'll be well on your way to eating clean.

When you follow these simple rules, you may notice that a lot of the foods you're used to buying are no longer on your grocery list. This switch in what you buy can take some time, but don't stress! You can ease into the process. Becoming aware of what you put in your shopping cart and bring into your house is the first, and most important, step.

Avoiding fast food

As you transition into an eating clean lifestyle, you must begin to consider and choose the foods you eat carefully. Although a fast-food meal is (relatively) inexpensive and quick, a constant diet of such food can have a very expensive and time-consuming effect on your health in the future in terms of medical bills and trips to the doctor.

To help you visualize just how different processed foods and clean foods are, take a look at Tables 4-1 and 4-2, which compare a meal composed of typical American fast foods with one made up of clean, whole foods. If you find yourself sliding back into old habits, just pull out these charts and compare the bottom line. (*Note:* In the tables, *g* stands for gram and *mg* stands for milligram.)

TABLE 4-1 **Fast-Food Meal**

Food	Fat	Carbs	Fiber	Sodium	Protein	Calories
12 ounces of soda	0 g	42 g	0 g	35 mg	0 g	150
1 fast-food cheeseburger	12 g	33 g	2 g	750 mg	15 g	300
1 serving of french fries	19 g	48 g	5 g	270 mg	4 g	380
3 tablespoons of ketchup	0 g	12 g	0 g	500 mg	1 g	45
Total	31 g	135 g	7 g	1,555 mg	20 g	875

TABLE 4-2 **Eating Clean Meal**

Food	Fat	Carbs	Fiber	Sodium	Protein	Calories
Chicken Lettuce Wraps	11 g	15 g	3 g	654 mg	23 g	250
Slow Cooker Tomato Barley Soup	1 g	27 g	6 g	512 mg	4 g	126
Frozen Yogurt Bar	1 g	5 g	1 g	12 mg	4 g	39
Total	13 g	47 g	10 g	1,178 mg	31 g	414

The fast-food meal shown in Table 4-1 may be enjoyable to eat, but you'll be hungry soon after eating it, you're not meeting your body's nutritional needs, and you're consuming too much sodium, fat, preservatives, and artificial flavors. The amount of sodium in this one meal is more than half of the daily recommended amount (which is 2,400 mg). The meal also provides almost half of the total calories you should consume in a day (which is 2,000) and is very high in fat.

The fast-food meal is also very low in nutrients. Although the ketchup and tomato on the cheeseburger do provide some vitamin C, you don't get a lot of vitamin D, calcium, or other micronutrients in this meal. In addition, the meal is most likely loaded with hormones from the meat and pesticides from the potatoes, tomato, and lettuce, which were most likely grown on a large factory farm.

REMEMBER

The meal in Table 4-2 uses clean recipes. Compare these two charts to look at the fat content, amount of fiber, sodium content, protein content, and total calories. The clean meal has good fats, including monounsaturated fats from olive oil and nuts, less sugar and sodium, and more fiber and protein. Plus, it fills you up, provides you with more nutrients, and keeps you feeling satisfied longer with fewer calories, preservatives, and artificial ingredients. The eating clean diet is one you can live with for life — quite likely a longer, more active, and healthier life, too!

Eating mini meals to combat hunger

Back in the 1980s, the term *grazing* applied to people as well as cows. Scientists thought that eating smaller meals throughout the day (rather than just three large meals) helped keep the body's metabolism going and prevented overeating by keeping blood sugar as stable as possible. When your blood sugar drops, all kinds of nasty things happen: You feel hungry and irritable, your willpower goes out the window, and you reach for any edible substance in sight.

Despite lots of research, scientists haven't found a clear-cut answer about whether eating mini meals offers all those benefits. But if you do eat more often, you may be less tempted to eat processed snack foods, which is one reason why the eating clean diet involves eating five or six smaller meals a day rather than the traditional large breakfast, lunch, and dinner. After all, if you know that you get to eat a turkey sandwich with homemade bread in an hour, that doughnut stand you pass on your coffee break will be much less tempting.

Don't forget the hunger rating system that is described in the earlier section "Decoding hunger cues." Eating smaller meals at regular intervals throughout the day prevents your hunger from dipping to 1 or 2 on the hunger scale, and eating smaller meals means you almost never reach a 9 or 10 on the fullness scale.

TIP

To get the most out of your mini meals, follow these guidelines:

>> **Make sure each mini meal includes complex carbohydrates, lean proteins, and healthy fats.** You find complex carbs in fruits, vegetables, and whole grains; lean proteins in chicken, fish, lean beef, and pork; and good fats in nuts and nut butters, olive oil, and lean meats.

>> **Always, always eat breakfast.** Eating healthy, filling foods within an hour of waking helps keep your blood sugar from plunging and spiking so that you feel more satisfied the rest of the day.

>> **Make sure the meals stay mini!** Even though you're eating more often, each meal should be smaller. You need to use a little bit of arithmetic to see where this guideline comes from. If you want to consume 2,000 calories a day, each mini meal should be approximately 320 calories. You can allot more calories to each meal and make your snacks a bit smaller, especially when you're just getting started.

>> **Prepare the foods yourself so that you can be sure they don't include any preservatives or additives.** Make your own snack mix or assemble a little wrap sandwich or fruit salad.

>> **Carry your food with you.** If you work outside the home, make sure to bring your morning snack, lunch, and afternoon snack with you.

>> **Drink lots of water or unsweetened tea throughout the day.** Remember that thirst can masquerade as hunger. Drinking lots of water helps keep your digestive system running smoothly.

>> **Establish fairly regular eating times.** When you eat at about the same time every day, your body uses the calories more efficiently. Because you're not overtaxing or starving your digestive system, you feel stronger.

REMEMBER

Thousands of years ago, when human beings had to scratch and fight for every bite of food, their bodies used hunger to prevent starvation. When you let your body get too hungry or eat too little, it literally goes into starvation mode, which means you burn fewer calories. Your body believes it won't get any more food so it has to protect you! Because your body literally lives in the moment, it can plan only for periods of starvation, not abundance. Eating mini meals every few hours on a regular basis helps your evolutionary survival system relax so that you can relax.

Combining clean eating with your daily routine

Converting your daily routine to the eating clean lifestyle is easier than you think. Sure, you have to spend more time planning, shopping, and preparing meals than you do now, but as with all new skills, you'll get faster as you get more experience.

Especially when you're just getting started, you can eat clean meals with a little help from the grocery store. Whole-grain crackers spread with nut butter or some cheese and a granola bar make for perfectly acceptable mini meals. You don't have to make everything from scratch.

Build your clean eating plan right into your daily routine. Eat breakfast within an hour of waking up. Then schedule a morning snack three hours later. Eat your lunch at the regular time. Then have a piece of fruit during a mid-afternoon break. Eat your dinner at the regular time, and have a snack a few hours later to help you wind down your day and get in the mood for bed.

TIP

You may want to start a journal of your favorite mini meals. Think of the snacks you enjoyed as a child and try to find ways to convert them into clean foods. For example, if you loved eating nacho chips with a soda, try to make your own crackers with nuts and seeds, and enjoy a few of them with some iced tea sweetened with agave nectar. Before you know it, you'll have a long list of snacks and mini meals that you enjoy eating. Check out the nearby sidebar "Keeping a food journal" for more details.

6
Scaling Back the Stress in Your Life

Contents at a Glance

CHAPTER 1: Getting a Handle on the Causes and Effects of Stress 389
Experiencing a Stress Epidemic? 389
Understanding Where All This Stress Is Coming From 390
Looking at the Signs and Symptoms of Stress 396
Understanding How Stress Can Make You Sick 397

CHAPTER 2: Relaxing Your Body 403
Stress Can Be a Pain in the Neck (And That's Just for Starters) ... 403
Breathing Away Your Tension 406
Tensing Your Way to Relaxation 413
Mind over Body: Using the Power of Suggestion 417
Stretching Away Your Stress 419
Massage? Ah, There's the Rub! 420
Taking a Three-Minute Energy Burst 422
More Ways to Relax. 423

CHAPTER 3: Finding More Time 425
Determining Whether You Struggle with Time Management. ... 426
Being Mindful of Your Time 426
Becoming a List Maker 431
Minimizing Your Distractions and Interruptions. 436
Getting around Psychological Roadblocks to Time Management 440
Letting Go: Discovering the Joys of Delegating 443
Buying Time 445

CHAPTER 4: Stress-Reducing Organizational Skills 447
Figuring Out Why Your Life Is So Disorganized. 448
Clearing Away the Clutter. 450
Organizing Your Space 456
Organizing Information 458
Keeping Your Life Organized 465

CHAPTER 5: De-Stressing at Work 467
Reading the Signs of Workplace Stress 467
Knowing What's Triggering Your Work Stress 468
Making Positive Changes to Control Your Workplace Stress 469
Taking Advantage of Company Perks. 482
Coming Home More Relaxed (And Staying That Way) 483

Chapter **1**

Getting a Handle on the Causes and Effects of Stress

Are you feeling more tired lately than you used to? Is your fuse a little shorter than normal? Are you worrying more? Enjoying life less? If you feel more stress in your life these days, you aren't alone. Count yourself among the ranks of the overstressed. Most people feel that their lives have too much stress. Your stress may come from your job or lack thereof, your money worries, your personal life, or simply not having enough time to do everything you have to do — or want to do. You could use some help. Thankfully, you can eliminate or at least minimize much of the stress in your life and better manage the stress that remains. This chapter helps you get started.

Experiencing a Stress Epidemic?

You probably can't make it through a single day without seeing or hearing the word *stress* someplace. Just glance at any magazine stand and you'll find numerous cover stories all about stress. In most larger bookstores, an entire section is devoted to books on stress. TV and radio talk shows regularly feature stories documenting the negative effects of stress in our lives. Why all the fuss? Hasn't stress been around forever? Wasn't it stress that Adam felt when he was caught red-handed with little bits of apple stuck between his teeth? Is all of this just media hype, or are people really experiencing more stress today?

One good way of finding out how much stress people are experiencing is to ask them about the stress in their lives. A 2020 Harris Interactive survey of more than 1,550 Americans found that 46 percent reported that their stress level is higher than it was five years ago. Eighty percent said they experienced medium or high stress levels at work. Sixty percent said they experienced these same levels at home.

Our lives, it seems, have indeed become far more stressful. But why? The next section provides some reasons.

Understanding Where All This Stress Is Coming From

In his prophetic book *Future Shock* (originally published in 1984), Alvin Toffler observed that people experience more stress whenever they are subjected to a lot of change in a short span of time. If anything characterizes our lives these days, it's an excess of change. We're in a continual state of flux. We have less control over our lives, we live with more uncertainty, and we often feel threatened and, at times, overwhelmed. The following sections explain some of the more common sources of stress in our lives.

Coping with the pandemic

More than any other stressor in modern times, the coronavirus pandemic has become the most pressing source of stress in peoples lives. A 2021 survey published by the American Psychological Association found that as a result of the pandemic, Americans were experiencing higher levels of stress than in previous years. With stay at home orders, school closings, social isolation, and the constant uncertainty of contracting the disease, the emotional impact of the pandemic was staggering. Day to day struggles can be overwhelming, especially for younger adults and parents.

The survey found that:

>> A majority of adults (61 percent) reported experiencing undesired weight changes since the start of the pandemic, with more than 2 in 5 (42 percent) saying they gained more weight than they intended.

>> Two in three Americans (67 percent) said they are sleeping more or less than they wanted to since the pandemic started.

>> One in three Americans (32 percent) said sometimes they are so stressed about the virus that they struggle to make even basic decisions, such as what to eat. Millennials were particularly likely to struggle with this when compared with other age groups.

>> A majority of Americans (59 percent) said they have changed some behaviors as a result of the pandemic. Most commonly the changes were avoiding social situations (24 percent), altering eating habits (23 percent), procrastinating or neglecting responsibilities (22 percent) or changing their physical activity levels (22 percent). Pandemic stress has contributed to widespread mental exhaustion, negative health impacts, and an overriding feeling of not being able to cope.

Our politics is stressing us out

In recent years, politics has become a growing source of our stress. A striking new survey (2021), published by political science professor Kevin B. Smith at the University of Nebraska, found that 40 percent of respondents said they're stressed about politics. A fifth or more reported losing sleep, being fatigued, or suffering from bouts of depression. As many as a quarter of survey respondents reported self-destructive or compulsive behaviors such as saying or writing things they later regret, making bad decisions, and ignoring other priorities. Smith found that, regardless of political affiliation, too many of us, even if we are not political junkies, are feeling ground down by our political environment.

Struggling in a struggling economy

Money may or may not be the root of all evil, but worrying about it certainly is a major source of stress. Balancing your checkbook at the end of the month (if you bother) reminds you that living is expensive. You remember that your parents bought their house for a pittance and now realize that today you couldn't afford to buy that same house if you wanted to. The mortgage, college tuition, braces for the kids' teeth, camp, travel, taxes, savings for retirement — it all adds up. Fears of inflation grow. And so does the stress.

Getting frazzled at work

Having a job may mean avoiding the stress that comes with unemployment, but it certainly doesn't guarantee a stress-free existence. For many people, jobs and careers are the biggest source of stress. Concerns about job security, killer hours, long commutes, unrealistic deadlines, bosses from hell, office politics, toxic coworkers, and testy clients are just a few of the many job-related stresses people experience. Workloads are heavier today than they were in the past, leaving less and less time for family and the rest of your life.

Adding to this list of ongoing stressors is the overriding presence and consequences of the pandemic. A 2021 study by the American Psychological Association titled *Work and Well-being* found that after more than a year of working during the pandemic, the American workforce reports compounding pressures that are impacting the stress they feel, and their ability to do their jobs. Its survey found several factors that were contributing to this added stress:

>> Inadequate compensations (56 percent, up from 49 percent in 2019)

>> Long hours (54 percent, up from 46 percent)

>> Lack of opportunity for growth or advancement (52 percent, up from 44 percent)

>> Too heavy a workload (50 percent, up from 44 percent)

>> Lack of involvement in decision-making (48 percent, up from 39 percent)

Overall, 71 percent of workers reported feeling tense or stressed during their workday. Only 20 percent didn't feel tense or stressed. Of those feeling stressed, nearly 3 in 5 employees felt that this stress has impacted their performance at work. This included decreased levels of motivation or energy (26 percent) and difficulty focusing (21 percent). More than 2 of 5 said that they were likely to change jobs in the coming year, a significant increase over previous years.

Feeling frazzled at home

After you leave work, you may start to realize that the rest of your life is not exactly stress-free. These days, life at home, relationships, and the pressure of juggling everything else that has to be done only add to the stress level.

STRESS FOR WOMEN ON THE JOB

If you're a woman, you may experience even more stress on the job. Despite all the hoopla about women's rights and sexual equality, women still face added pressures and limitations in the workplace. Women are paid less and promoted less frequently than their male counterparts, even though they may be more qualified. If a woman has children, her career may be shunted onto the "Mommy Track," a glass ceiling that limits career advancement.

More subtle pressures come from the prevailing notions of the roles and behaviors expected from men and women. Men and women can act in similar ways that may advance their careers — competitive, aggressive, and assertive — but a double standard is common. When such behavior comes from a woman, people often view the behavior negatively as unfeminine and inappropriate. But when that same behavior comes from a man, people see him as strong and in control.

Sexual harassment for women on the job is no small source of stress. A woman may find herself in the no-win situation of either openly complaining or silently enduring the abuse. Both options can be highly stressful. Women who belong to a racial or ethnic minority may experience even more stress. Hiring and promotional practices may act in subtle and not-so-subtle discriminatory ways. Even where affirmative action policies are in place, women may experience the stress of feeling that others see any hiring or advancement as unfairly legislated rather than legitimately deserved.

Life at home has become more pressured and demanding. These days, many more of us are working at home, and our children my be schooling at home, creating newer sources of stress. True, we now have microwaves, robotic vacuums, and take-out menus, but the effort and stress involved seem to be growing rather than lessening. Meals have to be prepared, the house tidied, the clothing cleaned, the bills paid, the chores completed, the shopping done, the lawn and garden tended, the car maintained and repaired, the phone calls and emails returned, the homework supervised, and the kids chauffeured. And that's for starters. And what about the dog?

TECHNICAL STUFF

In her insightful book *The Overworked American: The Unexpected Decline of Leisure*, economist Juliet Schor points out that, in spite of all the new innovations and contraptions that could make our lives easier, we still need about the same amount of time to do what has to be done at home. In the 1910s, a full-time housewife spent about 52 hours a week on housework. Sixty years later, in the 1970s, the figure was about the same. Yes, some activities did become less time consuming. Food preparation fell almost 10 hours a week, but this was offset by an increase in the time spent shopping and taking care of the home and kids. Contrary to everyone's predicted expectations, we have less leisure time now than we did 50 years ago.

"I need two more hours in the day!"

This plea is a commonly heard lament. The stress of not having enough time to do everything that has to be done is enormous. We overwork at home and at our jobs. The result? We just don't have enough time.

Ozzie and Harriet we ain't

Some of this stress comes from the ways in which families have changed over the years. In two-parent families, it's now common for both parents to work. One-parent families have even more stressors. These days, more women are the main earners in the home (almost 40 percent) or are bringing in essential income needed to maintain the family. Nearly half of all marriages end in divorce. The number of single-parent households is multiplying. Families tend be more fragmented, with relatives often living great distances away. Although in certain cases this situation can be stress-reducing (your annoying Aunt Agnes is moving to Dubuque?), more often it promotes a greater sense of disconnectedness and alienation.

A woman's work is never done

Forty years ago, one-third of all workers were women; now nearly half are. Add on the additional stress of being a mother with a family to manage at home, and you compound the level of stress. Women may find themselves in the not-so-unusual position of having to cope with the problems of aging and ailing parents in addition to the problems of their own children. Caught in this generational divide, this "stress sandwich" can be incredibly draining, both physically and emotionally. Although men give lip service to helping with the kids and the elderly (and they do, in fact, help more than their fathers or grandfathers did), woman are still the ones who most often take primary responsibility for these care-giving roles.

A 2009 study reported in *Time* magazine found that 55 percent of women strongly agree that in households where both partners have jobs, women take on more responsibilities for the home and family than their male partners do. The men in the study saw it differently: Only 28 percent agreed. Sixty-nine percent of women say that they are primarily responsible for taking care of their children; only 13 percent of men say this of themselves. As an old adage reminds us, "Father works from sun to sun, but Mother's work is never done."

Piling on new stresses with technology

People's lives have become stressful in ways they never would have imagined even a decade ago. Whoever said there is nothing new under the sun probably never searched online the name of a restaurant or texted a friend. Changes in technology have brought with them new pressures and new demands — in short, new sources of stress. For example, one study of more than 1,300 people found that those who regularly used their cellphones or portable devices for communication experienced an increase in psychological distress and a decrease in family satisfaction, compared with those who used these devices less often.

Imagine this implausible scenario: You've been in a coma for the last two decades or so. One day, out of the blue, you wake up and take the bus home from the hospital. You quickly notice that life has changed. Technology rules. On the bus you notice that everyone is pushing buttons on small devices. You ask the person next to you what's going on, and he looks at you strangely and explains what a smartphone is, what downloading means, and what email does. You reach your home and discover that your old television and computer have become relics. Everything is digital. Everything is portable. People are magically "downloading" movies and television shows on their telephones. Your cassette player is a joke, not to mention your record player. Just as quickly, you realize that you have no idea how to operate any of these digital tools. You have no idea what the words FaceTime, Netflix, Kindle, GPS, Facebook, Twitter, YouTube, podcast, Instagram, and eBay even mean. All this technology is beginning to drive you a bit crazy. Your next-door neighbor, who was never in a coma and yet is just as stressed as you are, is also trying to keep up with all this technological change.

Dealing with daily hassles (the little things add up)

When you think of stress, you usually think of the major stresses you may face: death, divorce, financial ruin, or a serious illness. And then of course there are those so-called moderate stresses: losing your wallet, denting the car, or catching a cold. Finally, you face the even smaller stresses: the mini-stresses and micro-stresses. These stresses are what are known as *hassles*.

Here is just a sample of the kinds of hassles you face every day (a complete list would be endless):

>> Noisy traffic

>> Loud neighbors

>> Rude salesclerks

>> Crowds

>> Long waits for telephone customer-service representatives

>> Deliveries promised "sometime between 9 and 5"

>> Computers that crash

>> Airport delays

>> Cellphones that go off in theaters and restaurants

REMEMBER

Yes, these things are relatively small. But the small things can add up. You can deal with one, maybe two, or even three of these at once. But when the number begins to rise, so does your stress level. When you reach a high enough level of stress, you overreact to the next hassle that comes along. And that results in even more stress. Alas, life is loaded with hassle. The funny part is, people usually deal fairly well with the bigger problems. Life's major stresses — the deaths, illnesses, divorces, and financial setbacks— somehow trigger hidden resources within us. We rise to each demand, summoning up some unrecognized inner strength, and we somehow manage to cope. What gets to us are the little things. It's the small stuff — the little annoyances, petty frustrations, and minor irritations — that ultimately lead to a continuing sense of stress.

Looking at the Signs and Symptoms of Stress

The signs and symptoms of stress range from the benign to the dramatic — from simply feeling tired at the end of the day to having a heart attack. The more serious stress-related problems come with intense and prolonged periods of stress. These disorders and diseases are covered later in this chapter. Here are some of the more benign, commonly experienced stress signs and symptoms. Many will be all too familiar to you.

WARNING

Physical signs of stress include the following:

>> Tiredness, fatigue, lethargy

>> Heart palpitations; racing pulse; rapid, shallow breathing

>> Muscle tension and aches

>> Shakiness, tremors, tics, twitches

>> Heartburn, indigestion, diarrhea, constipation

>> Nervousness

>> Dry mouth and throat

>> Excessive sweating, clammy hands, cold hands and/or feet

- » Rashes, hives, itching
- » Nail-biting, fidgeting, hair-twirling, hair-pulling
- » Frequent urination
- » Lowered libido
- » Overeating, loss of appetite
- » Sleep difficulties
- » Increased use of alcohol and/or drugs and medications

WARNING

Psychological signs of stress include the following:

- » Irritability, impatience, anger, hostility
- » Worry, anxiety, panic
- » Moodiness, sadness, feeling upset
- » Intrusive and/or racing thoughts
- » Memory lapses, difficulties in concentrating, indecision
- » Frequent absences from work, lowered productivity
- » Feeling overwhelmed
- » Loss of sense of humor

That's just for starters. Prolonged and/or intense stress can have more serious effects: It can make you sick, as you find out in the next section.

Understanding How Stress Can Make You Sick

Researchers estimate that 75 to 90 percent of all visits to primary-care physicians are for complaints and conditions that are, in some way, stress-related. About 50 percent of those surveyed said that stress was affecting their health. Every week, more than 100 million people take some form of medication for stress-related symptoms. This statistic isn't surprising given the wide-ranging physiological changes that accompany a stress response. Just about every bodily system or body part is affected by stress. Stress can exacerbate the symptoms of a wide variety of other disorders and illnesses as well. Stress is linked to the five leading causes of death: heart disease, cancer, lung disease, accidents, and suicide. The following sections illustrate some of the more important ways stress can negatively affect your health and wellbeing.

REMEMBER

All the symptoms, illnesses, and conditions mentioned in this section can result from a number of medical conditions, not just stress. And for many of the disorders and diseases mentioned, stress may not be the direct cause of the condition, but stress may make these conditions worse. If you're concerned about one or more of these symptoms, be sure to consult your physician. They are the best person to give you advice and guidance.

Understanding how stress can be a pain in the neck (and other places)

Your muscles are a prime target for stress. When you're under stress, your muscles contract and become tense. This muscle tension can affect your nerves, blood vessels, organs, skin, and bones. Chronically tense muscles can result in a variety of conditions and disorders, including muscle spasms, cramping, facial or jaw pain, bruxism (grinding your teeth), tremors, and shakiness. Many forms of headache, chest pain, and back pain are among the more common conditions that result from stress-induced muscle tension.

Taking stress to heart

Stress can play a role in circulatory diseases such as coronary heart disease, sudden cardiac death, and strokes. This fact is not surprising because stress can increase your blood pressure, constrict your blood vessels, raise your cholesterol level, trigger arrhythmias, and speed up the rate at which your blood clots.

A 2021 study published in JAMA, comparing the effects of physical stress and emotional stress, found that emotional or mental stress took a significantly greater toll on the hearts and lives in the patients studied than did physical stress. Those experiencing greater mental stress were more likely to have a nonfatal heart attack or die of cardiovascular disease later in life.

Psychosocial stress induces a physiological inflammatory response in blood vessels. When vessel walls are damaged, inflammatory cells come into the vessel walls. Among other things, they release chemicals that may cause further damage. If the stress is chronic, the result can be chronic inflammation. A growing number of studies show that individuals with higher amounts of psychosocial stress and depression display elevated C-reactive protein and IL-6 levels, both markers of inflammation.

Many researchers believe that stress, inflammation and heart disease are all linked. Stress is now considered a major risk factor in heart disease, right up there with smoking, being overweight, and not exercising. All this becomes very important when you consider that heart disease kills more men over the age of 50 and more women over the age of 65 than any other disease.

TECHNICAL STUFF

A study reported by the Mayo Clinic in 2010 found that extreme or sudden stress that may accompany a relationship breakup or the death of a loved one can lead to "Broken Heart Syndrome" (BHS), or stress cardiomyopathy (severe heart muscle weakness). The study notes that this condition happens rapidly, and usually in women. In Japan, BHS is called "octopus trap cardiomyopathy" because the left ventricle balloons out in a peculiar shape.

Hitting below the belt

Ever notice how your stress seems to finds its way to your stomach? Your gastrointestinal system can be a ready target for much of the stress in your life. Stress can affect the secretion of acid in your stomach and can speed up or slow down the process of peristalsis (the rhythmic contraction of the muscles in your intestines). Constipation, diarrhea, gas, bloating, and weight loss all can be stress-related. Stress can contribute to gastroesophageal reflux disease and can also play a role in exacerbating irritable bowel syndrome, colitis, and Crohn's disease.

Speaking of your belt, it's important to recognize that people under stress usually experience changes in their weight. Stress can affect you in two very different ways.

>> When you're highly stressed, you may find yourself eating less. You may even find yourself losing weight. This "stress diet" isn't the best way to lose weight, and if the stress is prolonged it can result in lower overall health.

>> For many others, though, stress, especially moderate stress, can result in overeating. In effect, you're "feeding your emotions." The intent, often unconscious, is to feel better — to distract yourself from the emotional distress. The trouble is that "good feeling" lasts for about 12 seconds before you need another fix. And that means putting another notch on your belt. But it's not just your caloric intake. When you're stressed, your body releases a hormone called cortisol, which causes fat to accumulate around your abdomen and also enlarges individual fat cells, leading to what researchers term "diseased" fat. See Chapter 4 in Book 5 for tips on how to avoid emotional eating.

WHAT ABOUT STRESS AND ULCERS?

Once considered the poster disease for stress, ulcers have lost much of their stress-related status in recent years. Stress is no longer considered the primary cause of ulcers. It now appears that a bacterium called Helicobacter pylori, or H. pylori for short, is the culprit.

However, the final word on the relationship between stress and ulcers has yet to be written. More recent thinking has begun to question whether stress plays some role after all. Stress can affect secretions in the stomach that may exacerbate ulcers. A majority of those who do carry the H. pylori bacterium do not develop an ulcer, and many who do not carry the bacterium still develop ulcers. And of course, there is that body of research that has linked stress to ulcers. For example, the bombing of London during World War II and the earthquake in Kobe, Japan, both precipitated outbreaks of ulcer disease. Stay tuned.

Compromising your immune system

In the last decade or so, growing evidence has supported the theory that stress affects your immune system. In fact, researchers have even coined a name for this new field of study: psychoneuroimmunology. Quite a mouthful! Scientists who choose to go into this field study the relationships between moods, emotional states, hormonal levels, and changes in the nervous system and immune system.

Without drowning you in detail, stress — particularly chronic stress — can compromise your immune system, rendering it less effective in resisting bacteria and viruses. Research has shown that stress may play a role in exacerbating a variety of immune system disorders such as HIV, AIDS, herpes, cancer metastasis, viral infection, rheumatoid arthritis, and certain allergies, as well as other auto-immune conditions. Some recent studies appear to confirm this.

STRESS CAN BE TAXING

A number of studies have shown that when you're under stress, your cholesterol level goes up. In one now-classic study, researchers looked at the stress levels of accountants before and after the month of April, a notoriously busy time for tax accountants. They also looked at cholesterol levels in corporate accountants, who had stressful deadlines in both April and January. The researchers found that for both groups, cholesterol levels rose significantly before the April deadline and fell after the deadline. They observed a second rise in cholesterol levels for the corporate accountants as their January deadline approached. Again, after the deadline passed, blood lipid levels fell back to normal.

The cold facts: Connecting stress and the sniffles

In that wonderful musical comedy *Guys and Dolls*, a lovelorn Adelaide laments that when your life is filled with stress, "a person can develop a cold." It looks like she just may be right. Research conducted by Dr. Sheldon Cohen, a psychologist at Carnegie Mellon University, concluded that stress really does lower your resistance to colds. Cohen and his associates found that the higher a person's stress score, the more likely they were to come down with a cold when exposed to a cold virus.

Chronic stress, lasting a month or more, was the most likely to result in catching a cold. Experiencing severe stress for more than a month but less than six months doubled a person's risk of coming down with a cold, compared with those who were experiencing only shorter-term stress. Stress lasting more than two years nearly quadrupled the risk. The study also found that being unemployed or underemployed, or having interpersonal difficulties with family or friends, had the greatest effect. The exact mechanism whereby stress weakens immune functioning is still unclear. Tissues, anyone?

"Not tonight, dear. I have a (stress) headache."

A headache is just one of the many ways stress can interfere with your sex life. For both men and women, stress can reduce and even eliminate the pleasure of physical intimacy. Stress can affect sexual performance and rob you of your libido. When you're feeling stress, feeling sexy may not be at the top of your to-do list. Disturbed sexual performance for men may appear in the form of premature ejaculation, delayed ejaculation, and erectile dysfunction. For women the most common effects of stress are a lowered level of sexual interest and difficulty in achieving orgasm. The irony is that sex can be a way of relieving stress. In fact, for some people, sexual activity increases when they feel stressed.

» **Recognizing your tension**

» **Breathing properly**

» **Using the power of suggestion to relax**

» **Stretching, massaging, and using other relaxation methods**

Chapter **2**

Relaxing Your Body

When we hear the word *relaxation,* we tend to think of activities that take our minds off the stresses in our lives: watching TV, curling up with a good book, playing a round of golf, taking a nap — anything that might take us out of our world of worry, fear, and concern. In this chapter, though, learning to relax means something different. It means acquiring specific relaxation skills that can help you reduce bodily tension in a direct and systematic way. Rather than simply distract you or providing you with some temporary pleasure, these approaches focus more directly on releasing muscle tension. You find strategies and techniques that can help you let go of tension and relax your body.

Stress Can Be a Pain in the Neck (And That's Just for Starters)

The following is a short — and only partial — list of some of the effects tension has on your body. Unfortunately, many of these symptoms are all too familiar:

» Neck pain

» Headaches

>> Stomach cramps

>> Lower-back pain

>> Clenched, painful jaw

>> Teeth grinding

>> Sore shoulders

>> Muscle spasms

>> Tremors or twitches

And that's just on the outside. Inside your body, other tension-related changes are happening. Here is a sampling of what else is quietly going on in your body when you feel tense:

>> Your blood pressure goes up.

>> Your stomach secretes more acid.

>> Your cholesterol goes up.

>> Your blood clots more quickly.

All in all, knowing how to prevent and eliminate bodily tension seems like a pretty healthy idea.

REMEMBER

Your mind and body are far more interconnected than you might think. Separating the two isn't easy. When your mind tells you "you're worried" or "you're feeling anxious" or "you're afraid," your body hears this, as well. In turn, your body can become anxious and fearful. Your emotional distress (in your mind) is converted to physical distress (in your body). So, if you're worried, your body may become more tense and jittery, and you may start breathing faster. This process can also work the other way around. If your body is stressed, say from that fourth cup of coffee or a too-strenuous workout at the gym, your mind can interpret those physical states as stress, and you can become agitated or worried. That's why relaxing your body reduces not only bodily tension but also mental distress.

Funny, I don't feel tense

The fact is, you may not know when your body is tense. You get so used to being tense that you usually don't notice that you're feeling tense. Muscle tension creeps up on you. Slowly and often imperceptibly, your muscles tighten, and voila, the tension sets in. You don't feel the tension until you get a headache or feel the soreness in your neck and shoulders.

The trick is to become aware of bodily tension before it builds up and does its damage. Tuning in to your body takes a bit of practice. The next section gives you a simple awareness technique that helps you recognize your tension before it becomes a bigger problem.

Invasion of the body scan

One of the best ways to recognize bodily tension is to use this simple one-minute scanning exercise.

Find a place where you can sit or lie down comfortably and be undisturbed for a moment or two (see Figure 2-1). Scan your body for any muscle tension. Start with the top of your head and work your way down to your toes. Ask yourself:

>> Am I furrowing my brow?

>> Am I knitting my eyebrows?

>> Am I clenching my jaw?

>> Am I pursing my lips?

>> Am I hunching my shoulders?

>> Am I feeling tension in my arms?

>> Am I feeling tightness in my thigh and calf muscles?

>> Am I curling my toes?

>> Do I notice any discomfort anywhere else in my body?

TIP

With a little practice, you can scan your body in less than a minute, finding your tension quickly. Once you have the hang of it, try the body scan while sitting at a desk or standing up. See if you can do a body scan three or four times a day. It's a great way of becoming aware of your stress.

When you find your stress, of course, you want to do something about it. The following sections give you some options.

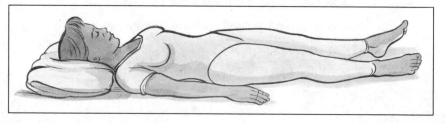

FIGURE 2-1:
A good position for body scanning.

Illustration by Pam Tanzey

Breathing Away Your Tension

Breathing properly is one of the simplest and best ways to drain your tension and relieve your stress. Simply by changing your breathing patterns, you can rapidly induce a state of greater relaxation. If you control the way you breathe, you have a powerful tool in reducing bodily tension. Just as important, you have a tool that helps prevent your body from becoming tense in the first place. This section shows you what you can do to incorporate a variety of stress-effective breathing techniques into your life.

Your breath is fine; it's your breathing that's bad

WARNING

"Bad breathing" can take a number of forms. You may be a chest and shoulder breather, bringing air into your lungs by expanding your chest cavity and raising your shoulders. This description certainly fits if you have more than a touch of vanity and opt for never sticking out your stomach when you breathe. You also may be a breath holder, stopping your breathing entirely when you're distracted or lost in thought. Both are inefficient, stress-producing forms of breathing. And when you're under stress, your breathing patterns deteriorate even more. To make things worse, once your breathing goes awry, you feel even more stressed. Quite a nasty cycle.

"Why change now? I've been breathing for years."

You probably take your breathing for granted. And why not? You've been breathing for most of your life; you'd think by now you would have figured out how to do it right. No such luck. When you're feeling stressed, your breathing becomes faster and shallower. When you breathe this way, your body reacts:

>> Less oxygen reaches your bloodstream.

>> Your blood vessels constrict.

>> Less oxygen reaches your brain.

>> Your heart rate and your blood pressure go up.

>> You feel light-headed, shaky, and tenser.

LOOKING UNDER THE HOOD

Breathing provides your body with oxygen and removes waste products — primarily carbon dioxide — from your blood. Your lungs carry out this gas exchange. Lungs, however, don't have their own muscles for breathing. Your diaphragm is the major muscle necessary for proper breathing. The diaphragm is a dome-shaped muscle that separates your chest cavity from your abdominal cavity and acts as a flexible floor for your lungs.

When you inhale, your diaphragm flattens downward, creating more space in the chest cavity and permitting the lungs to fill. You can see your stomach rising. When you exhale, your diaphragm returns to its dome shape. Diaphragmatic breathing, also called abdominal breathing, provides the most efficient way of exchanging oxygen and carbon dioxide.

Your diaphragm works automatically, but you can override the process, especially when you're under stress. And that's where problems can arise. Too often you neglect to use your diaphragm when you breathe, and you interfere with the proper exchange of gases in your system, which can result in greater tension, more fatigue, and more stress.

Our primitive ancestors knew how to breathe. They didn't have to deal with the IRS, stacks of unpaid bills, or the Boss from Hell. These days only opera singers, stage actors, musicians who play wind instruments, and a couple of dozen yoga instructors actually breathe effectively. The rest of us mess it up.

However, for a period of your life, you did get the whole breathing thing right. As a baby lying in your crib, you breathed serenely. Your little belly rose and fell in the most relaxed way. But then you grew up and blew it. Thankfully, all is not lost. You can re-teach yourself to breathe properly.

TECHNICAL STUFF

You probably think of breathing as a way of getting air into your lungs. However, in times past breathing was elevated to a more important status. Many religious groups and sects believed that a calming breath replenished the soul as well as soothed the body. In fact, the word *ruach* in Hebrew and the word *pneuma* in Greek have double meanings, connoting both breath and spirit. If you've read the Bible, the book of Genesis says that when God created Adam, he "breathed into his nostrils the breath of life, and man became a living soul."

Evaluating your breathing

REMEMBER

You may be one of the few people who actually breathe properly. But before you skip this section, read a little further. To find out whether the way you breathe is stress-reducing, take this simple test.

1. **Lie on your back.**

2. **Put your right hand on your belly and your left hand on your chest, as shown in Figure 2-2.**

   Try to become aware of the way you breathe. Check to see whether your breathing is smooth, slow, and regular. If you're breathing properly, the hand on your belly rises and falls rhythmically as you inhale and exhale. The hand on your chest should move very little, and if that hand does rise, it should follow the rise in your belly.

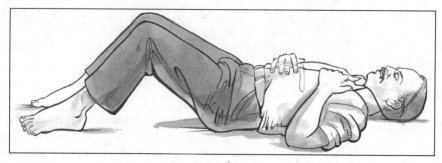

FIGURE 2-2:
Evaluating your
breathing.

Illustration by Pam Tanzey

Cutting yourself some slack

REMEMBER

It's common to find that people who want to adopt new patterns of breathing have a fervent desire to get it perfectly right. They frequently get so lost in body parts or lung mechanics that they wind up more stressed than they were before they started. Don't let this happen to you. And keep in mind that there's no one exactly right way to breathe all the time. Give yourself lots of room to experiment with your breathing. And don't overdo it. If you've been breathing inefficiently for all these years, changing gears may take some time. Above all, you're not taking a test. Don't grade yourself on how deeply you can breathe or how flat you can make your diaphragm. The goal is to reduce your stress, not add to it.

Changing the way you breathe, changing the way you feel

Sometimes, all it takes to make you feel better is one simple change. Changing the way you breathe can make all the difference in how you feel. The following exercises present various ways to alter your breathing. Try them and discover whether all you need is one simple change.

Breathing for starters

TIP

Here is one of the best and simplest ways of introducing yourself to stress-effective breathing:

1. **Either lying or sitting comfortably, put one hand on your belly and the other hand on your chest.**

2. **Inhale through your nose, making sure that the hand on your belly rises and the hand on your chest moves hardly at all.**

3. **As you inhale slowly, count silently to three.**

4. **As you exhale through your parted lips slowly, count silently to four, feeling the hand on your belly falling gently.**

   Pause slightly before your next breath. Continue to breathe like this until you feel completely relaxed.

Moving on to something more advanced: Taking a complete breath

TIP

Taking complete breaths (or doing Zen breathing, as it's often called) helps you breathe more deeply and more efficiently and helps you maximize your lung capacity. Follow these steps:

1. **Lie comfortably on a bed, in a reclining chair, or on a rug.**

   Keep your knees slightly apart and slightly bent. Close your eyes if you like. You may feel more comfortable placing a pillow under the small of your back to help relieve the pressure.

2. **Put one hand on your abdomen near your belly button and the other hand on your chest so that you follow the motion of your breathing.**

   Try to relax. Let go of any tension you may feel in your body.

3. **Begin by slowly inhaling through your nose, first filling the lower part of your lungs, then the middle part of your chest, and then the upper part of your chest.**

As you inhale, feel your diaphragm pushing down, gently extending your abdomen, making room for the newly inhaled air. Notice the hand on your abdomen rise slightly. The hand on your chest should move very little, and when it does, it should follow your abdomen. Don't use your shoulders to help you breathe.

4. **Exhale slowly through your parted lips, emptying your lungs from top to bottom.**

    Make a whooshing sound as the air passes through your lips, and notice the hand on your abdomen fall.

5. **Pause slightly and take in another breath, repeating this cycle.**

    Continue breathing this way for ten minutes or so — certainly until you feel more relaxed and peaceful. Practice this technique daily if you can. Try this exercise while sitting and then while standing.

With a little practice, this form of breathing comes more naturally and automatically. With some time and some practice, you may begin to breathe this way much more of the time. Stick with it.

Trying some "belly-button balloon" breathing

A simpler way of breathing more deeply and more evenly is to work with a visual image, in this case a balloon. Here's what you do:

1. **Imagine that a small balloon — about the size of a grapefruit — is replacing your stomach, just under your belly button, as shown in Figure 2-3.**

2. **As you inhale through your nose, imagine that you're actually inhaling through your belly button, inflating this once-empty balloon.**

    This balloon is small, so don't overinflate it. As the balloon gets larger, notice how your belly rises.

3. **Exhale slowly through your nose or mouth, again imagining that the air is leaving through your belly button.**

    Your balloon is now slowly and easily returning to its deflated state.

4. **Pause slightly before the next breath in and then repeat, gently and smoothly inflating your balloon to a comfortable size.**

    Repeat this exercise, as often as you can, whenever you can.

STANDING UP STRAIGHT

Your mother was right! When you're under stress, you have a tendency to hunch over, making your posture lousy and your breathing impaired. You then breathe less deeply, denying your system the proper supply of oxygen you need. As a result, your muscles get tense. When you stand or sit straight, you reverse this process. You needn't stand like a West Point cadet to correct bad posture. Overdoing it probably produces as much tension as you felt before. Just keep your shoulders from slouching forward. If you're unsure about what your posture looks like, ask your mother or a good friend.

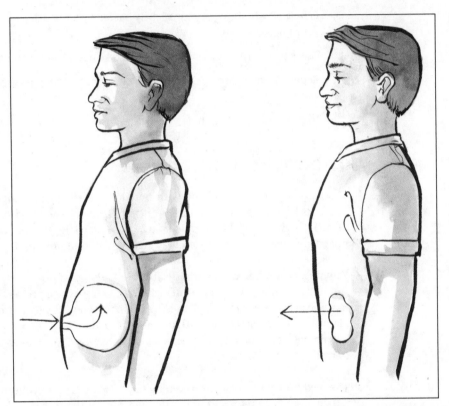

FIGURE 2-3:
Balloon
breathing.

Illustration by Pam Tanzey

Emergency breathing: How to breathe in the trenches

TIP

Breathing properly is no big deal when you're lying on your bed or sitting in front of the TV. But what's your breathing like when you're caught in gridlock, when you're facing down a deadline, or when the stock market drops 20 percent? You're now in crisis mode. You need another form of breathing. Here's what to do:

1. **Inhale slowly through your nostrils, taking in a very deep diaphragmatic breath, filling your lungs and filling your cheeks.**

2. **Hold that breath for about six seconds.**

3. **Exhale slowly through your slightly parted lips, releasing all the air in your lungs.**

   Pause at the end of this exhalation. Now take a few "normal" breaths.

4. **Repeat Steps 1 through 3 two or three times and then return to what you were doing.**

   This form of deep breathing should put you in a more relaxed state.

The yawn that refreshes

Yawning is usually associated with boredom. Business meetings you think will run well into the next millennium or painful telephone solicitors explaining (in detail) the virtues of their long-distance plan may trigger more than a few yawning gasps. However, your yawn may signal something more than boredom.

Yawning is another way Mother Nature tells you that your body is under stress. In fact, yawning helps relieve stress. When you yawn, more air — and therefore more oxygen — enters your lungs, revitalizing your bloodstream. Releasing that plaintive sound that comes with yawning is also tension reducing. Unfortunately, people have become a little over-socialized, making for wimpy yawns. You need to recapture this lost art.

The next time you feel a yawn coming on, go with it. Open your mouth widely and inhale more fully than you normally might. Take that breath all the way down to your belly. Exhale fully through your mouth, completely emptying your lungs. What a feeling! Enjoy it. So what if your friends don't call you anymore?

Tensing Your Way to Relaxation

After you master the art of breathing (see the exercises in the preceding section), you're ready to discover another way of relaxing your body. One of the better relaxation techniques derives from a method called *progressive relaxation* or *deep-muscle relaxation*. This method is based on the notion that you're not aware of what your muscles feel like when they're tensed. By purposely tensing your muscles, you're able to recognize what tension feels like and identify which muscles are creating that tension. This technique is highly effective and has proved to be a valuable tool for quickly reducing muscle tension and promoting relaxation.

Exploring how progressive relaxation works

You begin progressive relaxation by tensing a specific muscle or group of muscles (your arms, legs, shoulders, and so on). You notice the way the tension feels. You hold that tension for about ten seconds and then let it go, replacing that tension with something much more pleasant — relaxation. By the time you tense and relax most of your major muscle groups, you feel relaxed, at peace, and much less stressed. The following general guidelines set the stage for muscle-group-specific relaxation techniques later in this chapter:

1. **Lie down or sit, as comfortably as you can, and close your eyes.**

   Find a quiet, dimly lit place that gives you some privacy, at least for a while.

2. **Tense the muscles of a particular body part.**

   To practice, start by tensing your right hand and arm. Begin by simply making a fist. As you clench your fist, notice the tension and strain in your hand and forearm. Without releasing that tension, bend your right arm and flex your bicep, making a muscle the way you might to impress the kids in the schoolyard.

   REMEMBER

   Don't strain yourself in any of these muscle-tensing maneuvers; don't overdo it. When you tense a muscle group, don't tense as hard as you can. Tense to about 75 percent of what you can do. If you feel pain or soreness, ease up on the tension, and if you still hurt, defer your practice till another time.

3. **Hold the tension in the body part for about seven seconds.**

4. **Let go of the tension quickly, letting the muscles go limp.**

   Notice the difference in the way your hand and arm feel. Notice the difference between the sensations of tension and those of relaxation. Let these feelings of relaxation deepen for about 30 seconds.

5. **Repeat Steps 1 through 4, using the same muscle group.**

6. **Move to another muscle group.**

Simply repeat Steps 1 through 4, substituting a different muscle group each time. Continue with your left hand and arm and then work your way through the major muscle groups listed in the following section.

Relaxing your face and head

Wrinkle your forehead (creating all those lines that everybody hates) by raising your eyebrows as high as you can. Hold this tension for about five seconds and then let go, releasing all the tension in your forehead. Just let your forehead muscles become smooth. Notice the difference between the feelings of tension you felt and the more pleasant feelings of relaxation.

Now clench your jaw by biting down on your back teeth. At the same time, force a smile. Hold this uncomfortable position for about five seconds and then relax your jaw, letting your mouth fall slightly ajar.

Finally, purse your lips, pushing them together firmly. Hold that tension for a bit and then relax, letting your lips open slightly. Notice how relaxed your face and head feel. Enjoy this sensation and let this feeling deepen by letting go of any remaining sources of tension around your mouth and lips.

Relaxing your neck and shoulders

Bend your head forward as though you're going to touch your chest with your chin (you probably will). Feel the tension in the muscles of your neck. Hold that tension. Now tilt your head slightly, first to one side and then to another. Notice the tension at the side of your neck as you do so. Tilt your head back as if you're trying to touch your upper back. But don't force it or overdo it, stopping if you notice any pain and discomfort. Now relax, letting your head return to a more comfortable, natural position. Enjoy the relaxation for a moment or so.

Now scrunch up your shoulders as though you're trying to reach your ears. Hold it, feel the tension (again for about five seconds), and let your shoulders fall to a comfortable, relaxed position. Notice the feelings of relaxation that are spreading through your shoulders and neck.

Relaxing your back

Arch your back, being careful not to overdo it. Hold that tension for several seconds and then let your back and shoulders return to a more comfortable, relaxed position.

Relaxing your legs and feet

Either sitting or lying down, raise your right foot so that you feel some tension in your thigh and buttock. At the same time, push out your heel and point your toes toward your head, as shown in Figure 2-4. Hold this tension, notice what it feels like, and then let go, letting your leg fall to the bed or floor, releasing any remaining tension. Let that relaxation deepen for a while. Repeat this sequence with your other leg and foot.

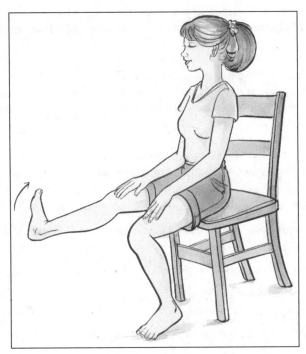

Illustration by Pam Tanzey

Relaxing your buttocks

Tense the muscles of your buttocks, noticing what that feels like. Hold that tension for several seconds. Slowly release that muscle tension, letting go, letting the muscles in your buttocks gently release. Notice those feelings of relaxation and let them deepen even further.

Relaxing your stomach

Take in a deep breath and hold that breath, tensing the muscles in your stomach. Imagine that you're preparing yourself for a punch in the stomach. Hold that tension. And relax, letting go of the tension.

After you finish this sequence, let your body sink into an even deeper state of relaxation. Let go more and more. Mentally go over the sensations you're feeling in your arms, face, neck, shoulders, back, stomach, and legs. Feel your body becoming looser and more relaxed. Savor the feeling.

Scrunching up like a pretzel

When pressed for time, you can do a quickie version of the progressive relaxation exercise that is described in the preceding section. Simply, this technique compresses all the muscle-tensing and relaxing sequences into one. Think of it as one gigantic scrunch.

To do this, you have to master the gradual version first. The success of this rapid form of relaxation depends on your ability to create and release muscle tension quickly, skills you master by slowly working through all of the muscle groups individually.

TIP

Here's what to do: Sit or lie comfortably in a room that is quiet and relatively free of distractions. Now, tense all the muscle groups listed here, simultaneously:

>> Clench both fists, bend both arms and tense your biceps. At the same time,

>> Lift both legs until you notice a moderate degree of tension and discomfort, and

>> Tense the muscles in your buttocks and hold that tension, and

>> Scrunch up your face, closing your eyes, furrowing your brow, clenching your jaws, and pursing your lips, and

>> Bring your shoulders as close as you can to your ears, while you

>> Tense your stomach muscles.

Hold this "total scrunch" for about five seconds and then release, letting go of any and all tension. Let your legs fall to the floor or bed and let your arms fall to your sides. Let the rest of your body return to a relaxed position. Repeat this sequence at various points throughout your day.

Mind over Body: Using the Power of Suggestion

Another important approach to bodily relaxation is called *autogenic training*, or AT for short. The word *autogenic* means self-generation or self-regulation. This method attempts to regulate your *autonomic nervous functions* and more specifically your *parasympathetic nervous system* (your heart rate, blood pressure, and breathing, among others) rather than relaxing your muscles. With autogenic training, you use your mind to regulate your body's internal stress levels.

AT relies on the power of suggestion to induce physiological changes. These suggestions are mental images that your subconscious picks up and transmits to your body. Just thinking about certain changes in your body produces those kinds of changes. As a result, you experience deep feelings of relaxation. AT may sound mysterious, but it isn't. After you master this technique, AT is a highly effective way of putting yourself in a more relaxed state.

TIP

The method described here is a more abbreviated form than the one originally devised. However, it's better suited to a busy lifestyle. Here's what you do:

1. **Get comfy.**

   Find a suitably quiet, not-too-hot, and not-too-cold place. You can sit or lie down, but make sure your body is well supported and as comfortable as possible. Try to breathe slowly and smoothly.

2. **Concentrate passively.**

   For this approach to be effective, you need to adopt a receptive, casual attitude of passive concentration. You want to be alert, not falling asleep but not asking your mind to work too hard. You can't force yourself to relax. Just let it happen. Be aware of your body and your mind, but don't actively analyze everything or worry about how you're doing. Should a distracting thought come your way, notice it and then let it go. If the relaxation doesn't come at first, don't worry. It comes with more practice.

3. **Allow various body parts to begin feeling warm and heavy.**

   Although autogenic training utilizes many suggestions and images, the two most effective images are warmth and heaviness. Start by focusing on your right arm. Now slowly and softly say to yourself:

   I am calm . . . I am at peace . . . My right arm is warm . . . and heavy . . . My right arm is warm . . . and heavy . . . My right arm is warm . . . and heavy . . . I can feel the warmth and heaviness flowing into my right arm . . . I can feel my right arm becoming warmer . . . and heavier . . . I can feel my right arm becoming warmer . . . and heavier . . . I can feel my right arm becoming warmer . . . and heavier . . . I am at peace . . . I am calm . . . I am at peace . . . I am calm.

Take the time to become aware of the feelings in your arm and hand. Notice that your arm is becoming warmer and heavier. Don't rush this process. Enjoy the changes your body is now beginning to experience.

4. **After you complete the phrases, remain silent and calm for about 30 seconds, letting the relaxation deepen; then focus on your left arm.**

   Repeat the same phrases again, this time substituting left arm for right arm. (Hopefully by now you've memorized these phrases and can close your eyes and not worry about a script.)

5. **Move to other parts of your body.**

   Focus on other areas, repeating the same phrases but substituting other parts of your body. Here is the complete sequence: right arm, left arm, both arms, right leg, left leg, both legs, neck and shoulders, chest and abdomen, and finally your entire body.

   Completing the entire sequence shouldn't take you more than a half hour or so. If you can fit in two or three autogenic sessions a day, all the better. You may need some time to master this technique, but the results are well worth the effort.

USE YOUR IMAGINATION? YOU'RE GETTING WARMER!

With autogenic training, you may find that using the "warm and heavy" suggestions and images isn't effective for you. You may need a different image to release the tension in your body. Here are alternate suggestive images that can induce feelings of warmth and heaviness:

- **Heat me up:** Imagine that the body part in question (arm, leg, and so on) is wrapped in a heating pad. Slowly but surely the heat permeates your body, relaxing your muscles more and more.

- **Get in hot water:** Imagine that you're immersing your arm or leg in soothing warm water.

- **Sunny side up:** Mentally direct a sun lamp to a particular part of your anatomy.

- **Heavy metal:** Visualize weights attached to your arm, leg, and so on.

- **Get the lead in:** Imagine that your limb is filled with lead.

Stretching Away Your Stress

Stretching is one of the ways your body naturally discharges excess bodily tension. You may notice that you automatically feel the need to stretch after waking up in the morning or just before retiring at night. But a good stretch can drain away much of your body's tension at other times, too. You may be desk-bound or otherwise required to sit for long periods of time during the day, causing your muscles to tense and tighten. Consider adopting one or more basic stretches and taking a stretch break at various points throughout the day. Cats do, dogs do, why not you?

TIP

Following are two tension-relieving stretches that are wonderful ways of draining off a lot of excess tension. They are simple and shouldn't evoke much comment or ridicule from friends or coworkers.

>> **The Twist:** This stretch is great for your upper body. Sitting or standing, put both your hands behind the back of your head, locking your fingers together. Move your elbows toward each other until you feel some moderate tension. Now twist your body slightly, first to the right for a few seconds and then slowly to the left. When you finish, let your arms fall to your sides.

>> **The Leg-lift:** This stretch is good for your lower body. Sitting in your chair, raise both your legs until you feel a comfortable level of tightness in them. Maintaining that tension, flex and point your toes toward your head. Hold that tension for about ten seconds and then let your legs fall to the floor. If doing this with both legs together is a wee bit uncomfortable, try it one leg at a time.

REMEMBER

Stretch slowly and don't overdo it. You're trying to relax your muscles, not punish them.

"ALL THIS RELAXING IS MAKING ME TENSE!"

Believe it or not, you may find that practicing relaxation can be stressful, at least at first.

Changing your breathing patterns, tensing and relaxing muscles, and exploring autogenic exercises can result in some strange side effects. You may notice some tingling or a feeling of restlessness and, paradoxically, an increase in tension. This is not unusual, and, although it's distracting, don't take this as a sign that you're doing something wrong. As you become more familiar with how your body feels when it's in a highly relaxed state, these sensations disappear.

Massage? Ah, There's the Rub!

Massage and other touch and pressure therapies are among the most popular ways of relieving muscle tension. These days you can get a massage almost as easily as you can get your hair cut. In the past, the idea of a massage usually conjured up an image of a liniment rubdown in a sweaty gym or pampered caresses in a swanky health spa. No more. Massage and related treatment have come of age.

The range and popularity of touch and pressure disciplines and therapies have grown enormously in recent years. A partial list of available methods and techniques include

>> Swedish massage

>> Reflexology

>> Shiatsu

>> Chiropractic

>> Acupressure

All these methods have their origins in early medicine and healing. Many claim spiritual as well as physical changes. Rather than go into each of these disciplines separately, this section discusses several of the simpler stress-relieving approaches from the preceding list that are particularly useful and easy to grasp.

You have several choices when it comes to massage. You can spend some bucks and get a professional to give you a massage. Or you can find someone who will give you a massage for free. Or you can give yourself a massage. This section starts with the last option, which is often the cheapest and doesn't require friends.

Massaging yourself

You can go two ways: high-tech or low-tech.

>> The high-tech route usually requires a wall socket or lots of batteries. Many specialty stores stock massage paraphernalia. One option is a mega-buck relaxation chair that transports you to relaxation heaven with the flick of a switch. On the less expensive side, a handheld vibrator massages those tight and tired muscles, leaving you much more relaxed.

>> Alternately, you can forego the batteries and the cash by letting your fingers do the work. Fingers are cheaper, easier to control, and readily available.

Following are a few simple ways to rub away your stress.

For your hands

Hold your left palm in front of you, fingers together. The fleshy spot between your thumb and index finger is a key acupressure point that should spread a sensation of relaxation when massaged. Using your right thumb, massage this spot in a circular motion for a slow count of 15. Switch hands and repeat.

For stress-related fatigue, pinch just below the first joint of your pinkie with the thumb and index finger of the opposite hand. (Pressure should be firm but not painful.) Increase the pressure slightly. Make small circular movements in a counterclockwise direction while maintaining pressure. Continue for 20 seconds. Release. Wait for ten seconds and repeat up to five times.

For your feet

Try this sole-soothing exercise. Take off your socks and shoes and sit comfortably with one leg crossed over the other. (The sole of your foot should be almost facing you.) With both hands, grasp the arches of your foot and apply pressure, especially with your thumbs. Now kneading (like you would bread dough, using your thumbs and fingers) every part of your foot, work your way from your heel right up to your toes. Give each of your toes a squeeze. Now massage the other foot in a similar way.

TIP

If crossing your legs is more stressful than it used to be, go to the kitchen and get your rolling pin. Sit in a chair and position the rolling pin next to your foot. Gently roll your bare foot back and forth slowly for two minutes or so. Then try it with the other foot. Now wash the pin. (If you don't own a rolling pin, work with a tennis ball. Put it under the arch of your bare foot, put some pressure on that foot, and move the ball backward and forward. Keep this rhythm going for about two minutes, and then switch to your other foot.)

For your neck and shoulders

Stress most often finds its way to your neck and shoulders. To dissipate that tension, take your left hand and firmly massage your right shoulder and the right side of your neck. Start with some gentle circular motions, rubbing the muscle with your index and pointer fingers. Then finish with a firmer massage, squeezing the shoulder and neck muscles between your thumb and other fingers. Now switch to the other side.

For your face

Start by placing both of your hands on your face with the tips of your fingers resting on your forehead and the heels of your palms resting just under your cheeks. Gently pull down the skin on your forehead with the tips of your fingers while pushing up the area under your palms. Rhythmically repeat this movement, contracting and releasing your fingers and palms. You can also try pulling on your ears in different directions.

Becoming the massage-er or massage-ee

Having someone else give you a massage certainly has its advantages. When someone else does all the work, you can completely let go: Sit or lie back and totally relax. And another person can reach places on your body that you could never reach. You can, of course, visit a massage therapist; you can also ask a friend to give you a massage. Of course, you may have to reciprocate. But even giving someone else a massage can relieve some of your tension. Here are some general hints and guidelines to get you started:

>> Use some massage oil or body lotion to add a relaxing aroma and smooth the massage process. (Warm the oil to room temperature so as not to shock your or your partner's system.)

>> Lower the lights to provide a soothing, relaxing atmosphere. Calming music also adds a nice touch.

>> Focus your massage on the lower back, neck, and shoulders — places stress tends to reside and cause the most discomfort.

>> Start by applying pressure lightly until the massage-ee is relaxed. Then increase the pressure, using your palms to knead the muscles.

>> Finish up with a lighter massage, and let your partner linger for a while after the massage to extend the sense of relaxation.

>> Don't overdo it. A good massage shouldn't have the massage-ee writhing in pain. A bad massage can cause more stress than it attempts to relieve.

Taking a Three-Minute Energy Burst

Any concentrated expenditure of energy produces more stress by tensing your muscles, speeding your heart rate, and quickening your breathing. However, after you stop expending energy, you find that your muscles relax and your heart rate and breathing slow down to a level that is lower than when you started. This energy boost can come from walking briskly, running for a short distance, doing jumping jacks, jumping rope, doing sit-ups or push-ups, running up steps — anything that gets your body going.

>> **Become a shaker.** Shaking off tension is fun. You can do this exercise either sitting or standing. Begin by holding your arms loosely in front of you and shaking your hands at the wrists. Now let your arms and shoulders join in the fun. Continue for a short while and taper off slowly, letting your arms fall comfortably to your sides. Now lift one leg and start shaking it. Then shift to the other leg. (If you're sitting, you can do both legs at the same time.) When you finish, notice the tingling sensations in your body and, more importantly, the feelings of relaxation. Admittedly, it looks a little strange, but it works.

>> **Soak up your stress.** Think of your bathroom as a mini health spa and your bathtub as a pool of relaxation. Besides, not only do you emerge relaxed and de-stressed, but you're also clean. Here's the recipe for that relaxing soak:

- A spare half hour

- A tub of hot, soapy water

- Soothing scents, such as lavender Epsom salts

- Soft lighting

- Relaxing music

- A phone that is turned off or at least silenced

More Ways to Relax

A few relaxation techniques from off the beaten path:

TIP

>> **Throw in the towel.** Barbers used to give their customers shaves along with haircuts. In those days, you felt marvelous as your barber carefully placed moist, hot towels on your face. These days, stylists only cut hair. And unless you fly first class to Europe or dine in an upscale Japanese restaurant, you're unlikely to experience the joy of a hot towel on your face — unless, of course, you put it there yourself. Simply take one or two washcloths and immerse them in hot water. Squeeze out the excess water, lie back, close your eyes, and put them on your face. Ah, nirvana.

And what if you don't have a towel or hot water? Use your hands. Rub them together till they feel warm. Place each hand on a side of your face. No, the feeling isn't quite as good as a moist, hot towel, but it can still help you relax.

>> **Jump into a hot tub.** If you have a hot tub, great, but keep in mind that many bathtubs have the same benefits.

HAVE A DRINK?

May you use an alcoholic beverage as an agent of relaxation? Yes and no.

For some time now, research literature has been supportive of the value of moderate drinking (that is, no more than one or two alcoholic drinks per day). At this level of intake, alcohol has been found to raise levels of HDL (the good cholesterol) and lessen the risk of heart disease. However, the risks from excessive drinking far outweigh these benefits. For many, drinking can be a slippery slope, with the cure becoming the disease.

The bottom line: Don't put alcohol at the top of your stress-reduction list. If you have successfully integrated a drink or the occasional use of a pill into your life, fine. But always remember, you can reduce your stress in better ways.

>> **Try some yoga.** Why reinvent the wheel when some marvelous relaxation approaches have been around for many years? Yoga has been practiced for 5,000 years. Yoga looks at health and wellbeing from a broad, holistic perspective that sees the mind and body as dynamically interconnected. This ancient Eastern tradition combines physical and postural exercises with meditation practices, breathing techniques, and mindfulness that can help you relax your body and calm your mind. Most people who have tried yoga swear by it. Find a good teacher and give it a try. (Ask friends about yoga classes in your community. See Chapter 4 in Book 4 for more about yoga.)

>> **Relax in the bedroom.** Sex can be a marvelous way of unwinding and letting go of physical tension. Including some form of mutual massage in your love-making can increase the relaxation benefits.

» **Making time for yourself**

» **Getting more done in less time**

» **Overcoming procrastination**

Chapter **3**

Finding More Time

H ave you noticed how quickly your days fill up? You often find yourself hurried, harried, and rushing to do all that you feel has to be done. Putting out fires, dealing with last-minute crises, and taking care of unending details leave little spare time for anything else. Add to that a busy job, a family, and at least a few other obligations, and you notice that your stress level is escalating. And something else is happening: You have less and less time to spend on the things that you really enjoy and that bring you satisfaction. Fortunately, managing your time more effectively is something you can master.

This chapter gives you direction and strategies to help you manage your time more efficiently and effectively, and reduce your time-related stress. For even more information on this topic, try the latest edition of *Successful Time Management For Dummies* by Dirk Zeller (Wiley).

REMEMBER

Effective time management is really all about managing your priorities. The trick is figuring out what those priorities are and making time for them to happen. Remember those wise words of Bertrand Russell: "The time you enjoy wasting is not wasted time."

Determining Whether You Struggle with Time Management

Maybe you don't experience time-related stress. Let's find out. Take a look at the following list and check off those items that seem to describe you:

>> I don't have enough time for myself, my family, or my friends.

>> I waste too much time.

>> I'm constantly rushing.

>> I don't have enough time to do the things I really enjoy.

>> I frequently miss deadlines or am late for appointments.

>> I spend almost no time planning my day.

>> I almost never work with some kind of prioritized to-do list.

>> I have difficulty saying no to others when they make demands on my time.

>> I rarely delegate tasks and responsibilities.

>> I procrastinate too often.

Checking off only one or two items on this list suggests that your time-management skills require only a tune-up. Checking off more than four of them suggests that your time-management skills may be in need of a major overhaul.

Being Mindful of Your Time

An important step in changing the way you manage your time is becoming aware of how you use your time. Without awareness, your time management can become a victim of your time-wasting patterns. Much of your life is lived on auto-pilot. You repeat the same patterns of thinking and behavior, failing to step away and consider how you're using your time. The price you pay ranges from the minor (lateness, procrastination, missed deadlines) to the more dramatic (missed opportunities and life experiences). The following sections show you how to be more mindful about time management to get the results you want.

Knowing where your time goes

TIP

For a short period of time, perhaps a day or two, keep a simple time log. A sheet of paper will do or, if you're more comfortable with your electronic device, use that. At convenient times during your day, enter what you did, or are doing, in the appropriate time slots. Don't become compulsive about this; you don't have to make it exact to the minute. However, be sure to record your electronic time usage — those times when you checked your email, made or received a phone call, texted, visited social-networking sites, or surfed the Internet. A sampling of a day or two should supply enough data to give you a rough picture of how you use — or misuse — your time. Use this simple rating code:

1 = Great use of my time

2 = Okay use of my time

3 = So-so use of my time

W = Waste of my time

Also add some comments that reflect how you feel about the way you used that time. Table 3-1 gives you a sample of what one day may look like.

TABLE 3-1   ## Time Log for Monday

Time Spent	Activity	Rating	Comments
7–7:20	Overslept	W	I didn't need it
7:20–7:45	Got ready for work	1	
7:45–8:05	Ate breakfast	1	
8:10–8:45	Commuted to work	1	
9–9:20	Read/answered email	2	Ten minutes would do it
9:20–9:40	Returned phone calls	2, but W	Could have been a lot shorter
10–10:45	Did productive work	1	
10:45–11	Took a coffee break	2	
11–12	Sat through a meeting	3	Unnecessary meeting
12–12:30	Read/answered email	2	
12:45–2	Lunch	1, but W	Too long
2:15–3:00	Did productive work (paying bills)	1	Good use of my time

(continued)

TABLE 3-1 *(continued)*

Time Spent	Activity	Rating	Comments
3–3:45	Read/answered email	2	Could have done it another time
3:45–4:00	Fiddled on computer	W	Dumb!
4–4:30	Did productive work	2	
4:30–5	Paid bills	2	Do at home?
5–5:30	Made phone calls	3	
5:45–6:20	Commuted home	1	Listen to news and music
6:30–6:50	Talked with spouse	1	Don't do it enough!
6:50–7:15	Read newspaper	2	
7:15–8	Ate dinner	1	Over too quickly
8–9	Watched TV	2	Love this program!
9–10	Watched TV	W	Not worth watching
10–10:30	Watched news	2	
10:30–11	Read in bed	2	

Figuring out what you want more time for

TIP

As an exercise, grab a sheet of paper and jot down activities that you would like to spend more time doing. This exercise helps you get in touch with those activities that you value and derive satisfaction from.

The following is a sample of general items you may want to consider. (You can, of course, add others.)

>> Spending time with your family and friends

>> Advancing your job or career

>> Pursuing a hobby or interest

>> Reading

>> Exercising

>> Nurturing your soul

>> Volunteering for community activities

>> Traveling

>> Sleeping

Knowing what you want to spend *less* time doing

Knowing what you want to spend more time doing is only half the battle. Knowing what you *don't* want to spend time doing is just as important. Here are some things you may wish you spent less time doing:

>> Working late at night and on weekends

>> Doing office paperwork

>> Attending events you don't enjoy

>> Cleaning the house

>> Doing laundry

>> Spending time with people you don't enjoy

>> Surfing the web

>> Watching so much television

REMEMBER

Your goal is to fill your life with more of the things you *want* to do — things that bring more meaning and joy to your life. This means knowing how to minimize time spent doing the things you *have* to do.

Minding your time with cues and prompts

One good way of becoming mindful of your time is to use naturally occurring cues and prompts as signals to stop for a moment, take a breath, and consider how you're using your time. A prompt or cue can take various forms. It can be as simple as turning on your computer or beginning a new task. These basic behaviors prompt you to mentally step away from what you're doing and take a more careful look at what you have done and what you will do.

You can also introduce cues or prompts that are not naturally occurring. Stick a small paper dot on your watch face or use that photograph of your last family vacation as reminders to become more mindful of what you're doing or not doing.

Here are some other possible cues and prompts that could act as reminders:

>> Hanging up after a phone call

>> Feeling the urge to check your email

>> Leaving your office or cubicle

>> Sending the kids off to school

>> Finishing a task

>> Taking a bathroom break

>> Ending a meal

>> Checking the time

>> Turning on the TV

>> Thinking of visiting your favorite social media site

So, instead of automatically checking your email every ten minutes or turning on the TV every time you're bored, use the behaviors as your cues to stop what you're about to do, step back mentally, take a breath or two, and gain some emotional distance. When you have that distance and awareness, ask yourself some pertinent questions that can help you evaluate how you're about to use your time.

Questioning your choices and changing behaviors

TIP

One great way of creating awareness is to have some questions ready to ask yourself. These can free you from the grip of auto-pilot and set a more productive course. Here are a few to help you get started:

>> "Am I making the best use of my time right now?"

>> "Am I procrastinating and avoiding doing something more important?"

>> "Could I be doing what I'm doing in a more efficient way?"

>> "Could I delegate or share this task with someone else?"

>> "Do I really need to check my email so frequently?"

>> "Do I really need to be on the Internet right now?"

>> "Should I really be watching TV right now?"

Rather than answer these questions with a simple yes or no, expand your answer to include additional material that either strengthens your rationale for doing what you plan to do or provides you with strong counter-arguments motivating you to spend your time doing something else. For example, your internal dialogue might sound something like this:

"Okay, I'm about to pick up the TV remote. Is there something on now that I really want to watch? Not really. I'm a little bored and am avoiding doing stuff that I really should be doing. Watching TV is fine, but not right now. What could I be doing now that could be more important, more satisfying, or even more fun? What about hitting the gym or finishing that article? Watch TV later when there's something good on, and use it as a reward for doing other things first."

By introducing this "wise voice," you create a strong ally that can defend or revise how you spend your time. This makes it more difficult to be seduced by your avoidant automatic behavior. This awareness and self-talk makes it more likely that your use of time will be productive and worthwhile.

Becoming a List Maker

Making lists might seem so obvious and sooo last century, yet lists can be one of your better time-management tools. You can work with three lists:

>> **A master to-do list:** This list is your source list, detailing all the tasks and involvements that you want to accomplish. This is your primary list.

>> **A will-do-today list:** This list details how you want to spend your time *today*.

>> **A will-do-later list:** This list enables you to schedule tasks in the *coming days or weeks*.

All these lists work together, providing you with a comprehensive time-management plan.

Starting with a master to-do list

You want to start with a master to-do list. Simply create a list of things you want to do or have to do either now or in the near future. Try to rank these items in order of importance, putting the more important ones first.

TIP

To help you rate the importance of the things on which you spend your time, try using this simple rating system:

1 = High priority (highly valued or important to me)

2 = Medium priority

3 = Low priority (not especially important to me)

D = Difficult or time-consuming

E = Easy or enjoyable

Q = Quick! Could do this in less than five minutes

Here is a sample of a master to-do list:

To Do	Priority/Rating
See my patients	1
Call plumber re: water heater	1
Pay estimated taxes	1
Pay phone bill	1-Q
Look into refinancing mortgage	1-D
Buy two books	2-E
Clean bedroom	2
Paint guest room	2
Get to the gym	2
Call Aunt Rose	2-E
Get a haircut	2
Do billing paperwork	2
Pick up printing paper	1-Q
Get plane tickets for trip	2
Pick up meds	2
Download photos	2-E
Download new music	3-E
Pick up lunch food	2-E

Review and update your list daily, adding items and tasks as they come up and removing tasks when they are completed or become irrelevant.

Creating a will-do-today list

When you have your master to-do list in hand, you're ready to create your more specific will-do-today list. Actually, this looks more like a daily planner than a usual list. It schedules how you want to spend your time *today*. This can be created the night before or first thing in the morning. You'll need a day planner, either paper or electronic. Both will work well.

Working from your master list, schedule your day. Enter the activities and tasks, work and personal, that you'd like to accomplish today. Table 3-2 shows a sample of what a "planned" day looks like.

TABLE 3-2

Will Do Today: Tuesday, January 5

Time	Task	Outcome
7:30	Create my daily to-do list; check email	✓
8	See patient A	✓
8:45	Make calls; send email	✓
9	See patient B	✓
9:45	Make calls; send email	✓
11	See patient C (cancelled but paid estimated taxes instead)	
12	See patient D	✓
12:45	Eat lunch	✓
1	See patient E	✓
1:45	Make calls (Aunt Rose); check email	✓
2	Do insurance billing (needs more time)	
2:45	Pay phone bill	✓
3	Go to the gym	✓
4	See patient F	✓
4:45	Buy plane tickets (try again tomorrow)	
5	See patient G	✓
5:45	Return phone calls	✓
6	See patient H	✓
7	Paint guest room at home	✓
8	Paint guest room at home	✓
8:30	Have dinner; watch news	✓
9	Have dinner; watch news	✓
9:30	Watch TV	✓
10	Read in bed	✓
11	Sleep	✓

Having a will-do-later list

TIP

As you look at your master to-do list and daily will-do-today list, you may decide that some items would be best done a day or two (or five) later. You need an extension of your will-do-today list where you can enter tasks to be done later on. Enter those tasks into your weekly or monthly planner. These may be tasks that can't be done until an earlier part is finished or until you obtain some additional information. It may be that the person you need to deal with won't be in the office until later in the week. It may simply be that you don't get around to it. Whatever the reason, keeping a longer-term list gives you more flexibility and comprehensiveness.

Keeping some tips in mind as you make your lists

TIP

Here are some suggestions and ideas to keep in mind as you put your daily lists together. Remember, not every idea works equally well for everybody. Give each suggestion some thought and give it a fair try. Ultimately you'll put together your own unique time-management ideas that best match your style and personality.

>> **Don't overdo it.** Don't make your to-do list so long that it becomes unwieldy. Watch the number of tasks you stick on that list.

>> **Don't schedule the "guaranteed to happen" stuff.** Don't include tasks you know for certain you'll be doing. For example, you don't need to include daily activities that will automatically be done, such as commuting to and from work and eating dinner. These tasks happen without prompting and don't require any special motivation or pre-planning. These are usually not time wasters. Again, come up with a daily plan that works best for you.

>> **Do the important tasks first.** Starting a new year, a new week, or even a new day often fills us with resolve. We begin our days with a higher level of motivation and determination. It probably makes sense to schedule the tougher, less desirable tasks first thing in your day. Pick a more difficult high-priority task first. Commit to staying with that task long enough to finish it or make a significant amount of progress.

>> **Be flexible with priorities.** When you write down your daily tasks, don't feel compelled to fill your day with all Level 1 items (the most difficult tasks). They *are* important and should have a place on your daily calendar. But don't be compulsive. Plan your day knowing yourself and what will work best for you. For some, doing a challenging, difficult task first thing makes sense; for others, later in the day might work better. You can mix it up a bit, juggling the difficult tasks with the easier ones.

» **Identify your best work times.** You may be a morning person. You may be a night owl. The hours right after lunch may be your least-effective working hours. Try to match your more-difficult, higher-priority tasks with your more-productive working times. Save easier tasks for times when you feel less motivated.

» **Don't over-commit.** Recognize that you may be less efficient than you expect to be. Be realistic. Be reasonable. If you do it all and have time to do more, that's great.

» **Break bigger tasks into smaller pieces**. If you're intimidated by the time it may take to do a major or complex task, break it up into smaller pieces and focus on one piece. It's hard to start a task that seems overwhelming. Create smaller chunks. For example:

- Clean up the house → Clean the kitchen

- Write the chapter → Write the outline

- Pay all the bills → Pay the high-priority bills

» **Schedule breaks.** Recognize that a break between tasks can give you a breather and even act as a reward for your impressive effort. These few minutes can be used to catch up on email, make some social calls, text a friend — whatever. You can also take a quick walk, do some stretches, or do one of the many relaxation exercises described in Chapter 2 of Book 6.

» **Do the "quickies" quickly.** During breaks or other down times, you may be able to knock off some easy tasks fairly quickly. Just do it. Anything that you've given a "Q" ranking (meaning it can be done in less than five minutes), do right away. Get it off your list.

» **Group similar tasks together.** Save yourself a great deal of time by doing similar tasks at the same time. Grouping tasks is much more efficient and much less stressful. You can, for example:

- **Pay all your bills at the same time.** Designate a time to go through the bills, write the checks, address the envelopes, and mail them. (Or pick a time to sit and pay all your bills online.)

- **Combine your errands.** Rather than running to the store for every little item, group errands together. Keep a "Things We Need or Will Need Soon" list in a handy place and refer to your list before you dash out for that single item. An even simpler way to do this is to photocopy a master list with the common items you usually need to replace and stick it on the fridge. Check off a needed item when you notice that you're running low. When you've checked off a bunch of items on the list, head to the store.

>> **Indicate outcome.** When something is completed, either cross it off your list or make a "done" comment in your outcome column. If you don't get around to starting or finishing something, make a note about when you plan to complete the task.

>> **Update your master list.** What you don't accomplish by the end of the day should be reassessed the next day. It stays on your master list until it's done or you deem it unimportant.

>> **Use the 80/20 rule.** Apply the Pareto principle, also known as the 80/20 rule, to your time-management analysis. Simply put, it states: Of the things you have to do, doing 20 percent of the most-valued tasks will provide you with 80 percent of the satisfaction you may have gotten by doing them all. In other words, skipping your lower-priority items doesn't really cost you a whole lot in the long run. Don't get fixated on those less-valued, less-productive activities. Ask yourself, "Would it really be so awful if I didn't do this task?"

Minimizing Your Distractions and Interruptions

It's not only the "too much to do in too little time" that creates stress; it's also how your time is wasted by others or yourself. Much of your time can be consumed by small interruptions or distractions that take you away from what you're doing and thereby lengthen the time spent on the task at hand. Your distractions and interruptions may take the form of obsessively checking your email while in the middle of doing something else or being sidetracked by a spouse or roommate who has "just one quick question." Here are some suggestions to help you avoid wasted time.

Managing electronic interruptions

TIP

Try the following tips to stay on top of electronic interruptions:

>> Whenever you can, "bundle." Make phone calls and emails in batches. Rather than interrupting your schedule to make or return noncritical phone calls or send emails, wait until you have several items and do them all at once.

>> Just because you receive a phone call, text, or email doesn't mean you have to respond to it at that moment (unless your job requires that you do!). Let things go to voicemail. Turn off the pop-up notification that alerts you to every new digital message. When you take a break or finish a task, *then* check your digital messages.

>> Respond to your messages during low-productivity times. If answering your messages is critical to what you're doing, put it on your to-do list. Build it in.

>> When you do check your messages, realize that you don't have to respond to everything. Filter out the more important messages and let the less urgent stuff go until you have more time.

>> Whenever possible (and appropriate), use email or texting rather than the telephone. It's far more efficient and gives you more control over your time. (On the other hand, use the phone when you care about the person on the other end!)

Losing the visitors

TIP

Other people can be pesky. These "others" may be family members, roommates, coworkers, or others who like to pop their heads into your space and chat whenever they get a chance. (To be fair, you may be the problem, distracting others while robbing yourself of productive time.) Some ideas:

>> **Be polite but firm** and tell your visitors that "this really isn't a good time to talk. I absolutely have to finish this task. But I'll get back to you."

>> **Hide.** If you can find a room or space that is off the beaten track and where you can do some solid work, give it a try. Sometimes a restaurant or coffee shop can work.

>> **Look unavailable.** If you have a door, keep it closed. If you have an empty chair, put something on it. It can be books, files, clothing — anything that may dissuade a would-be sitter.

>> **Try some headphones.** People tend to steer away from people with headphones on. Remember, you don't need to be listening to anything on your headphones. Just having them on should do the trick.

>> **Talk to your recurring interrupter.** Tell the person about your problem with distractions. The person may not realize that they are part of your problem.

Lowering the volume

TIP

Noise can be a subtle or not-so-subtle source of distraction. It may be a loud coworker or street noise. Shutting your door can help, but it may not be an option. Some other suggestions:

>> **Consider noise-canceling headphones.** Use them with or without some relaxing music. Quality ear-buds can have a similar effect without your looking so anti-social.

Finding More Time

>> **Get a white-noise machine,** which can mask a variety of distracting sounds (traffic in the street, the upstairs neighbors). You can download white-noise files and have them repeat on a playback loop.

>> **Leave.** If a task or project demands a high level of attentiveness, find a quieter place to work. Sometimes a conference room at work goes mostly unused. At home it may be another room, or possibly space in the basement or attic. Sometimes less obvious places can work. On fine days, try the park or a quiet section of a lobby in a nearby hotel. Be creative.

Limiting your breaks

TIP

Taking a break can be a sensible and necessary part of your day. It can give you the opportunity to re-group, refresh, and start your next task with a clearer head. The problem is taking too many breaks, or taking them at the wrong times. Some suggestions:

>> **Schedule your breaks to follow the completion of a task.** This can be your reward for finishing.

>> **Do something that is relaxing or even fun.** It can be browsing the Internet, shopping online, or playing a digital game. Of course, it can also be listening to music, watching a video, or reading an article or a few pages of your current book.

>> **Limit the time you take for a break.** The most common trap is socializing with others for far too long. After you've mingled for a bit, take your coffee with you back to your space.

Shifting your time

A more radical solution is to re-arrange the times you need to concentrate and think so as to avoid interruptions and distractions for at least part of your day. Can you get up earlier and start your day (either at home or at the office) sooner, before the distractions appear? Doing some work after the kids are in bed may be more productive than sitting at the dining-room table on a Saturday afternoon. Your office may be much quieter after most of your coworkers have left. Just consider it.

Turning it into a positive

Whenever possible, turn your interruptions into something positive. Use those interruptions as cues to step back, do some relaxing breathing, and refocus your thoughts and direction. This brief breather can be a useful reminder, making you more aware of what you were doing and what you should be doing.

Minimizing your TV time

TIP

Although some television is terrific, a lot of it is not terrific. It's clear that people waste too much time watching television. The quality of our lives would be greatly enriched if we watched less television. TV reduction tactics include the following:

>> **Try to cut back drastically on the time you spend watching TV.** Never just randomly channel surf or scroll through your favorite streaming platform, sticking with the least-objectionable program. Watch only those shows that you *really* want to watch. Try to keep your TV time down to less than two hours per night.

>> **Make one evening a week a no-TV night.** Instead of watching television, do something else. Read a book. Go to the gym. Make soup. Make love. Go to bed earlier. You can always watch that show at a later time.

>> **Avoid a TV pileup.** When you've collected more programs than you could possibly watch in one day of dedicated TV viewing, start winnowing. Begin deleting rather than adding to your growing collection. Use the one-month rule. If you haven't watched it within a month, delete it.

Winning the waiting game

You may find that much of your time is lost while waiting. It may be waiting 45 minutes for the doctor to see you; waiting for the cable guy to come for his promised 9:30 a.m. appointment (good luck with that!); waiting for your bus, subway, plane, or train to show up or depart; or waiting for that meeting to get started.

The trick to beating the waiting game is to *expect* that at various times you'll find yourself having to wait — and then to put that waiting time to good use. Have some form of involvement, task, or activity easily available. This time-filling activity doesn't have to be actual work, though it can be, but it should be something you pre-plan to do when you find yourself having to wait.

TIP

Many people automatically listen to music or play a video game on a digital device. Here are some less obvious ways of putting that wait time to better use:

>> **Read.** Have a book, newspaper, magazine, or digital counterpart with you at most times. Fun reading, work-related reading, whatever.

>> **Learn.** Podcasts are a welcome way to pass the time. Radio shows are usually available in podcast form, too.

>> **Play.** Do the crossword puzzle, challenge yourself to Sudoku, or, yes, even play a computer game.

>> **Breathe.** Take this time to do some relaxation and meditation. Focus on your breathing, introduce some relaxing imagery, and turn your waiting time into a mini-vacation.

>> **Email.** Work on your laptop, tablet, or smartphone to read and answer your email. You can also make phone calls, as long as you don't annoy your neighbors.

>> **Work.** Do actual work, whether it's that pesky little task your boss assigned or personal tasks such as balancing your checkbook.

>> **Update.** Update your to-do list and daily calendar.

>> **Sync.** You probably own more than one digital device. By syncing your computer with your phone and tablet, you can create a continuous link with your electronic life.

Getting around Psychological Roadblocks to Time Management

You probably recognize that simply knowing the tricks of time management doesn't guarantee that you'll put them into practice. You're human! Your emotional and psychological dynamics come into play and can act as barriers that slow or even halt your good time-management intentions. Identifying those self-defeating patterns becomes just as necessary to effectively managing your time as is your to-do list. This section covers two of the more common time-wasting patterns. See which ones fit you and what you can do to overcome them.

Getting over your desire to be perfect

The old adage "Anything worth doing is worth doing well" is misguided. There's nothing wrong with wanting to do something well, even very well. But when your standards are too high, and you aim for perfection, you will feel stress. Perfection is overrated. Being perfect for any longer than three minutes is hard. Whenever you strive for perfection, you fall into one of two time-wasting and stress-producing traps:

>> You spend more time on the task or activity than is warranted.

>> You avoid doing the task altogether for fear that you won't do it well enough.

REMEMBER

Strive for "pretty darn good" instead of "perfect." And, sometimes, let yourself strive for "just okay."

Overcoming procrastination

Procrastination may be one of the main time robbers and ultimate stress producers in your life. By avoiding the kinds of activities that are important and valued, you wind up spending a lot of time doing activities that are less valued and less satisfying. Procrastinating on writing that letter to a loved one, updating your resume, or making that phone call to a friend almost always leads to regret.

You probably procrastinate for one of four major reasons:

>> **Discomfort dodging:** Life often involves doing things that involve some degree of effort and discomfort. When you're experiencing low discomfort tolerance (LDT), you begin looking for ways to avoid doing that discomforting task.

>> **Fear of failure:** You're afraid that you may not be able to do the avoided task as well as you'd like. Fear of failure and feeling bad about yourself make it less likely that you'll do what you ought to be doing. You see failure as a reflection of your self-worth and believe that if you fail, you are a failure. You figure, mistakenly, that maybe if you avoid the task or situation, you won't have to deal with failure. Not a great game plan for life.

>> **Fear of disapproval:** As is the case with fear of failure, you're afraid that somebody will be displeased with your performance and disapprove of you. You over-value other people's opinions and equate that approval or disapproval with your self-worth. Misguidedly, you avoid doing what you ought to be doing to spare yourself the bad feelings you create when you think you will be disapproved.

>> **Anger or resentment:** You feel that you shouldn't have to do the task or activity, and you're angry at having to do it. You feel that the world, or some of the people in it, are not treating you fairly. You resent having to do that task or face that situation because of that anger and resentment.

Bite the bullet

If you find that dislike and discomfort are steering you away from doing what you should be doing, see whether you can challenge your assumptions. Ask yourself,

"Why must I always do the things I like and want to do?" The answer, of course, is that you don't have to avoid difficulty and discomfort. Just do it! Then ask yourself a second question: "Wouldn't I be better off putting up with some discomfort and getting it out of the way?" The answer: Absolutely!

Commit to a chunk of time

Set the timer app on your phone or computer to, say, 30 minutes. (Somebody once estimated that 25 to 30 minutes is the optimal attention period for maximum performance.) Commit to working on a project or task for those 30 minutes without stopping, without being distracted. When the alarm beeps, you can stop and take a brief five-minute break. Or, if you feel like you're on a roll, you can continue working on the task.

Motivate yourself

Sometimes your level of internal motivation doesn't get you where you need to go. You need external motivation. You can either reward yourself for doing something or penalize yourself for not doing it.

Try the reward approach first. Create your own motivational ladder by coming up with a list of rewards that can motivate you to get the job done. Then rank them in order of their importance to you. For example:

>> Treat yourself to a mini-vacation.

>> Buy yourself something big that you've been dying to get but have been denying yourself.

>> Treat yourself to a great meal or a dessert.

>> Go to the movies, see a play, or do something fun.

>> Buy yourself a small present.

However, being nice, even to yourself, doesn't always cut it. You may respond better to the threat of pain and suffering than to a positive reward. If pain is your thing, try creating a penalty for not completing a task:

>> Deny yourself a favorite pleasure for a day (TV, a movie, a dessert, going out, and so on).

>> Deny yourself a favorite pleasure for a week.

>> Send a donation to a political candidate you dislike.

>> Send cash anonymously to a person you know and dislike.

Use the smallest reward or penalty that gets the job done. If that doesn't work, move up to the next reward or penalty on your motivational ladder. Be creative.

To make sure that you do enforce a penalty, tell a friend about your plan and ask them to make sure that you follow through. This approach improves your chances of successfully breaking through procrastination. If money is involved, put it in an envelope, address it, put a stamp on it, and give it to a friend, telling them to mail it if you don't come through on your end of the deal.

Go public

Make a public commitment. Tell a good friend about a task that you want to get done and tell them when you will complete it. Better yet, tell a bunch of people, perhaps in your next tweet or status update. Be sure to remind that friend or friends to ask you if you have done what you said you would.

Become more selective and assertive

After you identify those activities and tasks that have a lower priority in your life, discover ways to reduce or even eliminate them. For example, social engagements can easily eat up a good deal of your time. You probably attend many engagements out of a sense of obligation or habit. But you don't have to attend absolutely every party or dinner you're invited to. Nor do you have to attend every meeting posted by your church, temple, school, or any other organization you're affiliated with. Go to those events that you truly want to attend, but be selective and assertive. Give yourself permission to say no to many other invitations. You won't end up being hated by others or ostracized from the community.

Letting Go: Discovering the Joys of Delegating

Remember that old slogan, "If you want something done right, do it yourself"? Yes, it holds some truth. However, by doing it all yourself, you quickly discover that your stress level shoots skyward. Delegating tasks and responsibilities can save you time and spare you a great deal of stress.

You may have a problem delegating for several reasons. Here are some of the more common ones:

>> You believe that no one else is competent enough to do the task.

>> You believe that no one else really understands the problem the way you do.

>> You believe that no one else is motivated quite the way you are.

>> You don't trust anyone else to be able to manage the responsibilities.

All these reasons can hold some truth. But in many cases, these reasons aren't accurate at all. The reality is that other people can be taught. You may be pleasantly surprised by the level of work others can bring to a task or responsibility.

REMEMBER

Even if you're right, and others don't do the job as well as you do, you're probably still better off delegating than taking on everything yourself and feeling incredibly stressed.

The fine art of delegating

TIP

You may be from the "Do this, and have it on my desk by tomorrow morning!" school of delegating. Here are some tips to help you delegate more effectively:

>> **Find the right person.** Make sure that your delegatees have the knowledge and skills to do the tasks asked of them. And if you can't find a person who has the knowledge and skills, consider investing the time in training someone. In the longer run, you'll be ahead of the game.

>> **Package your request for help in positive terms.** Tell the person why you selected them. Offer a genuine compliment reflecting that you recognize some ability or competence that makes that person right for the job.

>> **Be appreciative of that person's time.** Recognize that you're aware that the person has their own work to do, but that you would really be grateful if they could help you with this task.

>> **Don't micro-manage.** After you assign a task and carefully explain what needs to be done, let the person do it. Keep your hands off unless you clearly see that things are taking a wrong turn.

>> **Reward the effort.** If the person does a good job, say so. And if they don't do it quite the way you would have but still put a lot of effort into the task, let them know that you appreciate the effort.

Delegating begins at home

TIP

You may associate the word *delegating* with working in an office and handing off a project to an associate or assistant. However, delegating tasks and duties at home is a major way to save a lot of time. Here are some suggestions:

>> **Let one and all share in the fun.** Everyone in the family (that is, the members who are old enough to walk and talk) can, and should, have a role in sharing household duties and responsibilities.

>> **Start with a list.** Divvy up those less-desirable chores, such as washing dishes (or putting them in the dishwasher), doing laundry, cleaning up bedrooms, taking out the trash, and emptying the dishwasher.

>> **Start small.** Don't overwhelm your family right off the bat. Give them one or two assignments and then add on as appropriate.

>> **Don't feel guilty.** In the long run, your family will come to value the experience. (Recognize that it may be a very long run, however.)

Buying Time

You may subscribe to the old work ethic, "Never pay anyone to do something that you can readily do yourself." This is a mistake. Hiring someone to help you can give you more time for the things you want to do and, in the process, make your life simpler and less stressful.

Here are some questions to help you decide whether hiring someone else or paying for a service makes sense:

>> What chores do I absolutely hate?

>> Which chores constantly provoke a battle between me and my spouse or me and my roommate?

>> What chores do I merely dislike doing?

>> What chores do I not do very well?

>> What chores do I not mind doing, but really aren't worth my time and effort?

Tasks that you may want someone else to do for you include cleaning, doing laundry, grocery shopping, painting, handling pet care, mowing the lawn, and so on.

Avoid paying top dollar

Getting someone else to do less-than-desirable chores need not cost you a bundle. You probably don't need an expensive professional. Lots of people who are "between opportunities" will be willing to do chores for you if you pay them.

Go online. A number of Internet services can match you up with someone who is willing to help you out (for a fee, of course). Friends on social-networking sites can also be a source of referrals. Don't rule out non-digital sources — supermarket billboards, neighborhood circulars, or your local newspaper. (When you find someone, be sure to check their references.) And don't overlook high-school and college students. Schools often have an "employment-wanted" service, especially during the summer months. These students can be cheaper and surprisingly reliable.

REMEMBER

Realistically assess your financial ability to hire someone to do a few or many of the items on your list. Remember, too, that the emotional relief and the extra time you gain are well worth the money in many cases. Spend the bucks.

Strive for deliverance

These days, many of the things you need can be delivered. If you live in a good-sized city, almost everything can be delivered. You can save time by dialing the right series of digits or clicking the right places on the Internet. In addition to take-out food, items that you can have delivered to your door include the following:

>> Groceries

>> Clean laundry

>> Meats from the butcher

>> Sweets from the bakery

>> Liquor from the liquor store

>> Books

>> Actually, just about everything

IN THIS CHAPTER

» **Understanding your disorganization**

» **Clearing away clutter**

» **Motivating yourself**

» **Organizing electronically**

» **Staying organized**

Chapter **4**

Stress-Reducing Organizational Skills

I f you've ever felt like screaming or maybe tearing out some hair when at the last minute you can't find your keys or that paper napkin on which you wrote important information, you're probably sympathetic to the notion that disorganization can trigger a whole lot of stress.

Sure, a little bit of disorder doesn't rival developing a serious illness, getting fired, or having your house burn down. Yet being disorganized can fuel a long list of frustrations, delays, lost time, and missed opportunities — all accompanied by varying levels of anger and irritation.

Who needs it? Your stress level is already high enough. This chapter shows you how to get organized. It gives you the tools you need to overcome the disarray, chaos, and confusion in your life.

Figuring Out Why Your Life Is So Disorganized

Okay, so your life is not a model of order and organization. Being disorganized is nothing to be ashamed of. In fact, it's totally understandable. Our days are crammed with too much to do, with too little time to do it. Our possessions threaten to drown us.

The following sections help you get to the bottom of your organizational challenges so that you can take action.

Are you organizationally challenged?

TIP

Your first step in coming up with effective organizational strategies is recognizing that you may be truly disorganized. Take this unofficial "test" and see whether becoming better organized is an area you need to work on.

Read each of the following statements and see to what extent each statement describes you. Use the following ratings to help you better gauge how disorganized you are:

3 = Very much like me

2 = Somewhat like me

1 = A little like me

0 = Not at all like me

» Your home is filled with far too much stuff.

» Your closets, drawers, and cabinets are disorganized.

» You're frequently late for your appointments.

» You're a big procrastinator.

» You find that you spend lots of time looking for things you've misplaced.

» You're often late paying your bills.

» Your friends and family tell you that you have a problem with clutter.

» You feel stressed out by all the stuff in your home.

» Your computer files are generally disorganized.

» You rarely use lists to help you get organized.

>> You buy duplicates of things you already own because you can't find the originals.

>> Your desk or workspace is disorganized.

>> You feel you don't have enough time to get organized.

You probably answered with twos or threes for at least a few of these quiz items. However, if you identify strongly with many or most of these statements, poor organizational skills may be playing an important role in creating excessive stress in your life.

More important than determining a global organizational score is identifying your specific areas and patterns of disorganization. The categories in the next section help you do this.

Identifying your personal disorganization

Getting better organized means being aware of the areas in which you could use some help. Disorganization can be broken down to more discrete sub–groups. See which ones best describe your own forms of disorganization.

>> **You don't manage your time well.** If your time-management skills are wobbly, you find that you often run late, miss deadlines, work inefficiently, procrastinate, plan poorly, and feel overwhelmed by not having enough time. Too many things don't get done. Time management is such an important stress-reducing skill that it warrants its own chapter — Chapter 3 in Book 6, in fact.

>> **You're surrounded by clutter.** You own far too many things, and those things are way out of control. Your flat surfaces are invitations to put stuff on, preferably in piles. You have great difficulty getting rid of your stuff. It could be clothes, books, papers, out-of-date electronics, or broken just-about-anything. You feel like you're drowning in your stuff, and you're not terribly optimistic that the situation is going to change.

>> **Your home is in constant disarray.** Your storage spaces are randomly organized. Cabinets and closets are a mish-mash of organization. Finding anything is a hit-and-miss affair. You make poor use of containers, storage bags, shelves, and drawers. You rarely use labels.

>> **You lack a good system for keeping track of bills and other important information.** Your personal records, bills, passport, mortgage paperwork, and important files are somewhere, but you aren't sure just where. You have no filing system. You don't use your computer, tablet, or smartphone to help you organize your life.

If you struggle with any or all of these areas, the rest of this chapter provides specific guidance for getting your life (and your stuff) in order.

Clearing Away the Clutter

If you lived in a place with infinite space, had a live-in maid, and were independently wealthy, you could consider your clutter a charming quirk, an amusing oversight. But your clutter has probably become a pain and threatens to stress you out even more. De-cluttering can seem overwhelming. It's only a matter of time before you feel like you're lost in your clutter. You need help. You're ready to start. But where? The following sections walk you through the de-cluttering process.

Bust those clutter excuses

If you're going to war with clutter, it's important to know exactly what the enemy looks like. Here are ten reasons why people hang onto stuff. At times, giving up your prized possessions is harder than pulling teeth. When pressed, you may vigorously defend your decision to hold onto some small thing. All the following excuses contain at least a sliver of truth. And all guarantee that after your funeral, your relatives will hold the world's biggest garage sale. See whether you can recognize some of your favorite clutter excuses.

TIP

>> **"Someday I'll need it."** This clutter excuse can be compelling. After all, you *might* need it someday. This is where your "what-if-ing" comes into play. The odds of your actually needing this are probably very small. That unread article or outdated computer cord will most likely never be reused. Do a cost-benefit analysis and ask yourself: "Aren't I better off just getting rid of this stuff rather than keeping it on the very unlikely chance that I *may* use it?"

>> **"It was a present for my ninth birthday."** This is your sentimental clutter. Anything that reminds you of your past or has sentimental value can be tough to let go. This category of clutter can include every piece of artwork you or your child brought home from school. It can include every playbill from every play you have seen and every picture that was ever taken of you. Create a scrapbook of selected items and let the rest go. Better yet, scan into your computer all the items you want to save and keep only a select few original items. If you don't have a scanner, take pictures. Who says you can't have your cake and eat it too?

>> **"Somebody will want to buy this."** Good luck with this one! If this treasure really has eager buyers, list it on eBay or find another way to sell it. But make the decision: "I will put this up for sale now, or I will give it away, or I will chuck it."

>> **"I'm sure I'll find the matching one."** Usually this excuse is for orphaned socks or gloves. If you haven't found the matching item in three months, let it go. Besides, everybody knows that washing machines eat socks.

>> **"Yes, it's broken, but it can be fixed."** Fix it, give it away, or throw it out. These days it will probably cost you more to fix something electronic than to replace it, but if you feel it can be reasonably repaired, commit to locating a repair service this week.

>> **"If I just lose 30 pounds, I'll fit into this."** Losing weight is a difficult task for most people. Why not keep a few items of clothing that you absolutely love and donate all the rest? After you've shed those pounds, you can reward yourself with some serious shopping for smart new togs.

>> **"My kids will want to give it to their kids."** Kids rarely relish getting old stuff from adults. Ask your kids if they would like these objects. If they say yes, ask them to take possession of them now. If your kids are very young, don't hold your breath.

>> **"I got it on sale."** This is your bargain clutter. It's hard to resist a good deal. Half-price sale? No problem! Buy one get one free? Let's do it! Shopping at the big-box stores can be a trap. When you see something on sale, it becomes hard to resist. And if you buy it, it's hard to get rid of because it was a bargain. What you want to avoid is *impulse* buying. If you're seduced by a "bargain," whether you see it online, in print, or in a store, stop and ask yourself some pertinent questions:

- "Do I really need this?"

- "Would I ever buy this if it weren't on sale?"

- "Do I have a place to put this?"

If possible, give yourself time to reflect on whether you really think this is a smart purchase. Most sales give you some wiggle room to think before you buy. If the idea still seems right the next day, and you're still determined to buy it, go ahead. If you're in a store and it's now or never, do your other shopping first, and then ask yourself the preceding three questions. If the answer is "no" to any of these, take a pass. Even if you regret not making the purchase later on, you'll almost always have a second chance to buy it at a bargain price. And if you're still paralyzed with indecision, get another opinion from someone who knows you well.

>> **"It will be a collector's item one day."** If you've ever watched those *Antiques Roadshow* programs on PBS, you know that one man's garbage can be another man's treasure. Alas, the truth is, one man's garbage is usually another man's clutter. Get an objective appraisal from a trusted, neutral source. If the item is worth something, sell it now.

>> **"I plan on reading this."** This is the excuse that keeps you from ever throwing out a book you hope to read one day but probably never will. If you haven't read it by a reasonable time, you probably won't. Give your books to the school or library rummage sale. Your shelves will thank you. If an article is important to you, scan it and put it in an organized digital file.

Get yourself motivated

TIP

Sometimes good intentions alone just don't cut it. You may find that you need a kick in the pants or some other form of external motivation to get you to clean up. Here are a couple of field-tested ideas that can keep you on track:

>> **Schedule it.** When you schedule things, you have a better chance of getting them done. People generally show up for dentist and doctor appointments, business meetings, and other engagements that they purposefully schedule. The same tactic can work when it comes to getting things done around the house. Commit to a definite time and write down the "appointment" in your calendar, daily planner, or whatever you use to keep track of your life.

>> **Find your clutter threshold.** Frankly, some people don't mind a little clutter in their life. For them, those minimalist, absolutely-nothing-out-of-place living spaces are scary. They require a touch of clutter to make them feel emotionally comfortable. Yet anything more than just a little bit of clutter begins to stress them out. Other folks are totally clutter averse. For them, any clutter is too much. You have to find your own clutter threshold, below which you get twitchy and above which you feel stressed. Then work hard to keep your clutter level within that threshold.

Draw yourself a clutter roadmap

TIP

Rather than seeing all the clutter in your life-space as one massive pile, see it as a succession of tasks that you can chip away step by step. One way to decide where to start, and where to go after you start, is to create a clutter roadmap. Begin by choosing a number of areas of your life-space that desperately need organizing. These areas may be geographical (a specific room in your home, the yard, or the garage) or topical (your clothing, magazines, or toys). Then come up with a sequence of areas that you want to work on. After you deal with one bit of clutter on your list, move on to the second and then on to the next, and so on. Think of your map as a kind of sequential "to do" list. It takes you where you want to go.

A clutter roadmap gives you the feeling that you know where you're going — and also a pretty good idea of how far you've moved toward your final goal. For many people faced with overwhelming clutter, having this game plan creates a feeling of being in control, which can reduce much of the anxiety often associated with de-cluttering. Be sure to make each piece on your map relatively small and doable. Also start by choosing areas of your life-space that will give you a great deal of personal satisfaction after they're organized.

Get your feet wet

One good piece of self-help advice is that Nike slogan, "Just do it!" However, "just doing it" for most people is probably not going to do it. Perhaps a more realistic saying is "Just get started!" Deep down, you realize that you'll be better off if you get rid of much of that unneeded stuff. So jump in.

REMEMBER

Have you ever noticed that after you start something, the momentum of doing that thing keeps you going? This is especially true when you're de-cluttering. After you get yourself in de-cluttering mode, go with it. Don't stop just because you finish a small section. Keep going. Build on your success. You may be surprised at how much you can get done when you're into it.

Stop kidding yourself

It's easy to fool yourself. That's because some small part of you really does believe that you'll clean out the basement, put those old clothes in boxes and give them to a thrift shop, and throw out those magazines that you've been hanging onto forever.

REMEMBER

The reality is that unless you take your clutter seriously, it will continue to spread. If you're going to successfully de-clutter, you need to convince yourself that the quality of your life will improve measurably after you unload much, if not most, of those collected objects. It will also feel so nice when you find that long-lost birth certificate and all the mates to those single socks lying in your bedroom drawer.

Simplifying your life-space takes grit. Your attitude as you approach the task should be, "I'm sick and tired of this, and I'm not going to take it anymore!" You may find this approach a bit too merciless, but be clear: You're dealing with a powerful force. Give no ground. Take no prisoners. Ask yourself the following questions to help increase your de-cluttering grit:

>> Do I really want to spend the next 20 years living with this item?

>> If my place were on fire and I could save only half of what I own, would I save this particular item?

>> Would the quality of my life be seriously diminished if I didn't own this item?

>> Can someone else use this more than I can?

In 90 percent of the cases, the answers to these four questions are no, no, no, and yes.

Avoid discouragement

A mistake that many people make when de-cluttering is thinking that they can finish their de-cluttering in one short Saturday afternoon. They get discouraged when they realize just how much stuff they have and how much de-cluttering they still have to do.

REMEMBER

Face it: It took you years to amass all your wonderful possessions, so it's prudent to assume that reversing the process may take you some time. However, when you figure out how much time you can save by not having to look for misplaced items, you quickly realize that you'll be way ahead of the game after you finish. Accomplishing most anything in life that is worthwhile takes effort and persistence. Mastering golf or tennis, learning to ski, or figuring out how to get the most out of your computer doesn't happen overnight. Stick with it.

Get down to the nitty-gritty

TIP

Okay, you've psyched yourself up for some serious de-cluttering. When you get into the trenches, try using the following clutter-busting techniques:

>> **Pick any number from one to two.** When considering what to do with an item of clutter, remember that you have two basic options: Keep it or lose it. If you decide to keep it, you must figure out what to do with it. If you choose to lose it, you can throw it away or give it away. Clearly, the biggest obstacle to getting rid of anything is having to make this choice.

>> **Take a second look.** It's never too late to get rid of some of the stuff you decide to keep. Go back over your keeper pile and take a second look. Organizing even a small pile of things takes a lot of time. And although storage and filing play an important role in managing all the possessions that clutter your life, simply getting rid of stuff often makes more sense.

>> **Use the Triage Method of Clutter Control.** One useful approach in making difficult keep it/pitch it decisions is something called the Triage Method of Clutter Control. First, create three categories: Definitely Keep, Definitely Get Rid Of, and I'm Not Sure. Then throw out or give away everything in the last two categories. The upside of unloading much more of your clutter far outweighs the downside of making a mistake. Don't look back.

>> **Get a clutter buddy.** Whenever it's time to de-clutter, perhaps you come up with marvelous ideas for organizing your partner's side of the room. Or maybe you have even better ideas when it comes to your children's rooms. You're probably less sentimental, less ambivalent, and more determined when dealing with other people's clutter rather than your own. Make this concept work for you. Ask your mate or a friend to help you de-clutter. Listen to that person, and do what they tell you.

>> **Get some emotional support.** De-cluttering can be a lonely and emotionally taxing job. You may need someone more emotionally supportive than your clutter buddy. This should be someone you feel comfortable talking with — a family member, a good friend, a colleague you trust, or perhaps a therapist. This support can keep you going when the going gets tough and you start to feel discouraged.

>> **Play the dating game.** If you can't bring yourself to throw something out, put it in a box and put a date on the box that is exactly a year away. Don't list what's in the box — just the date. If the future date comes and goes without your needing anything in the box, take a quick look inside. If nothing critically important catches your eye, chuck it without a second look. Don't look back. If you *do* need an item from the box, find a better place to keep it.

>> **Use the three-month rule.** Take a look at the dates on your magazines, and if they are older than three months for monthly publications or three weeks for weekly ones, throw them out.

>> **Find a clutter recipient.** Getting rid of stuff is much easier when you know that it won't end up in the trash but rather in the hands of somebody who wants it and can use it. In fact, your rejects may be someone else's cup of tea. Clothing, sports equipment, books, and furniture are often welcomed by others. Give your relatives and friends first crack at your treasures (but give them a definite time limit to come, look, and take). The Salvation Army, Goodwill Industries, thrift shops, and charity drives will be delighted (usually) to take the stuff that your family and friends turn down. You can even get a tax deduction for donating to charitable organizations.

>> **Consider consignment**. Sometimes it's hard to give an object away because you really do believe it's worth something. And you may be right. Putting it up for consignment may just do the trick.

>> **If it doesn't work, toss it.** Look around your home for a broken toaster, blender, vacuum cleaner, radio, or clock — any small appliance that hasn't worked for a long while. Once you find one, ask yourself whether you truly need it. If you decide to fix it, fix it. If not, replace or discard it. These days you may find that replacing the item is cheaper than having it repaired. However, chances are good that if you haven't needed it in the last year, you probably don't need it at all.

- » **Whatever you do, don't leave the broken item in your home.** Throw it out or, better yet, give it to a charitable organization that will repair it and give it to someone who will use it.

- » **Handle things only once.** You may be in the habit of putting some things aside and saying you'll figure out later what to do with them. This just adds to the problem. Deal with it right in the moment. File it! Pay it! Delete it! Chuck it! Deal with it only once!

- » **Invest in doors and drawers.** If you absolutely must keep something, hide it. Unless the object in question is something you're very fond of or somehow adds to the visual aesthetic of your decor, keep it out of sight. Store things in cabinets, closets, bureau drawers, or file cabinets — anyplace that contributes to a sense of visual order. But keep in mind that the space things occupy behind doors is still space that you could use for something else.

  Whole stores are now dedicated exclusively to storage furniture and containers. Their catalogs are great fun to look through, but be sure not to make them a new part of your clutter.

- » **Take a sample.** You can't keep absolutely every piece of artwork, craft project, or report card that your children bring home. The solution? Get a large folder and take samples of the masterpieces you're especially fond of. Store this "art" folder in a closet. You can scan and electronically file the smaller masterpieces and mementos. When your children become famous "artistes," you'll cash in.

- » **Take a picture.** Often, items in your "I'm Not Sure" pile have sentimental value but are too big to keep around. You want the memories, but not necessarily the object. Take its picture. Pictures (especially the digital variety) take up far less space and still can bring a warm smile to your face. The photograph on your computer will collect far less dust. You may also want to include someone in the picture. Looking at your daughter squeezing Cuddles is a lot more satisfying than just looking at Cuddles by herself.

Organizing Your Space

TIP

Being organized is about more than just being neat and tidy. It also means having items and information in places where you can reliably find them, use them, and then put them back where they came from. Part of your problem may be that you don't know how to organize and store your things. Here are some guidelines and suggestions:

- » **Start big.** Rather than organize your stuff item by item, start with a more ambitious agenda. First pick an area you want to organize. Let's say it's your medicine cabinet. Take out everything and put it on the bathroom counter. Have a trash can handy. Give the cabinet a wipe and you're ready to go. Now group the cold medicines together and put them on a shelf. If you come across items that you never use or that are out of date, throw them into the trash can. Move on to another category. Put the stuff you use most in the most convenient locations. Label the items that are hard to spot or aren't clearly marked. When you've finished with the medicine cabinet, you can move on to your refrigerator, clothes closet, shoes . . . Remember, not everything has to be saved.

>> **Use containers.** Yes, you should go out and buy more stuff! *But not just yet.* First figure out which containers you need. Jars, hooks, plastic boxes, plastic bags, and even baskets can find their places in your reorganization planning. Your first step is determining what you want to store. Food containers should most often be clear with lids. Objects like crayons, small toys, and blocks all do well in see-through containers as well. To save space, go with square containers rather than round ones. Stackability is also a plus because it takes advantage of vertical space. Containers make cleaning up a lot easier by giving you definite places to return the things you use.

>> **Label it.** Whatever container you use, it helps to label the contents. For opaque containers and boxes, labeling becomes a must. On plastic bags, a permanent marker does the trick. An inexpensive labeler also proves useful when you can't write on a container.

>> **Categorize.** While it's true that if you stick all your books into a bookcase it will look orderly, it may not be the best organizational strategy. Come up with some basic categories without overdoing it. Start with fiction/nonfiction and add one or two more sub-categories. Similarly, in the kitchen, rather than having all your spices thrown together, use a simple A-F, G-N, and so on. Grouping can help you navigate. Labeled spice racks could do the trick as well. Just keep them where you can see them.

>> **Group.** Rather than having your electronic gadgets all over the house, create a drawer or shelf just for these alone. Have a container for the small stuff that might otherwise get lost. Put all your sports equipment into a bin labeled for each particular sport. Again, smaller sports items (balls, pucks, and tees) could go in a box or container within the bin. In your medicine cabinet, group your medicines, soaps, and razors in separate sections or on different shelves.

>> **Prioritize usage.** Some things you use frequently, others much less. In your refrigerator, keep the most-used items near the front and on the most accessible shelf. The same with clothing. Socks, underwear, and favorite shirts and pants should be where you can easily reach them. Put the once-in-a-blue-moon stuff in the back. Better yet, give it away.

>> **Put it back!** If you use it, put it back where you found it. Don't let all that organizational effort go to waste.

Organizing Information

Organizing the "stuff" in your life is only part of the problem. You may not know whether you have paprika in the back of that kitchen cabinet, but do you know where your birth certificate, mortgage or lease paperwork, and college transcripts are, not to mention that fabulous chicken recipe you cut out of last month's cooking magazine? To make things even more complicated, more and more information now comes to you electronically. You can be swamped by your emails, tweets, attachments, and more. Here are some suggestions to help you manage this information overload.

Losing the paper trail

When computers first began appearing, we were told that we would be living in a paperless world. We're not there quite yet. In fact, our use of paper has doubled in the last ten years. Those who have made the study of clutter their life's work say that paper is the real enemy. Your paper clutter can include everything from a toaster warranty to your last electric bill to the endless stream of circulars, catalogs, junk mail, instruction manuals, and other paper items that pass through your hands every day. Here's how to start organizing that proliferation of paper.

To merge or to purge? That is the question.

REMEMBER

The two secrets to managing the paper in your life are fairly simple. In fact, they are amazingly similar to the two options you have when considering what to do with your non-paper clutter. You can either throw out the paper if you don't need it or find an effective way to organize it if you do need it.

This approach to paper sounds pretty easy, but the problem lies in actually doing the throwing out and organizing. Sorting through all that paper takes time and effort, and who knows — you might really need that coupon for a ten-gallon jar of spaghetti sauce, or you might actually read that article on skiing in the Himalayas. Yeah, right! You need help.

Your snail mail: Cut 'em off at the pass

TIP

Finding a birthday card or letter from a friend in your mailbox is fun. Finding bills and junk mail? Not so much. Your mailbox can be an insidious force, feeding you an unstoppable river of solicitations, announcements, catalogs, and bills. You can slowly drown in this incoming sea of paper. The trick is to catch it early, before it has a chance to collect. Following are some tips for keeping your mail from becoming a huge problem:

>> **Junk the junk mail.** Keep a wastepaper basket near your front door. Throw out junk mail immediately. Do not open it. Do not be intrigued. Realize that no matter how much mail you receive telling you that you've probably won a million dollars, the chances of it actually happening are infinitesimal.

>> **Get yourself off mailing lists.** Perhaps you once subscribed to something and, when you received it, you noticed that they had spelled your name wrong. Then maybe you noticed that you were getting tons of other unwanted stuff in the mail with the same wrong name. Being on one list can quickly put you on many others. Get yourself taken off mailing lists. The Internet can make this task relatively easy. The World Privacy Forum research group offers a how-to list titled "Top Ten Opt Outs" (`www.worldprivacyforum.org/2015/08/consumer-tips-top-ten-opt-outs/`), which gives you a number of suggestions for cutting down on unwanted mail.

>> **Curb your catalog habit.** Leafing through a catalog and mentally shopping can be fun. And if you have an absolute favorite, keep it. But cancel the others. Virtually every catalog you receive in the mail can be viewed online. Peruse the web and save the paper. The website `https://catalogchoice.org/`, a service of TrustedID, and `https://dmachoice.org/`, created by the Direct Marketing Association, allow you to opt out of a particular company's catalogs. Both are free.

>> **Go electronic.** Ask that bills, credit-card statements, bank statements, investment information, catalogs, and magazines — just about anything, really — be sent to your computer, tablet, or smartphone. If possible, create a separate and secure email address for your important documents so they don't get lost in your email shuffle. Remember, you can pay many of your bills online without using a single sheet of paper. (You'll save money on stamps, too.)

Organizing the papers you do need to keep

The notion of having a method of organizing the paper in your life probably doesn't come as an earth-shatteringly new idea. Yet you probably still don't have one, or if you do, you use it inefficiently.

Coming up with a system of organization takes thought and planning. And making use of it requires time and effort. In the short run, letting papers pile up is a lot easier. But in the long run, doing so can turn into a major headache. Taking the time and effort to develop a systematic way of organizing your papers can result in a lot less stress and hassle. Try the following as you create your filing system.

Start simple

Come up with a filing system that's relatively easy to use. You don't want your filing system to be more stressful than the stress it's supposed to alleviate. You may not need a formal filing cabinet at home, but if you have the room, and if you have a lot of paper to file, it may not be a bad idea. Alternatively, you can work with desk drawers that hold files, or even plastic or cardboard filing boxes.

Be colorful — with your files and folders, that is

Files and folders of different colors, or tabs and labels of different colors, can not only turn your filing system into a work of art but also make it easier to find different subjects and interests. Make your files easy to recognize so you can identify the contents. Put those files you need most often in a place that is easy to access.

Keep important papers where you know how to access them

REMEMBER

Keep your original documents in a safe place, but make sure you can easily get hold of them when you need them. And back them up! Keep a digital copy that is easily findable. Lest you forget, here are some of the more important documents to keep track of:

>> Automobile registration, title, and insurance documents

>> Bank-account information

>> Birth certificates

>> Citizenship papers

>> Credit-card numbers

>> Bank-account numbers

>> Deeds, leases, and contracts

>> Mortgage documents

>> Important receipts

>> Instruction manuals

>> Insurance policies

>> Loan agreements

>> Marriage license

>> Divorce decrees

>> Estate-planning documents and wills

>> Adoption papers

>> Medical records

>> Passports

>> Power of attorney

>> Health proxies

>> IDs and passwords

>> PIN numbers

>> School transcripts

>> Service contracts

>> Tax returns

>> Warranties

>> Back-ups of important computer files

>> Photographs, letters, and other personal papers

>> Anything else you don't want to lose

REMEMBER

Some of these categories will warrant their own separate files. Some, such as your important account and PIN numbers, can be combined. For the more important documents, you may want to keep the originals in a fireproof safe or safe-deposit box and keep copies in your files. Storing them on your computer may be a better option and certainly a good back-up option. Storing them in the cloud makes it easier to access this information from any computer. If you choose to store information virtually, it's important that you consider the possible risk that others may obtain access to your files and documents.

Safeguarding your digital documents

TIP

It's more likely that someone will steal files and information from your computer than from your bottom dresser drawer. Although you may not care much if someone hacks into your computer and steals your Aunt Agnes's prized recipe for brisket, you probably will be much more distressed if someone steals your Social Security number, passport information, or personal IDs and passwords. Here are some steps to help you store your digital information more safely:

>> **Go to the cloud.** Find a cloud storage company that is well-regarded and has a solid reputation and clear security policies. This may take some research on your part, but the result is well worth the effort.

>> **Get encrypted.** Find out if your data and documents will be encrypted when stored in the cloud. With no encryption, anyone may be able to get access to your files. You want to ensure that files you don't want others to read are protected and accessible only by you.

>> **Pick a strong password.** Whether your personal documents are stored on your computer and/or in cloud storage, it's vital that you have a password that protects you. In general, the longer the password, the better. It's best to use seven or eight characters with at least two being numeric. Also try to include punctuation characters and mix in upper and lower-case letters.

>> **Stay away from "Whiskers."** Don't use personal information as your password. Don't use the names of any family members or pets. Don't use your telephone number, anybody's birth date, any part of your Social Security number, your driver's license number, or any of the preceding items spelled backwards.

>> **Have more than one.** Don't have just a single password for everything. If someone cracks that password, they have easy access to everything you've got.

>> **Store your passwords.** After you come up with these hack-resistant passwords, you need a place to put them. These days password-management systems store your passwords and other login info either on your computer on in the cloud. You can create a setup whereby your multiple passwords can be accessed only with the use of a master password. This master password is a lengthy, brilliantly conceived winner. (Some apps will do this for you.) If you want to go lower tech, and your computer is in your home, jot down your password and keep it in a safe place.

>> **Have a magic number.** As an added safeguard, create a PIN, a personal number (three or four digits) that is never written down, stays stored only in your head, and is memorable. Your new password is a combination of what you have written down or stored on your computer or in the cloud *plus* your PIN. Even if your written-down passwords are discovered, you have another layer of protection.

Never put all your papers in one basket

TIP

Organizational expert Stephanie Culp suggests that you have four baskets for your paper (in addition to the extremely important wastepaper basket):

>> **A "To Do" basket.** The wire see-through kind works best.

>> **A "To Pay" basket.** Again, wire works best here.

>> **A "To File" basket.** Use a larger wicker basket.

>> **A "To Read" basket.** Try an even larger wicker basket with handles.

Culp recommends that you stack your "To Do" basket on top of your "To Pay" basket on your desk. Keep the "To File" basket under your desk, out of the way of your more immediate paper needs. You can keep the "To Read" basket in a different part of your home — such as your bedroom or study (or bathroom!) — so that you can catch up on your reading whenever the opportunity arises.

Make filing a habit

Find a time during the week to empty your "To File" basket and file those needed papers away. This task really shouldn't take long; 15 or 20 minutes should do it.

Fine-tune later

At a later date, take a look at what's in your files. Usually, you find that a file is either underused or bulging. If you find that you have only one or two things in a file folder, find or create a file that's broader in scope. Alternatively, if you find that a folder is overflowing with contributions, create subcategories, either by topic or by dates.

Organizing electronically

When it comes to getting organized, your computer can be your best friend. It may not help you with your shirts or sports equipment, but it can be invaluable with records, papers, pictures, and other forms of information. An organized electronic filing system is the key to effective electronic organization. Without it you can find yourself spending lots of time trying to locate a document, article, or file you know you have — somewhere. If this sounds very much like finding your misplaced phone charger, you're absolutely right. The good news is that filing electronically uses the same principles as manual filing.

Decide what you want to keep electronically

Your first step is asking yourself what you want to store on your computer. Some of the more common choices include photos, recipes, music and video files, personal documents, movies, tax information, letters of recommendation, college transcripts, books, contacts, restaurant information, children's art, report cards, and so on. As you can see, the list of categories could be endless. Pick the ones that make sense for you.

Create folders

Your computer already has wonderful organizational tools built in. It starts you off with the more common organizational folders or categories. You'll probably need to create additional folders that are relevant to your needs. "My recipes" or "my taxes" are good examples. Create these categories or folders as concisely as you can, but make it clear what is in each folder.

Think hierarchically

Create sub-folders that fine-tune the information you have in the primary folder. For example, a folder for recipes can have sub-folders for desserts, soups, entrees, and so on. Similarly, a "travel" folder may have sub-folders for specific countries. Your "tax" folder may include individual years.

** Watch out for too many levels. Going deeper than a few sub-folders may cause confusion down the road. Come up with a digital organizing system that's relatively easy to use. You don't want your filing system to be more stressful than the stress it's supposed to alleviate.

Scan, scan, scan

A scanner can be an important tool in helping you become better organized. Yes, you should get *rid* of stuff, not buy new stuff. A scanner, however, can make your paper-filled life a lot easier. You can scan all of your important papers, articles, documents, receipts, children's artwork, report cards, business cards, and recipes into your computer, where they can be organized and shared with others without taking up any physical space. Just be sure to keep important originals in a safe place.

Back it up!

You may think your computer will never let you down. But it can, and at some point it will. You've heard this many times before: Always back up your important files on discs, flash drives, or external hard drives. Better safe than sorry. If you prefer (or are perpetually forgetful) some online backup services automatically create backup files for you.

Managing your email

Your email can be a source of delight or major stress depending on how many messages you get, whom they come from, and what the senders want from you. Not only do you have to read most email, but sometimes you even need to respond. You can easily feel overwhelmed. The following are some simple strategies to help you manage your inbox.

Check your email, but don't overdo it

Most people fall into one of two groups: They either under-check or over-check their email. Checking your email too infrequently can get you into trouble. When people send you an email, they expect that you will respond in a reasonable time frame. That time frame is usually mere hours, not days. Delaying responses to personal emails can trigger the ire of family and friends. The damage of tardy responses in work-related situations can be more serious. But you can also go too far in the other direction. Constantly looking at your email can resemble an addiction, becoming somewhat compulsive. It can disrupt the flow of your day and become an unwelcome source of distraction.

TIP

Find some set times when it's convenient for you to check your email. It could be in the morning with your coffee, before lunch, and toward the end of the day. This will ensure that your inbox doesn't overflow and that you respond to important emails in a timely manner. A good time to check your email is after you've completed some other chore or piece of work. You're ready for a break, and looking at your email gives you breathing space.

Be efficient

Reading your email can become a black hole that sucks up your time and attention. Minutes can turn into hours. Unless you have that free time or you just really enjoy the process of email correspondence, keep your time per email short and to the point. Remember that bit of sage advice: "Only handle your mail once." The same principle holds for email. If you read it, answer it right away as briefly as is necessary.

Have more than one email address

One effective way of organizing your email is to have a second email address. This will ensure that email regarding specific parts of your life can be separated. For example, if you rent a vacation property for several weeks a year, any email regarding this rental can be directed to a different email address.

Keeping Your Life Organized

Say you manage to reverse eons of disarray and disorganization and now, having applied much grit and determination, you have a clean slate. Rather than waiting for the disorganization to return, you can do a number of things to maintain the order and harmony that you've achieved.

Being proactive

TIP

Following is a list of tips to help you keep your life organized:

>> **Do it now.** Rather than postpone clearing up clutter, do it as soon as you create it.

>> **Do it every day.** Try to spend 15 to 30 minutes at the end of the day putting things away so that you can start tomorrow in a (relatively) organized place.

- » **Become aware.** Every time you come across an item or piece of paper, ask yourself two questions:

  - How long have I had this?

  - Do I really need this?

- » **Build it in.** Create patterns. Clean up the yard in the spring. Do the shopping on Saturday. Clean the house on Wednesdays. Create a routine that frees you from having to make decisions. You do it automatically. You do it because your calendar says so.

- » **Delegate.** You may not have to do all of this alone. Don't be bashful about getting others (your partner, your kids, your guests) to pitch in with the program.

Buying less

REMEMBER

One of the reasons your life becomes more stressful is that you probably have too many "things." Fewer possessions mean a less complicated life. You can really live happily without many of the things you buy. So before you pull out your wallet at the cash register or pick up the phone or computer mouse to order something, ask yourself the following questions:

- » Do I really need this item?

- » Would the quality of my life be seriously compromised if I passed this up?

- » How many of these do I already have?

If you're like most people, your answers to these questions probably are no, no, and enough.

Here are some other buying suggestions that you may want to consider:

- » Don't buy stuff just because it's on sale. It's not a good deal if you don't use it.

- » Don't buy in bulk unless you're sure that you'll use all of it.

- » Don't buy anything without considering where you're going to put it.

» **Understanding why your workday really starts the night before**

» **Taking the stress out of commuting**

» **Building stress management into your workday**

» **Creating a stress-resistant workspace**

» **Bringing less stress home with you**

Chapter **5**

De-Stressing at Work

If you feel that your job is stressful, you're not alone. Too many workers report that their job is a major source of stress in their lives. The specific sources of work stress can be job insecurity, low pay, impossible clients, a terrible boss, dreadful coworkers, ridiculous deadlines, nasty office gossip, or lost time with family members. So before you're a candidate for a job-burnout seminar (and certainly before you do something you may regret later), read this chapter. You find out how to regroup, get a grip, and minimize your stress at work.

Reading the Signs of Workplace Stress

Some people thrive on the adrenaline rush they get from diving into the "challenges" they face at work. But if you're not stimulated and feel that you're drowning instead, then work stress may be the problem. See whether you recognize the signs of work stress. Check off the symptoms that describe you while you're at work:

____	You're often irritable.
____	You have trouble concentrating.

___	You're tired.
___	You've lost much of your sense of humor.
___	You get into more arguments than you used to.
___	You get less done.
___	You get sick more often.
___	You care less about your work.
___	You struggle to get out of bed on workday mornings.
___	You have less interest in your life outside of work.

At some point in their professional lives, most people will check off one or two of these items. However, if you feel that items on this list *consistently* describe you, or if you feel they have become a major source of distress in your life, you may want to seek professional help. Start by making an appointment with your family physician.

Knowing What's Triggering Your Work Stress

All right, so you're stressed at work. One of the key steps in managing your work stress is knowing where the stress comes from. Simply check off any of the items below that you feel are a major source of your stress:

___	Work overload (too much to do)
___	Work under-load (too little to do)
___	Too much responsibility
___	Too little responsibility
___	Dissatisfaction with career/job choice
___	Dissatisfaction with current role or duties
___	Poor work environment (noise, isolation, danger, and so on)
___	Long hours
___	Lack of positive feedback or recognition

____	Job insecurity
____	Lousy pay
____	Excessive travel
____	Limited chances for promotion
____	Discrimination because of gender, race, religion, age, disability, or sexual orientation
____	Problems with the boss or management
____	Problems with clients
____	Problems with coworkers
____	Office politics
____	A grueling commute

You have others? Jot them down:

_____

_____

_____

_____

Researcher Robert Karasek and his colleagues at the University of Southern California found that the two most stressful aspects of a job are:

>> **Lots of pressure to perform:** Tight deadlines, limited resources, production quotas, severe consequences for failing to meet management's goals — any or all of these can result in a highly pressured work environment.

>> **A lack of control over the work process:** Stress often results when you have little or no input regarding how your job should be done.

Making Positive Changes to Control Your Workplace Stress

Pinpoint your stress triggers at work and then ask yourself to what extent you can remove or at least reduce the impact of that stress. In some cases, you don't have the ability to eliminate some of the sources of stress at work. You may have little control over whether you keep or lose your job. You may dislike what you're doing but feel you can't change jobs. Getting the boss transferred may take some doing, and asking for a raise the day after the company announces downsizing plans may not be in your best interest. What you can change, however, is you. You can manage your stress and reduce its consequences by applying some of the ideas in this section.

Overcoming SNS (Sunday night stress)

As the weekend winds to an end, you may find yourself dreading Monday morning. The real culprit is Sunday night and your anticipatory anxiety. The irony here is that most often, when you get to the office and spend a couple of hours on the job, your stress level actually lowers. You stop worrying about what your work problems might be, replacing those concerns with distracting involvement and action. You find that the reality is less distressing than your negative anticipation.

TIP

The trick is figuring out how to cope with the night *before*. Take in these tips:

>> Get to bed a little bit earlier Sunday night. (Many people find that their Sunday-night sleep is their worst sleep of the week.)

>> Avoid eating that late-night heartburn special, which is guaranteed to keep you up 'til Wednesday.

>> Plan something relaxing and enjoyable that you can look forward to on Sunday night — rent a movie, curl up with a good book, or take a bubble bath.

>> Try not to schedule something you dislike as the first thing to do on Monday.

>> If possible, make Monday a day with a lighter workload.

>> Plan something you can look forward to on Monday. (How about lunch with a friend?)

Starting your workday unstressed

TIP

Getting to your job in reasonable condition is half the battle. By the time you open your office door (if you have one), you don't want to feel as if you've already fought (and probably lost) several minor skirmishes. Get a leg up on your work stress. Hit the ground running. Start your day the night before. Here's how:

>> **Go to bed.** Not getting enough sleep the night before can be a real stress producer. Your stress threshold is lowered. You're more irritable and find it much harder to concentrate. People and situations that normally wouldn't get

to you, now do. Arriving at work tired is a guarantee that this isn't going to be one of your better stress days.

>> **Get up a tad earlier.** Getting out of bed even a few minutes earlier in the morning can give you enough of a safety net so that you don't find yourself rushing, looking for something at the last minute, and racing out the door with a powdered donut in your hand. Don't add to your stress by running late.

>> **Eat breakfast.** To manage your stress, getting off on the right nutritional foot is important. When you wake up in the morning, as many as 11 or 12 hours have passed since you last ate. Your body needs to refuel. You may feel fine skipping breakfast, but studies show that people who don't eat a reasonable breakfast more often report feelings of fatigue and more stress later in the day.

>> **Work out before you shower.** If you can manage it, getting some physical exercise before your workday starts can put you ahead of the game. Hitting the stationary bike, working the stair climber, or even walking briskly around the block can throw you into gear and get you ready for your day. Studies show that even short periods of exercise can speed up your heart rate, increase the amount of oxygen to your brain, and release endorphins, which can exert a calming effect. You're ready for anything your job might throw at you.

>> **Check your schedule.** When you get to the office, spend the first part of your morning organizing your day. Knowing that you're in control of what will get done reduces any uncertainty and anxiety. An important part of this is becoming more organized and managing your time effectively. (You may want to take a look at Chapters 3 and 4 in Book 6.)

Generally, most people feel that Monday is the most stressful day of the week. Studies show that you're more likely to have a stroke or heart attack on Monday morning than at any other time during the week.

Calming your daily commute

Commuting can be a major stressor. Following are some tips to help you reduce the stress of coming from and going to work:

>> **Practice some "auto" relaxation.** Try this simple technique while you're caught in traffic or even while stopped for a red light: Using both hands, squeeze the steering wheel with a medium-tight grip. At the same time, tense the muscles in your arms and shoulders, scrunching up your shoulders as if you're trying to have them touch your ears. Hold that tension for about three or four seconds. Then release all of that tension, letting go of any muscle

tightness anywhere in your body. Let this feeling of relaxation spread slowly throughout your entire body. Wait a few minutes and do it again.

» **Beat the crowd.** Often, leaving a little earlier or a little later can make a big difference in the quality of your commute. You may get a seat, you may find that the traffic is less congested, and you may find that what was horrific yesterday becomes a lot more endurable.

» **Amuse yourself.** Commuting can seem like a joyless endeavor. You can, however, make your time in your car (or on the subway, bus, or train) productive, entertaining, or at least pleasant.

Have some interesting reading material in your pocket or purse whenever you go out. It can be an amusing little paperback, your e-reader, or an article you've cut out or downloaded but haven't yet found the time to read.

You can also turn to your digital device for solace. These days the selection of music, video, audio books, and podcasts is incredibly wide.

Minimizing your travel stress

Your business travel may be more than getting to and from work. You may spend a lot of time on trains or planes. To many, the idea of travel may seem glamorous. Flying to Paris, Rome, or even Cleveland for work may sound like an adventurous outing, an escape from the stress of the office. But be careful what you wish for. Yes, a little travel can be a welcome change of pace. But traveling a lot is stressful. Just ask anyone who spends many hours in the air each month. A study by the World Bank Group found that nearly 75 percent of respondents said their stress levels were high or very high because of their business travel.

TIP

Here are some traps to watch out for and some ideas to help you tame that road-warrior distress:

» **Bad eating habits:** You can more easily control what and when you eat when you're at home. Sitting in business class (if you can swing it) tempts you with all kinds of wonderful yet not terribly healthful goodies. It can be hard to say no. A study by the Mailman School of Public Health at Columbia University found that those who travel more are more prone to obesity than those who travel less. And, as you know, when you're overweight, you're prone to a host of weight-related risks such as higher blood pressure, diabetes, and elevated cholesterol. The trick is to pre-think what you're going to eat *before* you get into that tempting situation or pick up that restaurant menu.

>> **Little exercise:** Business travel can be pretty sedentary. Obviously sitting on the plane for hours is confining. Get up and walk around from time to time, do some static exercises, and stretch on the flight. Even when you get off the plane, you may have little time for physical activity. Seasoned travelers have figured out how to build some exercise into their travel plans. These days you can find a health club, spa, or gym in every major hotel. Many hotels have exercise videos available. Even if you didn't bring your sneakers, the hotel can often provide you with work-out clothes.

>> **Poor sleep:** While some travelers swear they sleep best in a hotel, many more find that the quality of their sleep is worse. One obvious culprit is jet lag that finds you tossing and turning at 4 a.m. Another is the late nights spent entertaining clients. It may also be getting used to a new bed. A survey conducted by Westin Hotels and Resorts found that 55 percent of frequent business travelers experience sleep deprivation, and 22 percent experience some form of sleep disruption or insomnia.

If you can arrive at your destination a day or two earlier, this will help your body adjust. Try not to burn the candle at both ends. Get to bed as early as you can. Watch the alcohol and the caffeine. Some people swear that taking melatonin helps, but the jury is still out on its efficacy. Set your watch for the new time. This will help you adjust psychologically to the change. Drink water both during and after the flight to avoid dehydration. Take a hot bath before you go to bed. Finally, sometimes earplugs and an eye mask can help reduce distractions.

De-stressing during your workday

One of the secrets of effective stress management at work is finding ways to incorporate a variety of stress-reduction techniques into your workday. By using these methods on a regular basis you can catch your stress early — before it has a chance to turn into something painful or worrisome.

Take a look at the following surefire strategies to help you nip that stress in the bud.

Cut muscle tension off at the pass

A day at work is usually a day filled with problems, pressures, and demands, with little time to think about your newfound relaxation skills. Your stress builds, and much of that stress takes the form of tension in your muscles. Drain that tension before it becomes more of a problem using some of the techniques described in Chapter 2 of Book 6. This may include trying some relaxed breathing, rapid relaxation, differential relaxation, meditation, or imagery.

Some potential relaxation opportunities include the following:

>> When you finish a phone call

>> When someone leaves your office and closes the door

>> When you find yourself in a boring meeting

Collect some mileage points

Get up and walk away from your desk — get some coffee or water, or make copies. Walk around a lot, and at lunch be sure to get out of the office and take a quick stroll.

Stand up when you're on the telephone — or, at least some of the time you're on the phone. Walk around. This gives your body a chance to use different sets of muscles and interrupts any buildup of tension.

Stretching and reaching for the sky

For many of you, your days are characterized by long periods of sitting at a desk or stuck in a cramped work area, punctuated only by trips to the coffee or copy machine. Other folks are on their feet all day. In either case, stretching is a great way of releasing any tension that has accumulated in your muscles. The following sections cover some recommended ways to stretch. For more stretching ideas, take a look at Chapter 3 in Book 4, which has plenty of great ways you can stretch and release muscle tension.

When you find that your bodily tension is over the top (better yet, try this before you get to that point), pick up a tennis ball or other soft ball, squeeze it for eight to ten seconds, and then slowly release all the tension in your fingers and hand. Let that feeling of relaxation spread out to the rest of your body. Repeat several times throughout the day.

The cherry-picker

This stretch works well for your shoulders, arms, and back. Sit in your chair, with feet flat on the floor, or stand in place. Raise both of your arms over your head and point your fingers directly toward the ceiling. Now, pretend to reach and pick a cherry on a branch that's just a little higher than your right hand. Stretch that hand an inch or so, and then make a fist. Squeeze for two or three seconds. Relax your hand. Do the same with your left hand. If cherries aren't your thing, consider apples.

The pec stretch and squeeze

This move is good for relieving tightness in your pectoral and deltoid muscles and upper back. Sitting at your desk, or standing up straight, put both of your hands behind your head with your fingers interlaced. Bring your elbows back as far as you can. (See Figure 5-1.) Hold that tension for five to ten seconds, release the tension, and then do it a second and third time. Find various times in your day when you can repeat this stretch.

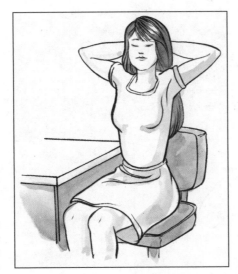

Illustration by Pam Tanzy

The leg lift

This stretch relieves tension in your quadriceps (in the thighs) and strengthens your abdominal muscles. Sitting in a chair, lift both of your legs straight in front of you. At the same time, curl your toes toward you. (See Figure 5-2.) Hold that tension for five to ten seconds and then let your feet fall to the floor. Repeat two or three times, and at other points in your day.

The upper-back stretch

This stretch is great for relieving any tension in your upper back. Put your finger-tips on your shoulders, with elbows out to the side. Raise your elbows until they are in line with your shoulders (see Figure 5-3). Now bring your elbows forward until they touch or almost touch each other. Hold that position for five to ten seconds and then let your arms fall comfortably to your side. Repeat two or three times, and also at different times in your day.

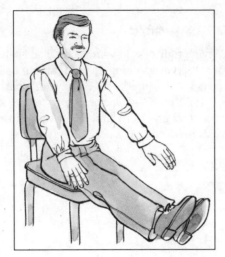

FIGURE 5-2:
The leg lift works your quadriceps and abdominal muscles.

Illustration by Pam Tanzy

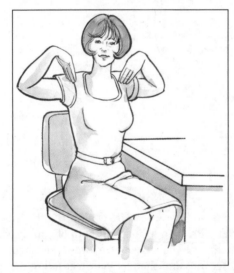

FIGURE 5-3:
Use some elbow grease to ease tension in your upper back.

Illustration by Pam Tanzy

Creating a stress-resistant workspace

You may not be able to control every single aspect of your job, but you probably have the power to control your personal work area. Your workspace can (literally) give you a pain in the neck, straining your muscles and tiring your body. The culprit may be an awkwardly placed computer monitor, uncomfortable seating, poor lighting, or simply a totally cluttered desk that's hiding that memo you remember writing and now urgently need. Your life is stressful enough as it is. You don't need your workspace adding to your daily dose of stress. This section shows you a few ways to make your workspace a lot more stress-resistant.

Organizing your desk

How can a neater desk reduce stress? Well, because the source of many types of stress comes from a feeling of being out of control, of being overwhelmed. When your work area looks like a battlefield, you feel the tension growing. And when you can't find that report you need, your stress level soars even higher. By organizing your files and piles, you get a sense (perhaps mistakenly) that there is some order in all the chaos. So, at the end of your workday, straighten up things. Doing so takes only a few minutes, but the rewards are large.

Lights! Sound! Action!: Creating a more pleasant workspace

Here are a few ways to take some of the stress out of your workspace. Your employer may not be entirely supportive of all your stress-reducing efforts. And if you share a tiny cubicle with three others, it may be hard for you to burn incense, move in a couch, or install a multi-speaker stereo system and personal video player. Nevertheless, see what you can do with some of the following ideas:

>> **Soothe yourself with sound.** If you can orchestrate it, listening to calming music at your workspace can unruffle your feathers. Your smartphone or radio can be the source of relaxing music. Classical music, especially Bach and Mozart, works nicely. If these composers are too highbrow for your tastes, try one of the "lite" radio stations.

TECHNICAL STUFF

Recent studies at the University of California found that listening to Mozart, particularly the piano sonatas, can significantly improve a person's ability to reason abstractly. Not only do stress levels go down, but IQ goes up. On the other hand, listening to Philip Glass or Metallica didn't enhance anything.

>> **Lighten up.** Although a naked, 300-watt bulb dangling from your office ceiling can provide you with more than enough light, you want more than "just enough light." The right lighting in your workspace can reduce eyestrain and make your environment a more pleasant place to work. Go for soft and indirect lighting. Just make sure you have enough light.

>> **Create visual resting spots.** Give your eyes — and your mind — a break. At regular intervals, look away from your computer screen or paperwork and focus on a distant object to "stretch your eyes." You can also create visual relief in your office by adding a few interesting objects. For example:

- Strategically place one or more photographs of those you care about to bring a warm glow to your heart. Better yet, have the picture include a scene — a vacation, a gathering — that reminds you of a happy experience.

- Place a plant or flowers in your workspace to add an air of beauty and relaxation to your workday. Some plants (such as English ivy and spider plants) are even said to help clean the air of indoor pollutants — an added bonus!

- Hang some artwork that you find calming and peaceful.

» **Be scent-sible.** Fill a bowl with green apples to add a relaxing scent to your office. Be careful, though. Many people are scent sensitive and may be allergic to your favorite smells. If you share your workspace, ask before you scent.

» **Have more than one dumbbell in your office.** Keep a set of weights or mini barbells in your office. In a spare moment or two you can rip through a set of reps and feel a bit more relaxed. Alternately, keep an elastic stretcher in your desk that you can use for both your arms and legs.

» **Keep a toy chest.** What's an office without a few toys? (Balls that knock into each other . . . a game on your computer . . . that peg-jumping triangle game . . .)

» **Don't get tied down.** One of those headsets that attaches to your telephone can free up your hands to do other things, such as look through your email, lift those weights, or play that computer game. The better ones are wireless and let you really move around your office so that you can file, play Nerf basketball, or rearrange your books in order of their color.

Becoming EC (ergonomically correct)

Your desk or workspace can cause stress for other reasons besides disorganization. The problem is, your body wasn't designed to sit and work in one place for long periods of time. When you sit in a stationary position, your muscle groups contract. The blood flow to these muscles may become reduced, resulting in oxygen-deprived muscles. This can lead to pain, strain, muscle aches, and fatigue.

Here are some suggestions that can help you avoid that ergonomic pain in the neck:

» **If you spend long periods of time typing at your computer, where and how you sit becomes important.** The height of your chair in relationship to your keyboard and monitor are important variables to consider in avoiding excessive muscle tension and fatigue in your shoulders, neck, and upper back. You don't want to be straining your neck while looking at your monitor.

Adjustability is the key. If your chair or table is too high or too low, replace it. Better yet, find an adjustable chair and table. Seat heights should range from 15 to 22 inches, depending on what your dimensions look like.

» **You should also have some padded support for your lumbar (lower back) region.** The backrest should be full-length, extending some 18 to 20 inches higher than the seat of your chair. If your lower back isn't supported sufficiently, consider a lumbar roll — a cylindrical pillow that fits nicely in the small of your back.

» **Your keyboard should be approximately at elbow level when you're seated.** When using your keyboard, make sure your fingers are lower than your wrists. To avoid repetitive-stress injuries (such as carpal tunnel syndrome), you may want to consider an ergonomically designed keyboard that reduces the strain on your wrists. You should also consider a support for your wrist when you're using your mouse.

» **Having a foot rest is a good way of taking some of the strain off your legs and back, especially if you're short.**

TECHNICAL STUFF

A study carried out by AT&T on its telephone operators found that switching to easily adjustable tables and chairs resulted in a significant reduction in reported discomfort, particularly in the back, shoulders, and legs.

» **Not all writing instruments are ergonomically equal.** Find a pen that is particularly comfortable to work with. The grip should not result in your fingers becoming easily fatigued.

» **If you spend a lot of time on your feet, finding the correct footwear becomes a necessity.** If you find you have to trade some style for greater comfort, go for the comfort.

LISTEN TO YOUR MOTHER: SIT UP STRAIGHT!

Sometimes your stress comes from the most unlikely of places — your chair, for example. Sitting improperly for long periods of time can result in bodily fatigue, tension, and, ultimately, pain. Sitting actually puts more pressure on your spinal discs than does standing. When you slump or hunch forward, the pressure is even greater.

Sit back in your chair with your spine straight. Your lungs now have room to expand, and you place less strain on your back. You may find that you have to invest in a more supportive chair. Spend the bucks — a good chair is well worth the money.

Managing your work time

TIP

Having too little time is often cited as a major work stress. In the current economy, time-related stress is magnified by having fewer people to do the same amount of work. Deadlines introduce even more stress. If getting organized is near the top of your list of stress reducers, time management is way up there as well. Chapter 3 in Book 6 describes a number of effective ideas and strategies to help you manage your time. Here are some work-related time-management highlights:

» Work with lists and calendars.

» Prioritize your tasks.

» Batch your emails and phone calls.

» Divide and conquer by breaking larger tasks into smaller parts.

» Don't over-commit.

» Delegate when you can.

Nourishing your body (and spirit)

What goes into your mouth from 9 to 5 (or from 8 to 7) can make a big difference in your stress level. Eating the wrong foods, or even eating the right foods in the wrong amounts or at the wrong times, can make it harder for you to cope with the stress in your life. Also, when you eat poorly, your body doesn't work as efficiently as it should. Low levels of blood sugar can result in feelings of anxiety and irritability. Poor eating habits can also leave you unnecessarily fatigued. Over-eating during the workday can leave you lethargic and sleepy.

All of this means that you're not in the best position to handle all the pressures and demands you must face at work. Here are some ideas and suggestions that can help make what you eat an ally in your battle against stress, and not the enemy.

Do lunch (with a difference)

Although the days of the three-martini lunch are gone, you can still find the harried worker overloading his or her plate with the kinds of food that ensure a high stress level for the rest of the day. Some suggestions for powering up your body (and not creating a meltdown) for the afternoon:

» Never skip lunch — no matter how busy your day gets.

» Eat less at your midday meal — no seconds.

>> Eat stress-reducing foods.

>> Don't drink any alcohol.

>> Skip dessert.

Make your lunch break a stress break

TIP

Lunchtime isn't only about eating; it's a great time to work on lowering your stress. Try to get out of your work environment at lunch. Even if the outing is as simple as going for a walk around the block, go. Better yet, find a park, library, waterfront — anything relaxing — that can put you (however temporarily) into a different frame of mind. Find your lunchtime oasis.

Work it out

If you can swing it, one of the better things to do on your lunch break is to hit the gym or health club. Many are conveniently located near work sites. Work up a sweat, take a shower, and then have a quick but nourishing bite to eat.

THE COFFEE-FREE COFFEE BREAK

The caffeine in two cups of coffee can increase your heart rate by as much as 15 beats per minute. It can also make you irritable and nervous. So forgo that third or fourth cup of coffee (and donut). Instead, eat something that adds to your body's ability to cope, such as a

- Cup of low-fat yogurt.
- Cup of fruit salad.
- Handful of mixed nuts.
- Piece of chocolate (one piece!).
- Piece of fruit.
- Cup of herbal tea.
- Glass of water. (You need to hydrate!)

And, if you must have that nth cup of coffee, at least try going the unleaded (decaffeinated) route.

Avoid the (jelly) beans

WARNING

Many people remember Ronald Reagan for his accomplishments as president. What others may remember, however, are those jars of jelly beans strategically positioned in his office. While they are admittedly colorful, having gobs of candy at hand may not help you with your stress. A sugar fix energizes you in the short run but leaves you flagging later in the day. You're better off avoiding this and any other candy. If you need a pick-me-up, try to choose something from the list in the nearby sidebar "The coffee-free coffee break."

Taking Advantage of Company Perks

These days, larger companies and organizations offer a number of services and benefits that can help reduce your stress level. If you're not aware of such perks, ask around or check with your HR office to learn more. Here are some possibilities that might be available to you.

Gyms and health clubs

Exercise is an important source of stress reduction. The tough part is actually *getting to* the gym or health club. Convenience and accessibility make this more likely to happen. If it's close, you're more likely to show up. Many employers have workout facilities right on their premises. This makes it easier for you to show up before work, during your lunch hour, or after work. Even on the coldest, rainiest day, you can manage to take the elevator to the building's health club and get a workout.

Many companies and organizations that don't have exercise facilities on their premises offer corporate discounts at nearby gyms or health clubs.

Flextime

Trying to fit your busy schedule into someone else's can be a major source of work stress. A number of work settings give employees the option of determining which hours they want to work rather than the normal "9 to 5." This may take the form of working a condensed week or working a regular week but starting work and leaving work at a preferred hour. The clear benefit to employees is greater control over their time and more flexibility balancing work with home and family. The result is that employees working on a more flexible schedule report being more satisfied with their work experience and less stressed.

Working from home

Many employees feel that their work stress is lessened when they're allowed to work from home even for a small part of their week. The good news is, more and more companies are allowing their employees to work one or more days a week at home (especially since the start of the COVID-19 pandemic). Given the rapid developments in technology, working on your computer or phone at home might not be a negative for the company. Again, the clear advantage for the employee is flexibility and greater control over your time. The result is increased job satisfaction, higher autonomy, less work–family conflict, and less stress.

Employee assistance programs

Most large employers now offer a variety of personal services. This can range from exercise and weight-loss programs to personal and financial counseling (even stress management!). The individual needs don't necessarily have to involve the workplace. You may need help dealing with your aging parents, overcoming substance abuse, handling a crisis, or addressing legal concerns. And of course you may need help with issues at work. Often employers contract with third-party companies that manage the service. Confidentiality is assured, and your boss need not know what you're up to.

Coming Home More Relaxed (And Staying That Way)

You've had a long, long day. You're tired and dragging your tush. The last thing you want to do is take your work stress home with you. Consider these guidelines to make sure you arrive home in better shape than when you left work:

>> **After work, work out.** If early mornings or lunchtimes are impractical times to hit the gym or health club, consider exercising right after work. Take out your frustrations and worries on the stair climber or in a step class. Not only is this mode of venting healthier, you'll still have your job in the morning!

>> **Leave your work at work.** One of the more common stress traps is to take your work-related stress and spread it around so that the other parts of your life become stressful. You probably have enough stress at home without importing more stress from your work. If you find that you absolutely have to take work home, be very specific about what you want to accomplish and how much time you want to spend doing it.

Never take work home routinely. And try not to go to work on the weekends unless it's absolutely necessary.

Ah, home sweet home! But is it? Even if your ride home has been relatively non-stressful, opening your front door can lead to a whole new set of challenges. Walking straight into these stressors can catch you off guard and put you into a foul mood. When you get home, be sure to build in a short period of relative quiet — say 15 or 20 minutes — that can help you make the transition into your second world.

Following are some suggestions for low-stress work-home transitions:

>> Take a relaxing bath or shower.

>> Sit in your favorite chair and simply veg.

>> Listen to some relaxing music.

>> Read a chapter from a good book.

>> Work out.

>> Take a relaxing walk.

If, when you open your door, chaos descends, and it's clear that none of these activities are even remotely possible, you may want to consider implementing some of these relaxing segues before you reach home. Perhaps sipping a latte and doing the crossword puzzle at the local coffee shop near your home can work for you. You can take that walk or spend a few minutes in a local park (with a good book?) before you open your door. You are now ready to cope with the chaos.

ALL WORK AND NO PLAY . . .

When your job is stressful, you may need something positive to look forward to. It can be a quiet dinner at home with family, a night out with friends, a restaurant dinner, a movie, or a concert. It can be as simple as sitting on your couch and catching up on your favorite TV series. It just has to be something that adds a measure of contentment to your life.

An upcoming vacation can also provide a source of positive excitement. Planning that trip can (hopefully) be part of the pleasure. Finding out where to go and what to do can be involving and satisfying. Your trip need not be a long vacation; it can be a mini-vacation where for a day or two you get away. Weekends are especially important times for you to recharge and introduce positive experiences into your life.

7

Reining In Online Activities

Contents at a Glance

CHAPTER 1: Defining and Overcoming Internet Addiction in a Nutshell 487

Defining Behavioral Addiction 488

Understanding How and Why People Get Addicted to Screens and the Internet 489

Digging into Digital Devices and the Internet 491

Recognizing the Threats 492

Identifying the Signs and Symptoms of Internet and Screen Addiction 494

Recovering from Internet and Screen Addiction 496

Balancing Technology with Real-Time Living 498

CHAPTER 2: Discovering What Makes the Internet and Smartphones So Addictive 499

Eyes on the Prize: Factors Involving Focus on a Screen 500

The Good (or Bad) Stuff: Factors Involving Content 502

This Must Be the Place: The Internet as the Car, Map, and Destination 505

The Human Factor: The Internet as a Digital Drug 508

CHAPTER 3: Examining the Addictive Nature of Social Media 511

A Social Network: A Rose by Any Other Name 512

Recognizing What Makes You Come Back to Social Media for More 513

Seeking Communication and Self-Esteem — But at a Price 517

Seeing Why Social Media Can Be Counter-Social 519

Finding Relief: Life beyond Social Media 522

CHAPTER 4: The Endless Stream: Binge Watching TV and Online Entertainment 523

Missing Your Life While Being Entertained: The Ease of the Binge 524

Looking at Other Problems of Watching TV All the Time 529

It's a Choice: Screening the Stream 532

CHAPTER 5: Adopting Self-Help Strategies 533

Remembering That Life Isn't Lived on a Screen 534

Disrupting Your Tech Habits with a Digital Detox 537

Monitoring and Limiting Your Time and Content on Screens 539

Establishing Values-Based Tech Use 541

Removing Notifications and Addictive Apps 544

Filling Your Life with Real-Time Activities 545

» Knowing the difference between an addiction and dependence

» Surveying the important traits of Internet addiction

» Taking steps to address an Internet addiction

Chapter **1**

Defining and Overcoming Internet Addiction in a Nutshell

The interesting thing about the word *addiction* is that technically it isn't really a medical term or diagnosis. Although used by nearly everyone, both clinicians and the public, it's more of a popularized term used to describe a set of behaviors or a syndrome. Official diagnostic terms for substance and behavioral addictions include *substance use disorder, alcohol use disorder, pathological gambling,* and *Internet gaming disorder.* For the purposes of this book, the term *addiction* is used for ease and simplicity.

Most people confuse an addiction with physical dependence. Physical dependence occurs when the body gets used to a substance, be it alcohol or drugs. It is characterized by a tolerance to that substance and then withdrawal when the substance is discontinued. Essentially, the body's receptors for that drug become accustomed to having it in the system. When it's no longer available, there are physical and psychological symptoms that we call withdrawal.

Addiction is more typically defined as a pathological or compulsive use disorder. This means that when you use a substance or engage in a repetitive behavior (such as Internet use or video gaming), significant negative effects are created in your life. Despite these negative effects, the user cannot easily stop or may not think they need to stop. This distortion of reality is often inherent to addiction and is also known as denial.

We all engage in pleasurable behaviors and at times take substances that are pleasure inducing. Take alcohol, for instance. Alcohol is a legal psychoactive substance that has long been associated with pleasurable sensations, but unfortunately, it is also known for its addictive potential. Many pleasurable substances and behaviors can produce an addictive response due to their activation of the reward circuitry in the brain.

There is some confusion over whether *intoxication* and/or *withdrawal* described in alcohol or substance use is also experienced in behavioral addictions such as gambling, food, sex, or the Internet. Clarifying this issue isn't necessary to recognize behavioral addictions, however. Addiction is not simply the intoxication or withdrawal we get from a substance or behavior. It is the creation of a potential set of behaviors and life-impacting consequences reflecting a complex biopsychosocial process. We call it *biopsychosocial* because it affects our physical health as well as our social and emotional life.

This chapter introduces you to Internet and screen addiction, how to recognize it, and how to get help.

Defining Behavioral Addiction

There is some confusion about what causes an addiction; this confusion often occurs because of the physiological response of tolerance and withdrawal from drugs or alcohol. But what about gambling? With gambling, you aren't ingesting anything, yet you see all the same markers and consequences of addiction, including an impact on social relationships and psychological functioning, as well as on work, legal issues, finances, health, or academic performance.

Gambling addiction (the official medical diagnosis is *pathological gambling*) is part of a group of addictions called *process* or *behavioral addictions;* the American Society of Addiction Medicine, in part, defines addiction as the use of a substance or behavior that causes *negative* and *deleterious* life consequences:

Addiction is characterized by inability to consistently abstain, impairment in behavioral control, craving, diminished recognition of significant problems with one's behaviors and interpersonal relationships, and a dysfunctional emotional response. Like other chronic diseases, addiction often involves cycles of relapse and remission.

REMEMBER

The complex process of addiction almost always involves disruption of reward patterns, motivation, compulsion, executive function, and judgment, but it may not include the physical withdrawal symptoms seen in drug or alcohol dependence.

Understanding How and Why People Get Addicted to Screens and the Internet

So, what about the Internet? And how exactly do you become addicted to a digital screen connected to the Internet? Well, the answer is not all that different from how you become addicted to other behaviors and substances. Part of what happens with screen use (when linked to the Internet) is that you're accessing content that is stimulating and rewarding to you, but because the delivery mechanism of this digital drug is variable (meaning you don't know what you will get, when you will get it, and how desirable it will be for you), your brain receives a variably rewarding experience. Each time you get a reward, you receive a small hit of dopamine in your mid-brain (also called the limbic system). This unpredictability, or *maybe* factor, is very resistant to extinction or, putting it another way, addictive.

This is the same way that addiction to gambling works, and that is why you can think of the Internet as the "world's largest slot machine." Each time you pull the handle on a slot machine or click your mouse, you might win; with gambling, you might win some money — on the Internet, you might win some form of desirable content.

Screen technology is essentially doing the same thing that drugs, alcohol, and gambling do. Obviously, there are differences between the various types of addictions, but the underlying neurobiology is essentially the same. You tend to repeat behaviors that are pleasurable, and the perception of that pleasure is often unconscious and largely biological; the impacts these addictive patterns have are more often behavioral and psychological, but the underpinnings of all addictions are neurobiological.

Many people can experience the excitement and rewards of the Internet and most forms of digital content with few problems, although you will frequently hear people complain about how *addicted* they feel to their smartphones, Facebook, TikTok, Instagram, Snapchat, Reddit, Twitter, pornography, video games,

YouTube, and even streaming sites such as Amazon Prime, Hulu, and Netflix. The reality is that some people are unable to limit their use of these forms of online content, and because the Internet delivery system operates on a variable reinforcement schedule, the brain gets used to the *maybe* factor that helps produce the addictive response. The pleasure part of the brain responds with increases in dopamine, and the unpredictability of *what, how much,* and *when* helps create a digital addictive experience. Obviously, the content you might *like* and respond *favorably to* will vary, but the Internet has *so much* available content that it is easy to understand why many people feel addicted to their screens (the reality is that many people are overusing their screens, but may not be addicted).

REMEMBER

It's perhaps important to note here that feeling addicted to your screen may not mean that you are. Many of us are aware of our overuse of our screens, but it may not have risen to a point that meets addiction criteria. Nevertheless, it can be a lifestyle problem that you should address by making some changes in *how* and *when* you use your Internet technology. Find out about signs and symptoms of Internet and screen addiction later in this chapter.

REMEMBER

Addiction represents an extreme problem with a drug or behavior, but it has different levels of severity just like any illness or behavioral health problem. The levels of addiction can range from mild to severe, with each level representing more significant negative impacts on your behavior and functioning. At the lowest level of impact, you might be overusing your technology and screens to a point where you're eating up too much time and energy that might be better spent on other tasks and activities. At the most extreme level, there are people whose lives have been severely impacted and limited by their screen use. It is perhaps fair to say that most of us (at times) fall into some level of overuse, abuse, or addiction to Internet technology.

TECHNICAL STUFF

The American Society of Addiction Medicine gives the following more complete definition of addiction:

Addiction is a primary, chronic disease of brain reward, motivation, memory, and related circuitry. Dysfunction in these circuits leads to characteristic biological, psychological, social, and spiritual manifestations. This is reflected in an individual pathologically pursuing reward and/or relief by substance use and other behaviors. Addiction is characterized by inability to consistently abstain, impairment in behavioral control, craving, diminished recognition of significant problems with one's behaviors and interpersonal relationships, and a dysfunctional emotional response. Like other chronic diseases, addiction often involves cycles of relapse and remission. Without treatment or engagement in recovery activities, addiction is progressive and can result in disability or premature death.

Digging into Digital Devices and the Internet

Today, digital screen devices reflect a wide range of technologies and include iPhones and Android smartphones; iPads, Kindles, and other tablets; laptop and desktop computers; and streaming devices and smart TVs. These days, it's very difficult to find something that isn't directly or wirelessly linked to the Internet. You likely almost always have easy access to an Internet connection portal, which increases your overall risk for developing an addiction or unhealthy Internet use habits.

WARNING

All digital devices have the power to rob you of your time and attention, and this imbalance creates problems.

The power of, and attraction to, the Internet comes from its ability to connect people with other people, information, and services. This has essentially changed the way we live our lives; however, the most powerful aspect of the Internet is its addictive potential. The way the Internet works can lead to increases in the amount of time you spend online, irrespective of the specific content you consume.

REMEMBER

The Internet is neither good nor bad — it's amoral. It has no feelings in its power to captivate you. However, you should always keep in mind that the only goal of everything online is to *capture* and *hold your attention*. It's not necessarily a nefarious intention, but nevertheless, it's a potent force whose purpose is to keep you screen-bound (for largely economic reasons). The only way out of the black hole of the Internet is to take back control of your time and attention.

REMEMBER

Smartphones are the world's smallest slot machines. Their ease of access and availability make them highly addictive Internet access portals. And making smartphones even more addictive are the *notifications* they provide you. Each time you receive a notification of some type, your brain registers a triggering signal that a desirable message, information, or content is waiting for you. This facilitates your continually picking up and checking your phone all day long. There are estimates that many of you pick up your phone a hundred times or more a day! The activation of possibly finding something pleasurable when you're checking is *even more* rewarding than the content itself. Nothing is more intoxicating than *maybe*.

See Chapter 2 in Book 7 for more information on the addictiveness of smartphones and the Internet.

Recognizing the Threats

How do you know whether your *digital device* has become your *digital vice?* This isn't an easy question to answer, as everyone has their own personal values about time and everyone is different in terms of how much disruption is tolerable in their lives. Your technology use is often in part determined by your values around how you use your time and the consciousness you bring to your Internet screen use.

The idea that your screen use typically occurs below your conscious radar is well established. *Time distortion* and *dissociation* are common when you are on your screen, so it's very likely that you don't actually know how much time passes when you're staring at your Instagram or Facebook account, or circling down the rabbit hole on Reddit, or caught in an endless YouTube playlist or Netflix binge.

The first step in recognizing your Internet use is to become conscious of how much *content* you're consuming, and to become aware of exactly how much *time* you have unknowingly surrendered to your device. This is perhaps easier said than done, in that most of the time on your device may be spent without a thought, with little awareness that you have begun a slow descent into the electronic sink-hole of the Internet.

The following sections briefly cover addictive platforms and technologies.

Social media

What exactly is social media? Chapter 3 in Book 7 explains that *social media* is a broad category of applications and websites that are structured around the idea of connecting people, organizations, or businesses around themes, content, or interest areas. Although there are several well-known social media sites, the definition of social media has also expanded to include newer apps and websites that attract users' time and attention. Some examples of social media sites are Facebook, Instagram, LinkedIn, TikTok, Reddit, Snapchat, Vine, Twitter, and YouTube, and even travel sites such as Waze and Yelp have a social media component; undoubtedly, countless social applications are integrated into other apps and websites, as businesses have found that *social sells.*

Some social sites are integrated around news and communication, others focus on video and text, and still others are simply about photos and user life updates, posts, and sharing. Some integrate all of these features. Most are without fees to the user; however, none are free. Most accept advertising, and many sell your user data to others for a variety of purposes.

Make no mistake: If you think there are no obvious payment of costs connected to social media, then *you* are the payment! Your eyes and attention form the economic engine that drives social media, and many of these platforms have proven to be both addictive and negatively impactful on a variety of psychological levels.

Streaming audio and video

Consuming audio and video content (including music, podcasts, and audiobooks) has become commonplace; in fact, most of what you consume in terms of music, TV, movies, Netflix, Amazon Prime, Hulu, podcasts, YouTube, Kindle, and so on is essentially in streaming format. Even software is streamed or downloaded, and your data is increasingly held in the cloud (on a company's server) instead of on your devices. Streaming means that information and content is pushed to your device in real time, and you watch, read, or listen to it as it is streamed. Sometimes you can download it onto your device and store it for later use.

Although no one would argue against the convenience of consuming your digital entertainment in this manner, there are some inherent problems. One major problem is that many of these streaming sites have default settings, called *autoplay,* for audio or video content to keep going to the next movie, TV show, podcast, or YouTube clip — unless you deliberately turn off that feature. The net effect (no pun intended) is that you can end up watching or listening to a lot more content than you intended to or have time for. The automatic "pushed" nature of the content is equivalent to eating out of a large dish with no ability to measure the portion of food (or digital *content*) you are consuming. See Chapter 4 in Book 7 for more about streaming content.

Video games

Of all the content areas that are consumed on the Internet, video gaming is perhaps the most problematic in terms of negative life consequences. That doesn't mean that video gaming is bad or inherently dangerous; in fact, most people who use video games have no significant problem with them and are able to use games with little or no negative life impact. In other words, they can use them in a moderated manner. However, a small percentage of users (studies suggest between 1 and 10 percent) cannot self-regulate their use and spend inordinate amounts of time on gaming platforms, including handheld devices, consoles, and PC-based systems. Many people have problems with PC-based or console games.

Video games incorporate some very attractive factors that contribute to their addictive potential:

>> They provide stimulating content that is novel, interactive, and dynamic. Games are always evolving, through updates and modifications, to keep the novelty and challenge factor high.

>> When playing a video game, you can experience a level of growing mastery that often creates a sense of accomplishment; you might develop greater efficacy in your skills and a higher ranking in comparison to other users.

>> The game provides a sophisticated variable ratio reinforcement and reward structure (the *maybe* factor), and this structure is modified and changed to maintain user interest and to maximize the dopamine/pleasure response.

All forms of Internet communication facilitate some degree of social connection and group interaction, albeit in a two-dimensional online format, but many video game users find the social component of video gaming to be quite compelling. Many times, gamers are communicating verbally (on a headset) via apps such as Discord or others, and the conversations may not only be about the game being played.

Identifying the Signs and Symptoms of Internet and Screen Addiction

Following is a general list of things to look out for to determine whether you may be suffering from an addiction to the Internet. Sometimes just developing an awareness of what you're doing can increase your self-consciousness enough to cause you to change your habits and patterns. This is a good place to start. Generally, small changes can be valuable, but you can make those changes only if you are really aware of what you're doing.

REMEMBER

Every accomplishment starts with a *goal*, followed by an *assessment* of where you are, and a *plan* for where you want to be:

1. Do you spend more time online on your screen devices (computer, laptop, tablet, smartphone, or smart TV) than you realize?

2. Do you mindlessly pass time on a regular basis by staring at your smartphone, tablet, computer, or smart TV, even when you know there might be better or more productive things to do?

3. Do you seem to lose track of time when on any of your screen devices?

4. Are you spending more time with "virtual friends" as opposed to real people nearby? (Obviously, during the COVID pandemic this is a difficult question.)

5. Has the amount of time you spend on your smartphone or the Internet been increasing?

6. Do you secretly wish you could be a little less wired or connected to your screen devices?

7. Do you regularly sleep with your smartphone under your pillow or next to your bed?

8. Do you find yourself viewing and answering texts, tweets, snaps, posts, comments, likes, IMs, DMs, and emails at all hours of the day and night — even when it means interrupting other things you are doing?

9. Do you text, email, tweet, snap, IM, DM, post, comment, or surf while driving or doing other similar activities that require your focused attention and concentration?

10. Do you at times feel your use of technology decreases your productivity?

11. Do you feel uncomfortable when you accidentally leave your phone or other Internet screen device in your car or at home, if you have no service, or if it is broken?

12. Do you feel reluctant to be without your smartphone or other screen device, even for a short time?

13. When you leave the house, do you typically have your smartphone or other screen device with you?

14. When you eat meals, is your smartphone always part of the table setting?

15. Do you find yourself distracted by your smartphone or other screen devices?

If you answer yes to 50 percent (7 or 8) or more of these questions, then you may want to examine your Internet and screen use.

REMEMBER

Here's an important disclaimer: It should be noted that no medical or psychiatric diagnosis can be made solely from a written test or screening tool. These Internet and screen addiction diagnostic criteria are intended for educational and informational purposes only and are not a substitute for professional medical advice. If you are concerned about your smartphone, Internet, or screen use, you may want to consult with a licensed mental health or addiction professional with expertise in Internet and technology addiction.

REMEMBER

The main thing to look out for is an *overall lack of awareness* of how much time you are spending on your screens. *The more time, the more likely your life will be out of balance.* The content or app is not the most important thing here; rather, it is the amount of *time* you are diverting from balanced real-time living. The power of the Internet, in part, comes from its ability to dissociate you from real life and to become a digital drug by impacting dopamine levels in your brain.

Recovering from Internet and Screen Addiction

You cannot change anything in your life unless you have honest self-appraisal and feedback. The problem with addiction is that often, *self cannot accurately see self,* and people have a great capacity for denial and self-deception when engaging in addictive behaviors that impact their brain reward centers.

Recovery always begins with honest self-evaluation, often with some objective data to help you accurately see what you're doing online. With substance as well as behavioral addiction, there are well-established methods for assessing overuse and life impacts from an addiction. However, there is no simple answer for how much is too much, nor is there an easy fix. Addiction is complex and involves mind, body, and spirit — impacting many aspects of your functioning; that said, everyone has a different *bottom line* where they can no longer ignore the fact that their screen addiction is hurting their life in some way. The following sections introduce two options for recovery: self-help and professional help.

TIP

One thing you do have with Internet addiction is a *digital footprint;* that is, everything you do online and on your smartphone can be tracked, and you can see how much time you spend, what websites and apps you use, and what content areas you seem to have a problem with. This feedback can be critical in helping you start the process of recovery by seeing what you're doing, much like keeping a record of the foods you eat when attempting to eat better or lose weight. There are many aftermarket apps and programs that can record, track, block, and monitor your Internet and screen use. Most cellphone manufacturers and service providers have apps that offer a great deal of detailed information on your use. Several companies also produce software that you or an IT professional can install on all your screen devices that can give you accurate and detailed data, which provides you with total usage information and any problem content areas.

REMEMBER

Don't be surprised when you look at your usage information and find that it is much greater than you recall it being or that you were aware of. This is normal and is part of that dissociation and time distortion that is discussed earlier in this chapter. It's essential that you get accurate feedback about your use; otherwise, you'll be unable to take control of your screen time.

Exploring self-help options

Self-help options (covered in Chapter 5 of Book 7) have always been a substantive part of any addiction recovery and treatment plan. The most well-known is Alcoholics Anonymous, but there are 12-step and recovery/support programs for nearly every addiction; there are even specific support groups for pornography and sex addiction, including Sex and Love Addicts Anonymous, Sex Addicts Anonymous, and Sexaholics Anonymous. There are also many support and self-help groups for Internet and technology addiction. Groups such as Game Quitters, OLG-Anon (On-Line Gamers Anonymous), and others that focus on video gaming and other forms of screen use can be useful, but beware that many of these groups *are themselves* online. Some might argue that this defeats the purpose, but some help is always better than no help, even if it's online. (COVID also gave us new reliance on the utility of telemedicine mental health and addiction treatment.)

Self-help books and resources can be invaluable in making desired changes in any behavior or addiction. In the late 1990s, only one self-help book (*Caught in the Net*, published in 1998 by Dr. Kimberly Young) was available. Now, literally dozens of books and resources have been written, and a great deal of medical and scientific research has been conducted on the subject. A lot more is known about this addiction today than 25 years ago.

Getting professional help

REMEMBER

Sometimes self-help and support groups aren't enough to make the changes you need in your life. Breaking an addiction can be hard, and any behavior change can sometimes be made easier with professional help. Our recommendation would be to find a psychologist, psychiatrist, or therapist who has experience in addiction and addiction medicine, preferably with a background in Internet, video game, or screen addiction. Don't be afraid to ask questions regarding their experience (and expertise) in this area, and be wary of any doctor or therapist who underplays the issue and tells you it isn't a real problem.

Balancing Technology with Real-Time Living

Anything in excess can produce negative health issues, and the Internet and screen technologies are no exception. Health issues relating to screen use have been well established and may involve reduced and poor sleep, increased stress and elevated cortisol, repetitive motion injury, and neck and back problems. There have been reports of thumb, finger, and upper-back problems from excessive screen use, as well as eye strain and difficulties focusing. Some reports of more serious medical issues include elevated blood pressure, blood clots, weight gain from sedentary behavior, and heart-rate issues from dehydration; in extreme cases, people have died.

Health is in large part determined by *balance* in your life; screens and all the content you endlessly consume online may interfere with that balance. But balance is key. It can be hard to maintain because it involves conscious choices, but it is necessary for healthy living. Screen technology is anything but *benign*. It eats up your attention and can rob you of the most important resource in your life — your time — without your even knowing it.

People constantly embrace new technology: faster smartphones, faster processors, bigger and better screens, more apps, and more devices connected to the cloud and running their daily lives. This in some ways represents progress, but in many ways, it is a setback. All this technology requires more and more time and attention to manage, maintain, and learn how to use. How many times have you had to troubleshoot a problem with some digital device, install a new app, or just change your password for the millionth time? It takes time. It takes energy. It takes attention from other, perhaps more meaningful and satisfying parts of your life. All of this attention to tech adds up.

REMEMBER

Sure, all this convenience is wonderful, but is it really making life happier and satisfying? Has all your screen and Internet use really added quality to your life? Just because you can hook up everything in your life to the Internet does not *literally* mean it will improve the quality of your life; you always must ask yourself the question "Will the cost (time) really be worth the ultimate *benefit?*"

Chapter **2**

Discovering What Makes the Internet and Smartphones So Addictive

The Internet is no longer new. In the mid- to late 1990s, the Internet was still the digital Wild West. Twenty-five years ago, few understood that this new, miraculous modality of communication and commerce could be addictive, but we did understand that it was very appealing. Because the Internet was so new (and Wall Street was in love with its financial promise), most people did not see that all was not perfect in cyberspace.

In the early to mid-1990s, we were still using dial-up Internet that worked at a snail's pace, but it was still exciting. Back then, online shopping and commerce were barely in their infancy; these were pre-Amazon days (if you can imagine that), and there wasn't a lot happening online back then. But even before social media, Wi-Fi, smartphones, and high-speed Internet, you could feel how captivating this technology was.

In this chapter, you discover the common features and factors that make this technology so addictive.

Eyes on the Prize: Factors Involving Focus on a Screen

Why do we like looking at our screens so much? It may seem intuitively obvious why video gaming is addictive. After all, it is stimulating, endlessly variable, rewarding (the fancy medical term is *dopaminergic*), easily accessible — and fun. But many areas of Internet screen use are addictive as well. These include video platforms such as YouTube, social media, video gaming, Reddit, online shopping, online gambling, information scrolling and surfing (kind of equivalent to TV channel surfing from the old days), and, of course, pornography. This section looks at the main reasons why people can't help focusing on their screens.

WHAT IS GAMING DISORDER?

According to the WHO, *gaming disorder* is a subcategory of addictive behavior and is defined in the 11th revision of the International Classification of Diseases (ICD-11) as a pattern of gaming behavior ("digital-gaming" or "video-gaming") characterized by impaired control over gaming; increasing priority is given to gaming over other activities to the extent that gaming takes precedence over other interests and daily activities, and there is a continuation or escalation of gaming, despite the occurrence of negative life consequences.

For gaming disorder to be diagnosed, the behavior pattern must be of sufficient severity to result in significant impairment in personal, family, social, educational, occupational, or other important areas of functioning and would normally have been evident for at least 12 months.

Examining ease of access and near-constant availability

Ease of access has always been an enabling factor in addiction. In substance-based addictions, the availability of certain drugs or alcohol could often predict use, abuse, or relapse. With Internet and screen use, this is also a significant factor in that the Internet has become ever-present and easily accessible. Wi-Fi, high-speed Internet, smartphones, fast mobile service, tablets, and smart TVs have all brought the Internet to our fingertips. It's possible that 5G (the newest generation of mobile service networks) will only increase the addiction potential of the Internet and our devices, but especially the smartphone. The smartphone is essentially an *always-on* Internet portal that allows the Internet to be easily accessible, which may account for some of the Internet addiction cases over the last ten years.

Availability is like ease of access, but it speaks to the fact that Internet access is nearly *always* available, as smartphones, hardwired broadband home or office access, LAN, Wi-Fi, or access through your cell service makes the Internet nearly always available. More rural areas may be an exception to this unfettered access, but with satellite and fiber optics, this is also changing. In fact, many of us will soon rarely be without access to the Internet, which just increases the allure and temptation of checking that app or website, viewing that post, sending a text, or playing the latest version of your favorite game. It seems that there is no easy way to avoid easily accessing this digital drug.

REMEMBER

When an addictive behavior is easily accessible and available, it increases the likelihood of addictive use. It's also important to remember that a big part of why addictive use of Internet technology is problematic is because of the amount of time it steals from our lives without our being aware of it.

Talking about time distortion

Perhaps one of the most powerful drug-like effects of screen use is the time distortion that occurs online. One of the hallmarks of any substance or intoxicating behavior is that it can alter mood or consciousness, thus creating a time-distorting experience. A 1999 study found that a large majority of users reported the time-distorting effect of the Internet. Perhaps you yourself have noticed losing track of time when you're online? The immersive and dopamine rewarding experience of the Internet clearly impacts our perception of the passage of time.

REMEMBER

What time distortion tells us is that the Internet digital drug is powerful and can alter our perceptions. The reason for this appears to be, in part, that the Internet and screens hyper-focus our attention while interactively distracting us — and transmitting stimulating and intoxicating content at the same time. When you couple all of this with variable rewards, you can see how a person can become stuck online and get lost in cyberspace.

Digital drug delivery is very similar to the way drugs are consumed and metabolized in our bodies. The shorter the time between introducing an intoxicating drug or behavior into our nervous system and subsequent intoxication, the more addictive that drug or behavior is. This is because our nervous system is very responsive to the brevity of time between stimulation and intoxication — in essence, this is classical conditioning. The shorter the time that passes between when you click and then see, find, or play something online that is desirable to you, the more addictive potential it has. This speed factor likely means there are potential negative implications to faster processor speeds and high-speed Internet access connections — in this sense, faster may not always be better.

Giving you the world online: The illusion of online productivity

The Internet seems to create an illusion of productivity. Perhaps this is in part because we use our screens so much for school and work (and during the COVID pandemic, even more so). The problem is that the Internet doesn't actually increase productivity when you factor in all the wasted and unproductive time we spend on our screens. This is not to mention all the glitches, lost passwords, Internet outages, and other technical difficulties that we experience. There are estimates that 80 percent of the time we spend online is *not* for productive purposes, and much of the time we spend online is related to surfing or scrolling around, social media, pornography, video gaming, sports, shopping, or other intoxicating behaviors that devour time and attention without our being aware of it.

The Good (or Bad) Stuff: Factors Involving Content

Part of the appeal in accounting for the addictive nature of the Internet is an interaction between stimulating *content* and the *process* of Internet delivery of that content. It seems that the interaction between the attractiveness of any content can be amplified using the Internet modality. Think of this as *synergistic amplification* (a mouthful). It is as if online content were the drug, and the Internet delivery mechanism was the hypodermic delivering that drug to our nervous system. It is this amplification that gives the Internet some of its power and potency, as you find out in this section.

Finding out about content intoxication

What is content intoxication? This involves understanding how varying forms of content, when consumed via the Internet, have greater power to elevate mood and instigate changes in the reward center of the brain. Many of these forms of content, such as shopping, stock trading, gambling, video gaming, and porn, existed prior to the Internet and were quite pleasurable (and potentially addictive), but when consumed through the Internet medium, they become even more intoxicating and addictive.

For example, pornography has been around for quite some time and certainly existed before the Internet. It was always stimulating to look at it, when viewing it in books, magazines, films, photos, or on videotapes and DVDs. But when the Internet became more widely available in the early to mid-1990s, it was a new ball game. The ease of access, availability, anonymity, disinhibition, and convenience all coalesced to produce an immersive experience unlike previous forms of media or communication. The Internet allows for endless variety, privacy, and interactivity in a way never seen before. This was content on steroids, and thus began an entirely new type of addiction.

REMEMBER

The Internet amplifies the power of anything it broadcasts in a new and different way, and it happens without your knowing that your brain is slowly being conditioned — just as if you were playing a slot machine. Rewarding and stimulating behaviors are one thing, but when provided via an Internet platform, they become quite another.

Mixing stimulating content and digital devices

Why would a video game be more addictive when played on a computer or gaming platform connected to the Internet? In a word or two: *variability* and *interactivity.* The Internet allows people to play games with other people, and this, along with speed, variation, privacy, and ease of access, makes it entirely new. Digital devices, when connected to the Internet, make content much more personally accessible — to a point where the line between normal and excessive use can easily become blurred.

All forms of content consumed on the Internet are amplified and intensified. This is true whether we're talking about shopping, investing in stocks, gambling, video gaming, and most certainly pornography. Even searching for information becomes a new experience that you can call *infotainment.* Who would have thought that surfing YouTube, Reddit, Wikipedia, or a variety of apps or websites could be fun? But the interactivity, speed, perceived anonymity, and ease of access put simple information on *steroids.* The variability of finding what you want and not knowing when you will get it gamifies the process, and at the same time you're getting intermittent hits of dopamine when you find something you like, and even higher hits when you think that *maybe* you found or will find something you will like.

Understanding instant gratification

The Internet allows for a near-instant reflex, where a click or screen tap enables you to find just what you're looking for. There is very little lag between the impulse to look for something, play a game, or respond to a notification and the act of doing it. The shorter the time between clicking and viewing the content, the more addictive it becomes. The shortened lag also produces a sense of instant or near-instant gratification and reinforces your inability to delay gratification. What this ends up looking like is that you never really have to wait for anything. Everything is instantly experienced, from a whim to satisfaction.

Sometimes waiting can build our tolerance to address aspects of life that are not instantly satisfied or that require sustained attention and effort. At times we might even learn to endure boredom for a few short minutes, without reaching for a screen, but the Internet seems to facilitate the opposite.

WARNING

Data seems to show that the ability of younger people to delay gratification and maintain sustained effort has waned over the last 25-plus years. Add to the equation that we're carrying an Internet portal everywhere we go, and we can see how our smartphone erases the last vestiges of our willpower by allowing us to instantly satisfy every impulse. Every social media update or notification we receive becomes a trigger to pick up our phone and look. Every question, curiosity, or text we have becomes another glance at our phone. The problem is that it never ends, and any boundary between screen life and real-time life evaporates. There is no off button, no downtime to enjoy without the pull of our phones and the lure of that instant dopamine hit.

Did you know that the anticipation of finding or seeing something desirable or stimulating (dopamine-releasing) is stronger than the actual pleasure itself? In other words, the *anticipation* of seeing something you *might* like will produce even *higher* levels of dopamine. Just like in gambling, it's the expectation or belief that you *might win* that is most intoxicating. So, if you post something on social media and see notifications come in, they will be more dopamine-elevating than looking at your phone and seeing that your post was liked or commented on. To your brain, being in the game is more powerful than winning the game — but winning also provides an additional secondary hit of dopamine.

Facebook uses this anticipation factor in the form of staggered posting of your received likes or comments, and then delivering them to you *randomly* to keep you looking at your page over and over.

Defining infotainment

The term *infotainment* describes what we all do to some extent with the Internet, and especially our smartphones. Information has taken on an entertaining quality, and it can keep our eyes onscreen for content providers to data-mine and to sell us things. Social media has this quality, driving our excessive use. This is new stimulation to our brain, and our limbic reward center is scanning for novel and stimulating pieces of information.

TECHNICAL STUFF

Digital drug delivery is very similar to how drugs are *metabolized* in our bodies.

This Must Be the Place: The Internet as the Car, Map, and Destination

The Internet is a unique form of technology; it's not just a communication or information tool, but it's also a *place to go* in and of itself, as you discover in this section. Early in its history, we assumed that the Internet was like many earlier communication modalities such as the telephone, radio, movies, and television, and that the Internet would simply be another tool to connect and entertain. Although e-commerce was seen early on as a possible use for the Internet, no one could have imagined how quickly it would morph into not just a means to connect, but a *destination* to connect to as well.

What do we mean by a destination? The Internet is a place to virtually hang out, not just on chat sites, but to shop, trade stocks, game, gamble, or hang out on a social media site such as TikTok, Reddit, Twitter, Snapchat, Instagram, or Facebook. The Internet is not simply a means to an end, but it has become an end to itself. It was a new place to go, and it has only increased in this capacity to entertain and captivate. In fact, there is such a small boundary between real-time and virtual these days that many of us don't differentiate between the time we are online and the time we are offline. (Even though essentially, we are never offline anymore with our smartphones always in our pockets.)

Unlike when the Internet made its debut and we had to dial up to get online (kind of like getting in the car to go somewhere), the Internet connection is now *always* live with high-speed DSL, cable, satellite, fiber-optic, and fast smartphone connections. Even a slower DSL connection is always on, and a seamless highway is always open on your desktop, laptop, smartphone, or TV. This connected factor is in part what makes the Internet so powerful — and there is something intoxicating about having the world's information and people at your fingertips.

Getting the word in and out: Broadcast intoxication

One of the things we discovered early on with the Internet was *broadcast intoxication*. This is essentially a recognition that it is stimulating to broadcast to others (as well as receive broadcasts) through various platforms, but especially on social media. Chapter 3 of Book 7 discusses in detail how social media creates an intoxicating experience when you broadcast your status, updates, posts, photos, videos, or virtually anything. Likely, this intoxication is in part caused by the anticipation of a *like, comment, follow,* or *DM* (direct message) to your post. The response by other people creates a social validation loop whereby there is a dopamine elevation from the social validation. Part of the reason for our intoxication from this validation is that we are all hardwired for social connection and social approval. The Internet, and especially social media, may capitalize on a very basic human quality: the desire to be liked and appreciated.

Weaving a web: A story without an end

All forms of communication and media have boundaries. A book, TV show, newspaper, magazine, movie, and even a text or phone conversation all have boundaries. They all have a beginning, middle, and end, with markers that tell you where you are in the entertainment, information, and communication process.

The Internet, however, is an entirely different matter. Whenever you go online to do anything, there are no markers for where you are and how long you might be there. In fact, there is a purposeful attempt to eliminate such markers, just as a casino removes clocks or windows to obscure time passage. There are a myriad of cross links, back links, hypertexts, live photo links, click-bait, and feeds that take you down endless rabbit holes, which have you later emerging from your journey without a clue as to how this occurred. *No boundaries equal no markers for time passage.*

The Internet is a completely dynamic, active, and interactive system. It isn't linear, but rather a networked and almost circular set of interactive data. It in some sense operates more like our brain than a book. But without markers for time or space, the Internet can take you on a journey far beyond where you intended to go.

Obviously, online content providers and Internet companies love how this lack of boundaries creates captive audiences of you and me.

REMEMBER

The Internet and digital screen technologies are amoral. They have no agenda in and of themselves, and service providers, content developers, and app and software creators all have the same goal: your attention and your eyes onscreen. This is a battle for how you spend your time, but your time is a non-renewable resource, and technology must always be balanced in terms of how it ultimately serves us, not simply for a promised better life.

Apprehending the myth of multi-tasking

There is perhaps no better example of the purported benefits of screen technologies than the power of multi-tasking. Multi-tasking is a very misunderstood concept, and there has been much research on the neuroscience of attention; the overwhelming conclusion is simply that there is no such thing as multi-tasking.

WARNING

What is often seen as multi-tasking is rapid *attention-shifting* and moving your focus in an alternating fashion. What this means is that you're quickly shifting your attention from one screen or activity to another, and although it feels seamless and simultaneous, it isn't. There is no way for the human brain to attend to and process two stimuli at the same time. So, the next time your teenager has a laptop, tablet, TV, textbook, and smartphone open in front of them (while they are listening to music) and then tells you they are attending to all of them at once, they are kidding themselves (and you!). They may believe they are attending to all these activities simultaneously, but what the research shows is that the amount of comprehension of each stimulus is basically reduced by a factor of how many other sources of input you have going on at once. So, if you are doing homework while doing other activities, it will simply take you longer to get it done and/or there will be less comprehension of what you worked on. Internet and screen technology does not actually increase efficiency; it increases the functional organization of how we manage information, but even this benefit must be weighed against the amount of *distraction* it creates along the way.

Telling a social story: The net effect on people

The big question is this: How does Internet and screen technology affect human relationships and our overall health and wellbeing? From its early adoption, the Internet been touted for its ability to connect people; initially social media was hailed as an important way to stay connected with our friends, family, work, and school. There is little argument that the Internet is a useful tool, and the COVID pandemic has offered further evidence of how amazing and useful this technology is. It has allowed us to continue our work and school from home and to shop and stay connected to our friends and loved ones. There is no debating the utility of this technology, but what about the quality of some of those activities and social connections made online?

There is little disagreement as to the mixed quality of online social connection and questionable satisfaction (and efficacy) of attending school online. Why is that? Why is it that social behavior online seems decidedly two-dimensional? Why has online schooling during COVID been seen as a failure? Why is online intimacy and social connection generally rated as inferior to real-time interaction? Even Zoom, which may be one of the heroes emerging from COVID, can leave people feeling hungry for more real-time, physical contact and connection. From the COVID experience, we see that our children, who have been schooled virtually, report increasing depression, social isolation, and dissatisfaction from the online academic experience — and some are experiencing other increased mental health issues as well.

These experiences aren't a coincidence. They are reflections of some of the weaknesses of Internet interactions for social and academic communication. The Internet is best at connecting people with information and services, but it leaves people yearning for more depth and breadth when all is said and done. Perhaps it is best said that our expectations for a two-dimensional experience may be higher than what an Internet screen can deliver.

The Human Factor: The Internet as a Digital Drug

People sometimes want to know how the Internet and digital screens can be addictive. After all, how can you get addicted to a screen behavior? Part of the reason for this question is that it evolves from the idea that addiction is about ingesting a substance and that it is the *substance* itself that creates the addiction through the body's physical dependence on it.

REMEMBER

The problem with this analysis is that it's wrong. This isn't how addiction really works. Yes, the body can become physiologically dependent on a substance (drugs or alcohol), but if that is what solely created an addiction, then once people detox from the substance, the addiction should be gone. However, this is not what typically happens. Addiction is the combination of many variables that involve learning, memory, emotions, social factors, physiology, behavior, and neurobiology.

Often there are co-occurring psychiatric problems that contribute to an addiction, or the addiction may be a way to deal with emotional pain or negative circumstances. Let's face it: Addictive behaviors can be an escape.

With addiction, there is always a *disruption* of the reward system in the brain, but the addictive substance or behavior (in this case, Internet use) is not really the primary issue. It is certainly a factor, but the addiction process is as much about learning to deal with triggers and to manage one's emotions as anything else, and what we see with excessive screen use is like what we see in many addictions: Addictive behaviors start out as a solution that then becomes another problem.

WARNING

Being online is a pleasurable and stimulating activity that impacts the brain's reward system and elevates dopamine; it has a similar potential to create an addictive experience as drugs and alcohol, although physiological dependence is less of an issue.

Grasping the power of "maybe"

The Internet is the world's biggest slot machine. The slot machine operates on the power of *maybe,* and this explains the neurobiology of gambling, and most addictions, in some ways. So how does *maybe* work in our brains? When you pull the handle of a slot machine, your brain knows that it is going to *win* something. What it does not know is *when* and *how much,* but it *does* know that eventually there will be a reward of some kind. It learns to expect this reward. This system of reinforcement (or dopamine reward) is called *variable ratio reinforcement.*

So why wouldn't you just give someone a win each time they pull the handle or after they pull it a certain number of times? The answer is simply *boredom* (also called *extinction*). B.F. Skinner did groundbreaking research on operant conditioning and found out that unpredictable (variable) rewards create longer-lasting response habits (which is another fancy way of saying addiction). If a reward is given variably and unpredictably, then your brain engages in this activity like nobody's business.

So how does this work with Internet use? Whenever you go online (or on your smartphone), you never really know *what* you're going to find or *when* you're going to find it. This is true for email, information surfing, scrolling, gaming, social media, shopping, and porn; virtually anything you search for online has a variability to it — a *maybe* factor. In essence, the Internet operates on the same variable reinforcement schedule that a slot machine does, and people are neurobiologically conditioned by their devices without really knowing it.

Not only does the brain love *maybe,* but it also loves *newness.* Novelty resets our attention and interest. And there is perhaps no better source of information that provides endless variability and novelty than the Internet. Every time you go online (and in a sense, we are always online with our devices), it can feel like a new experience each time you click or tap through your latest impulse.

Seeing how dynamic interaction keeps people coming back for more

Dynamic is a way of saying changeable and interactive — and being able to interact with our devices puts some psychological skin in the game for us. It's dynamic in that we are driving the interactive process by our clicks, and the cycle is complete when we are *responded* to by our screens. We self-guide our web adventure, and regardless of whether we are on our smartphone, laptop, tablet, or other device, our Internet journey feels like a dialogue. The AI (artificial intelligence) interfaces by Amazon and Google provide a voice to this interactive exchange, giving the cyber experience a very compelling feel. We now experience the Internet not simply as a source of information, but as having lifelike qualities, and the line between simplistic Internet algorithms and AI is fast eroding. Consider Alexa on an Amazon Echo. We know full well that she is just a machine-learning interface, but she feels real and is thus imbued with the dynamism of humanity.

REMEMBER

Most of us would be hard-pressed to admit that we love being online, but the fact is that many of us do. Some of us may find ourselves becoming addicted to a point that our lives are impacted, while others of us may overuse at times. Much of this is *not* conscious. We are virtually swept away in a tidal wave of intensity, stimulation, interactivity, and endless intermittent reward. The problem with tidal waves, however, is that they can hurt us, and our excessive Internet use can subtly rob us of many aspects of quality living. In more extreme circumstances, once addicted, we see our lives becoming impacted in negative ways that we did not fully appreciate. It is this lack of awareness that blinds us to the slow erosion of our most cherished values, and excessive Internet use can mindlessly peel away our time and attention to a point that we forget what real-time living feels like.

IN THIS CHAPTER

» **Breaking down the phrase** *social network*

» **Demonstrating the power of social validation looping**

» **Checking out social media's effects on communication and self-esteem**

» **Looking at the counter-social aspects of social media**

» **Finding relief from social media**

Chapter **3**

Examining the Addictive Nature of Social Media

What exactly is social media? We scarcely go a day without hearing the term, and it seems everyone is using Facebook, Instagram, Snapchat, Twitter, TikTok, Reddit, YouTube, LinkedIn, and endless other platforms. Social media has invaded almost *every* aspect of our lives, including shopping, politics, data collection, entertainment, influencing and marketing, news, and — in perhaps some ways — social connection.

Social media was initially created to connect people online. It has since morphed to including topics, interests, and being part of a local or wide "friend" network; photos, videos, and other personal information can be shared, rated, liked, and commented on. Facebook (with 2.85 billion users worldwide at the time of writing) was one of the earliest social media platforms, but others such as Myspace share an even earlier pedigree. More recently, social media has morphed into a colossal media machine and e-commerce platform, giving birth to social economics and social commerce, where advertising, sales, and marketing are all integrated.

For many users, social media, in all its iterations, has become a way to communicate regularly with friends and family by posting and scrolling through posts to view news, photos, and information about their lives and often to pass time. Social media represents a huge amount of time on our screens, and advertisers and marketing companies don't waste a second of that social capital. Although many social media websites and apps have the proposed goal of connecting people in some way, the quality of these connections is ultimately questionable. Is social media simply a convenient shadow of real-time social connection? The truth is probably mixed, as there is no doubt that many people experience connection and support from social media, but whether this can serve as a comprehensive substitute for real-time social interaction seems unlikely.

Typically, social media websites and apps are free to users (at least, on a direct monetary level); the companies typically make money through advertising and sales of data and metrics about you. If you doubt the financial profitability of social media sites, just check the stock market prices on some of your favorites, and you'll see just how profitable they are.

The initial impetus behind social media might have been to connect users, but it soon became apparent that it was necessary (and desirable) to financially support these services by capitalizing on the one key asset that social media companies have — you. Your eyes-on-screen were the currency that ultimately became the funding to support social media sites. The illusion that social media is free could not be further from the truth. If something online ever appears to be free, then your attention and demographic data pay for the service with the most precious commodity of all — your time and attention.

This chapter digs into social media's addictive nature, its effects on communication and self-esteem, its counter-social attributes, and much more.

A Social Network: A Rose by Any Other Name

Take a moment to dissect the phrase *social network*. In essence, what we have is a network of interconnected online users who engage interactively in some fashion. This may seem like a loose definition of social connection, but if you visit any social media site, you can see that the level of social *interaction* seems somewhat superficial, and it is a poor substitute for real-time social interaction.

This is not to say that people do not connect via social media platforms (can you imagine not having Instagram, Facebook, or other platforms during the COVID pandemic?). Today's youth, starting in grammar school to well beyond their college years, utilize social media systems to communicate and express themselves to their peers. The fastest-growing segment of social media users, however, are adults (even older adults), and as tweens, teens, and college-age kids have abandoned more established social media sites such as Facebook, they have migrated to other newer sites, such as Instagram, Snapchat, TikTok, and others.

REMEMBER

It's important to note that social media was originally intended as a *social connection platform*, but at this point it's difficult to separate the social and economic aspects of these sites. As social media has become increasingly monetized through ads, sales, and marketing, it seems there is less emphasis on social community and more of being on a marketing platform. You may even question whether the term *social media* is misleading, in that the only reason why these apps or websites seem to thrive is because your profile and viewing activity are potential revenue sources.

Recognizing What Makes You Come Back to Social Media for More

Imagine having a conversation with a friend; she is leaning forward, moving her head in response to your words, showing facial expressions that are indicative of someone who is listening and engaged in what you're saying. You behave similarly in return, and this interaction becomes the basis of the natural ebb and flow of communication. This is an example of *social connection,* and we are hardwired biologically to positively respond to such interactions. Social connections, such as what is described here, are highly rewarding, pleasurable, and health enhancing — especially when sharing is mutual. And because these experiences are pleasurable, these interactions are reflected by an increase in dopamine in your brain.

Social media operates much like this, but instead of real-time conversation, we use posts, instant messages (IMs) or direct messages (DMs), comments, photos, and videos that are responded to with *likes, comments,* and *follows.* The following sections explain two concepts in more detail: *social validation looping* and *variable reinforcement.*

TECHNICAL STUFF

Some evidence suggests that the use of alcohol and drugs has decreased in recent years for adolescents, and Dr. Nora Volkow from NIDA (National Institute on Drug Abuse) noted that this could be occurring because screen use may be providing the dopamine hits that were previously obtained from substance-based intoxication. In some sense, social media and screen use may be providing some of the fun and excitement previously obtained pharmacologically. Our screens, and in particular our smartphones, offer easy access and availability, and therefore can serve to "medicate" moods, emotions, and frustrations. It's like carrying a portable dopamine pump in your pocket, and we know that the more readily accessible a substance or behavior is, the more likely we'll use and, at times, overuse it.

Looking at social validation looping

REMEMBER

Every time we get a *positive social reinforcer* such as a *like, comment,* or *follow,* we tend to receive a small hit of dopamine; the fact that these positive social media responses are unpredictable and variable enhances the potential to produce a pattern of repetitive behavior. We are *rewarded* for our posts (through our likes, comments, follows, shares, and retweets), and so we post and check *again* to obtain *more* positive responses. Each positive response we receive elevates our dopamine level in a small way, and the unpredictability of the responses we get keeps us coming back again and again. This dopamine elevation is essentially based on the naturally rewarding (and hardwired) aspects of feeling socially validated and desired. This process is referred to as *social validation looping,* where there is a cycle of expression (posting) followed by responses (likes, follows, and comments), again followed by more posting, which starts the cycle over again — hence, social validation looping.

It becomes even more insidious because even the *anticipation* of a positive response from others can elevate our dopamine level; posting alone can *cue* the reward centers in our brain to anticipate a response, and this cycle can continue indefinitely if we get an occasional reward in the form of a *like, comment,* or *follow.*

We use the term *social validation* because social media providers are utilizing our inherent desire for social interaction and social connection — to be validated socially — to shape our behavior on social media apps and websites. The word *looping* refers to the fact that this behavior creates a repetitive cycle. Everyone feels good when what they post is acknowledged, and the likes and comments let us know we are being appreciated and valued. All these forms of social validation from our social media posts *variably reinforce* us in powerful ways. The likes, comments, and follows that we end up with produce that same slot machine–like addictive phenomenon that we see with many aspects of Internet behavior. Social validation loops are what motivate the endless wheel of posting and checking for *likes* and *reactions* and then posting again and again.

TECHNICAL STUFF

Part of what makes our brains so efficient and adaptive, from an evolutionary biology standpoint, is our ability to organize and categorize various forms of input that we then recognize as patterns; this allows us to predict potential outcomes that help increase safety and efficiency (thus increasing our survival potential).

REMEMBER

If our brains *neurobiologically expect* certain behaviors will be rewarded, it is an efficient shortcut to anticipate the outcome and consequence. All addictive behavior has its origins in the hijacking of survival-based reward pathways, so addiction has a functional place in our biology, even if it can ultimately lead to negative consequences.

Understanding the big deal about variable reinforcement

Any habit or behavior that is reinforced (rewarded) intermittently and unpredictably will last a long time because the brain likes *maybe.* If you have any doubts, look at the lines of people buying lottery tickets, watching TikTok, sitting in front of slot machines, betting on athletic events, investing in the stock market, or even surfing the Internet. Watch how people use eBay or other auction sites — it's the chase, the possibility, the *maybe,* that makes all of this appealing. *Variable reinforcement* is just what it sounds like: When our behaviors are intermittently reinforced in some way, they are much more likely to continue for long periods of time. We call this *extinction resistance,* and it's what helps create a *habit* or an *addiction,* depending on circumstances and life impact.

In the beginning, Facebook shares and posts were routinely made available for the public or friends to view. It worked well, but it was not until one Facebook employee created the *Like* button that things really took off. People began to post like crazy, and more posting meant more time onscreen. The *Like* button was the critical ingredient that was needed to produce social validation looping (see the previous section). Getting those *likes* (especially variably) really made users pay attention to their profile and the site and led them to keep checking it over and over. Doling out *likes* and comments in a delayed and intermittent or random format takes further advantage of the power of variable reinforcement. Soon after Facebook installed the *Like* button, users began posting and checking to see what people *may have said* about their latest post or comment, and this was a social media game changer.

REMEMBER

Social media creates the impression that living life is not rewarding in and of itself, but rather it is the *recording* and *sharing* of your life that makes it meaningful. (See the nearby sidebar "The risk of selfies" for details on a popular method for sharing your life.) Posting your experiences via photos, words, and video allows others to respond to your life and, in a sense, creates a form of *reflected self-esteem.* You feel good about what you did, not because of your experience, but because of *how others rated* your experience. You are no longer simply living and experiencing your life, but rather, you are experiencing it as a form of validation from others. This cycle only leads to disappointment, as you always end up comparing yourself to others in the process.

WARNING

You can never achieve self-satisfaction when using *social, material,* or *physical comparison* as your basis for self-esteem. Social comparison, which social media apps base their popularity on (especially for younger users), allows for superficial comparison of physical and other attributes of success as a valid reality and means of deriving identity.

The problem is that most people *do not* necessarily post accurate, honest, or complete portrayals of themselves (many users alter their personal images) and typically post only the best photos, videos, or circumstances that further propagate the idea that *life is the way it looks on social media.* However, nothing could be further from the truth. Social media portrays a two-dimensional view of who we are, and often leaves out our most human and humane qualities. Children, tweens, teens, and young adults are the most susceptible to these distortions and to unrealistic social comparison, but adults are susceptible, too.

THE RISK OF SELFIES

Taking photos of oneself — *selfies* — and posting them on social media is a very popular behavior among teens and young adults, but it may be practiced by younger children and adults as well. In essence, it is the same behavior no matter who is doing it.

Taking a photo or video (preferably an interesting one) and posting it is all about the *likes, comments,* and potential *compliments* you might receive once you post it. In extreme cases, this can lead to almost obsessional levels of photo-taking activity. There have been numerous instances where injuries and deaths have occurred in the process of trying to take the best and most exciting selfie possible, as sometimes these photos involved risky locations and situations. The desire to achieve likes, comments, and positive feedback drives people to take risks to get the best shot possible. In some cases, great care will also be taken to touch up photos to make them even more perfect.

The sad irony here is that all this effort to achieve external recognition offers limited real benefit. The net effect (there's that pun again) is to keep trying to capture more and more novel and exciting photos to continue to achieve the desired effect and to receive external validation (another example of social validation looping).

Taking selfies can be dangerous to your health and can even kill you. In 2019 there were a reported 259 selfie-related deaths (and these were the reported ones). Many of these photo ops were taken in obviously dangerous situations that went wrong. Taking a photo hanging off the edge of the Grand Canyon is never a good idea.

Seeking Communication and Self-Esteem — But at a Price

Can you use social media to connect, build, or maintain social intimacy? Well, this is the question of the day, and the answer is mixed. Some studies have looked at how social media use translates to deeper and more conventional aspects of socialization and relationships. The best we can glean so far is that social media is a very different form of communication and may in fact represent a completely new type of social interaction.

The Internet is a new medium (relatively speaking), but frankly, when the telephone was invented, people initially thought it would have no usefulness. Now, with texting, chatting, IMs, DMs, Snapchat, Twitter, and other forms of social media, some might say we really have no need for the telephone, but there is probably room for all modes of communication. However (and the data seems to support this), social media is *not* a replacement for real-time social connection.

Because most social media interactions utilize written messages as well as photos and video clips, there seems to be a difference in how messages are transmitted, received, and ultimately encoded in our brains. Typed messaging allows more distance (but less nuance) than does verbal communication, and the one-way and delayed effect of a photo or video message is quite different from an immediate, interactive video chat using an app such as Zoom, Skype, or FaceTime.

Research seems to support the idea that social media communications may lack sufficient social cues and nuance, and that if social media is the dominant modality by which you communicate, it can produce a perspective that lacks social empathy and depth. This may, in part, be due to the long-distance way in which information is shared — even if that information is of a personal nature. Social media communication is a less *nutritive* form of connection, but frankly, we do not have any long-term studies that look at how social media use impacts interpersonal and social development in the long term. The preliminary evidence suggests that there are some deficiencies relative to this type of communication. Social media technology is still relatively new, and we have only about two generations who have been raised on it and who are just now entering mature adulthood. Newer iterations of social media will undoubtedly be different, but one thing is for sure: These companies will need *your eyes onscreen* to monetize their platforms.

WARNING

The superficial aspects of social media, when it is used to communicate to a wider and larger audience outside of immediate friends and family, leads to an interesting phenomenon. The idea that you can attract a large cadre of followers and that you can influence people (or be influenced by them) may have its own intoxicating effects, with or without potential economic rewards. The satisfaction and excitement associated with having *likes, comments,* and many *followers* on any platform of social media is notable, but it is questionable that it offers any ultimate value beyond ego validation. There are numerous examples of YouTube, Instagram, and TikTok stars who are famous within these mediums. This may be akin to being a popular person at school or work, but a concern is that this lack of depth can lead to a risk of supporting superficial social exchange. It is not either/or, but it seems important that a balance be achieved.

Self-esteem that is connected to the perception that one's posts and communications via social media are well received, or received at all, is potentially problematic. There is an inherent risk that you can post something and have *no one* see it, or worse, that people will read it but *not* like or comment on it. The token of social exchange within the social media world is *some reaction* that is then communicated back to the user who initially posted it. This interaction can become a two-way social exchange, albeit with some delay, but it is not a guarantee.

WARNING

When self-esteem is tied to how your audience or online friends react, this leaves you vulnerable to only using *reflected* assessments in deriving your self-definition. Social interaction is a significant aspect of creating your sense of self, but it is questionable to what extent social media interactions can provide deeper (and psychologically necessary) levels of human connection; the term *social-lite* may be an apt description of such interactions.

REMEMBER

The best that might be said about social media is that it has produced a new form of communication, and just like other new forms of communication in the past (such as the telephone, radio, movies, and television), there are always adaptations and growing pains when fitting them into balanced living. The difference with the Internet and social media is that they can clearly produce addictive behavior, whereas other modalities don't seem to possess that level of power. Addictive behavior operates on a continuum, and many people use social media, as well other aspects of the Internet, with little or no ill effect.

WARNING

A fact that seems to be well established is that social empathy does not appear to be enhanced by social media. Social empathy scores are lower among heavy users of social media. The reasons for this are unclear, but it seems reasonable to assume that the cues for enhancing social empathy are somehow blunted when receiving information through social media modalities. This has significant potential implications when it comes to cyberbullying or trolling, and other negative uses of social media that shame or negate individuals via a social platform.

Seeing Why Social Media Can Be Counter-Social

This section doesn't use the term *counter-social* in a traditional psychiatric sense. Rather, we're saying that social media communication may run contrary to facilitating intimate connections. Clearly, social media *is* a form of communication, but the argument here is that it doesn't seem to live up to its name, as it is only *sort of social*.

There have been many anecdotal reports of individuals who have discontinued their use of social media and reported feeling a sense of relief. They described feeling enlivened by getting out of the validation loop of posting, reading, and posting again. If you or a loved one uses social media regularly, you may be on a merry-go-round of posting and checking (all the while getting caught in the whack-a-mole of ads, cute cat videos, and a myriad of other distractions) and are trapped by the addictive nature of social media.

Broadcast intoxication on social media

Broadcast intoxication, discussed in Chapter 2 of Book 7, is defined as the dopaminergic rewarding aspects of self-expression via the Internet and social media. Social media use carries with it many potential negatives, but the largest by far is how quickly we can become addicted to intoxicating effects of constantly posting and sharing our lives online. It promotes the illusion of social connection and intimacy, but in a buffered version. What we share via social media platforms probably reflects more of *what we want* the world to see about our lives and often consists only of socially desirable experiences. In other words, what we post is more a reflection of what we *think* may be interesting to others (and hence *likeable*), and might accumulate positive reviews, comments, and *likes.* The idea that social media is an expression of who we really are may be inaccurate because who we are on social media is at least partially shaped by the reactions we receive to what we post.

WARNING

The real challenge of social media is in learning how to be ourselves and to experience our daily lives without the impact of how our experiences might appear once we recount them to others via social media. Social relationships ideally promote not filtering what we do through how others will react and rate our experiences; this further disconnects us from ourselves and prevents us from experiencing our lives in the present moment, without the drive to photograph, video, and post our lives. *It is difficult to be fully present in our own experiences when we are evaluating how others will react to them.* The separation between living our lives and broadcasting ourselves has narrowed to a point where we have lost some of the ability to experience life *without* sharing it for potential review. This cycle is addictive and separates us both from ourselves and from real-time connection.

This is not to say that social media is all bad, but rather that social media is a potent time-sink and can easily suck you into a rabbit hole, eating your time, energy, and ability to live a balanced life. The allure of staying within this cycle is powerful, but the freedom that you can experience by breaking this pattern can provide that much more time and energy to devote toward internally gratifying pursuits and rewarding real-time relationships. This technology can *shallow our relationships* and separate us from ourselves, as the paramount focus is instead on the reactions of others.

Cyberbullying

When it comes to screen use, and especially social media, the adage should be *convenience* is the mother of invention, not *necessity.* The power of social media, and for that matter all things Internet, is the power to connect people to information as well as to other people. The purported purpose of social media is connection, but the reality is that large amounts of time are wasted and destructively expended. Cyberbullying is one of those dysfunctional and counter-social (perhaps antisocial) uses of the Internet.

This power to connect people, or to express thoughts and feelings about others, is what cyberbullying is about — albeit in a negative manner. There is a perception of anonymity when communicating online, and original research, going back to the late 1990s, showed that people often experienced the Internet as anonymous. *When communicating online, there is a perception of distance both from those you are communicating with, and from those you are communicating about.* This perceived separation insulates us from the impact of what we say, and how what we say might affect others. In addition, there is no *social threshold* to cross, and no one's eyes to avert. The electronic distance allows us to say things in a more *socially disinhibited* manner.

Emboldened by social distance and the efficient bully pulpit that social media provides, cyberbullying has become all too common. Social media is a safe place to speak the unspeakable and say the unsayable, and these platforms often involve children and adolescents who are vulnerable to the powerful impact of peer-based opinions. The 2019 Youth Risk Behavior Surveillance System (a survey conducted by the Centers for Disease Control and Prevention) indicates that an estimated 15.7 percent of high school students were electronically bullied in the 12 months prior to the survey. Fifty-nine percent of U.S. teens have been cyberbullied or harassed online, according to the Pew Research Center (2018).

WARNING

The potential negative impact of this power can be devastating. Bullying is always impactful, but cyberbullying may be even more so; there is an indelible footprint of every word uttered online and a record of everything said. Even if not on the front of our formal social media feeds, it is still always searchable, and some bullies will elect to save these posts to allow them to resurface another day. For those who are bullied, there is little defense. How can you defend yourself from a disembodied cyberbully who can say anything about you with an audience of your peers? The psychological impact is very real and damaging, often requiring psychiatric intervention in the form of counseling or therapy to help manage it. In some tragic circumstances, suicides have occurred because of cyberbullying.

It is all too easy, with the press of a button, to say things that cannot be retracted and that leave an indelible mark in cyberspace and on the psyches of those who fall victim to this prevalent behavior. Part of the Internet's biggest strength, its functional simplicity, allows the damaging, antisocial aspects of cyberbullying to flourish.

REMEMBER

The footprint of anything written on social media is essentially indelible; its effect is immediate, and in some cases the damage can be permanent.

Cyberstalking and trolling

Cyberstalking and trolling the Internet and social media platforms is a common activity. There are estimates that upwards of 50 percent of the demographic and identifying information present online is a lie, and original research found these numbers to be consistent with the 17,000 people surveyed.

What is cyberstalking and trolling? It is basically what it sounds like. It's a virtual version of following, monitoring, viewing photos and videos of, and attempting to communicate with people online or on social media. Typically, this monitoring or communication is unsolicited and unwanted and can be very frightening and upsetting to the victim. Often, undesired communications can severely disrupt the victim's life, again resulting in needed counseling or therapy.

It is exceedingly easy to cyberstalk or troll someone on social media or the Internet because some information always leaves a public trail that can be followed or trolled. The best recommendation is *not* to use public settings for any of your social media, but unfortunately many teens and young adults (and fully grown adults) leave their profile open (and public) to make it easier for people to find and follow them.

Finding Relief: Life beyond Social Media

Perhaps some of the most convincing evidence to support using less social media comes from those individuals who stopped or greatly reduced their use, and the sense of relief and increased time and energy they experienced. Most of them were reluctant to let the habit go, and all of them felt uncomfortable and ill at ease when breaking the *social validation loop* (see the earlier section "Looking at social validation looping"). However, after several weeks without social media, most, if not all, of those interviewed felt a sense of relief and renewed energy to pursue life. No one expected this, but in story after story, even though getting off social media was often promoted as a temporary experiment, most decided not to return to regular use.

Ardent social media users need content (often the content is themselves) to attract the *likes* and *comments* (and possible financial rewards) they desire, which then provides the pleasurable dopamine hits; unless they are a content creator, their broadcasted lives become the content, and all consumers of social media pay for access to social media with their time and attention. Social media is now a dominant force in influence marketing, social economics, and the social e-commerce business, and our eyes-on-screen are the currency that keeps this engine running.

The illusion is that social media is somehow about the user, and perhaps to some extent that is true, but the reality is that companies that develop and market these sites and apps *are making money from you* either directly or indirectly. This is not to say that one cannot experience a sense of community and connection with those they interact with on social media. After all, social media is a vehicle that uses the power of the Internet, which offers the ability to connect mutually interested consumers of information with a supply of that information; social media can excel at this in that social activities, business, interest groups, dating, and social and cultural activities all have a home on social media platforms.

REMEMBER

Much good can be done in connecting like-minded people who share an interest or circumstances and need a platform to facilitate the self-disclosure process. Care should be taken, however, in that social media sites can be quite compelling, and all things Internet can eat up your time. Choices must be made in how you spend the *one commodity* in your life that is essentially priceless (and irreplaceable) — your time. Social media has the capacity to entertain, sell products, and in some ways, connect people. Head to Chapter 5 in Book 7 for self-help strategies on living a balanced life, with the Internet and technology in its proper place.

Chapter **4**

The Endless Stream: Binge Watching TV and Online Entertainment

Television has really changed in the last decade or so. You've probably heard in the past about the impending transformation of television and how it's going to become interactive, but it wasn't until Netflix's streaming revolution in 2007 that a confluence of factors occurred, finally cementing the marriage of the Internet and TV.

The advent of user-friendly smart TVs and aftermarket devices such as Apple TV and Amazon's Fire TV Stick to access streaming apps and alternative program sources has been a game changer — and more accessible broadband Internet provided the final ingredient for the streaming formula. For better or for worse, these changes have allowed television to finally be free of the constraints of scheduled programming, where you built your viewing around what the networks or cable companies provided. Although you could previously record your programs with a VCR or DVR, the ability to watch entire seasons of TV programs all at once, at any time, in any order, is a new phenomenon. However, these innovations have produced darker screen issues in the form of binge watching. Like all things consumed via the Internet medium, television is amped up to potentially addictive levels when integrated with the Internet.

A *binge* is the repeated and unconscious use of something that may have a detrimental effect on you. You often hear about binge eating, where a person eats compulsively, often to a point of hurting themselves. The same might be applied to binge TV watching. The ability to turn on your TV and stream ten episodes of an already-released season can be very appealing at best but negatively impacting at worst — the main negative impact being loss of sleep and not getting other things done.

You can't binge without something powerful shutting down your conscious judgment and awareness. Only potent and addictive substances or activities can accomplish this. Pleasurable activities can trick your brain into experiencing what you're doing as good for you (enhancing life and survival potential) when, in reality, these potentially addictive behaviors are stealing your valuable time and energy. In this chapter, you discover the pitfalls of watching too much TV and what you can do about it.

Missing Your Life While Being Entertained: The Ease of the Binge

There are perhaps two clear saving graces that the Internet and screens have given us during the COVID pandemic. The first is Zoom, which allowed people to socialize, work, and attend school virtually, and the second is streaming entertainment services such as Netflix, Amazon Prime, Hulu, and others. These services have provided people with entertainment solace at a time when they *really needed the digital distraction.* These are wins for Internet tech, and they are good examples of the many benefits that online communication and entertainment can provide.

However, prior to this unexpected need for online content, people had other issues with their tendency to consume too much of a good thing. The *streaming binge* is a relatively new phenomenon that's been created by the move from live or recorded media to a content feed that is offered on an as-desired basis. This was as much a game changer as the VCR and the DVR, in that it supercharged the concept of convenience to an entirely new level. Now you could enjoy a movie or favorite TV show right away without driving to your local Blockbuster video store (remember them?) or having to order a DVD by mail like in the earlier days of Netflix. Those older methods seem so far away now — almost a different era. But it was not all that long ago. In the realm of technology, time indeed moves at light speed.

WARNING

Enter streaming — a feed of digital bits and bytes that make up your favorite video entertainment. What could be bad about this? Well, the ability *to get what you want, as much as you want, and when you want it* is not always a great thing. And if this sounds familiar, it is because it describes the same dynamics that help make the Internet so desirable and at times addictive.

REMEMBER

As you find out in the following sections, streaming offers endless choices, along with ease of access and stimulating content. It also lacks something that most other forms of communication and entertainment have — *boundaries.* Boundaries remind you of natural limits and where a story begins and ends. They serve as markers to help you set limits on your consumption, and the fewer the boundaries, the more likely you'll just keep watching. Streaming content developers count on this fact. They want you to keep watching (keep in mind that the profit engine of the Internet is eyes-on-screen). This is the reason why the default option on YouTube, Netflix, Amazon Prime, and others is the *autoplay* feature that automatically takes you to the next episode. It will even lead you to a similar show if you've finished the one you were watching and then start it automatically. The other change is that many TV shows and series are released all at once, so you have an additional impetus to binge, although some shows are still released weekly. This is equivalent to opening a bag of potato chips and eating them until you hit the bottom of the bag. After all, who can just eat one?

Understanding the allure of endless choice

So, what is it about *endless choice* that is so darn compelling? On the surface, having endless choice seems like a good thing. After all, what could be bad about having tons of choices? Well, let's look at a brief analogy. Think about going into a convenience store to get a cup of coffee. Say that you're in a rush, so all you want to do is run in and run out quickly. Well, no such luck. First, you have to decide on what size cup and choose from *five* different options, followed by *eight* types of coffee; then there are the creamers, *twelve* in all; then, the *six* types of sweeteners. Well, it may be hard to believe, but all those valuable choices produced nearly 3,000 possible combinations and options. All you want is a cup of coffee, not a life decision, yet that is where you end up.

You assume that *more is always better,* that more options mean more opportunity for satisfaction. But too much choice can produce complexity and stress. This is exactly why some people like shopping in small grocery stores — fewer options to choose from. This leads to a simpler experience and thus less time wasted, and less stress.

The same is true for the endless opportunity of watching 600 channels of cable, and if you add in the two dozen streaming sites and services, you have even more choices. Your brain doesn't really need this much choice, and when you have too much online content to choose from, it can add to what is called *Tech Stress Syndrome.* Sometimes, *more* is *not* necessarily better. Maybe you're reminded of the four or five TV stations that you had when you were a kid; maybe you often said to your parents that there was nothing on TV. Can you even imagine hearing that today?

Endless choice compels your brain to think there is always a different potential option. Options are good sometimes, but when it comes to digital content, you can easily become mired in the lure of promised entertaining experiences to keep you satisfied, but this satisfaction comes at a price — your time and attention.

Finding the power of instant access

There is nothing fun about waiting for content to load while staring at a buffering screen. But faster speeds mean a faster life, more choices, and potentially more stress. These increases in speed are a double-edged sword, as there is always a dark side to all tech advances.

The power of instant access is complicated by the fact that instant gratification capitalizes on a basic addiction and pharmacology principle. The shorter the period between when you click something online and when it shows up on your screen (and arouses your nervous system through elevation of dopamine), the more addictive that behavior is. This is the same with substance use. Drugs taken intravenously (the fastest route of administration) have greater addictive potential than if taken via another way, such as snorting or smoking. Faster devices, faster processors, and faster Internet all equal potentially greater risk of Internet and technology addiction; even if you aren't addicted, it can contribute to a greater tendency to abuse or overuse your screen technology.

There is a benefit in delaying your gratification through instant access; delay gives you the ability to think through your choices and make decisions based on executive skills and reasoning that are often inaccessible when engaging in an intoxicating and immediately gratifying experience. There is a lot of power and distraction potential from the instant access that streaming provides; the ability to satisfy your instant desires without interruption makes endless digital content easy to overuse and at times addictive.

Recognizing the pitfalls of effortless starting

Effortless starting (autoplay) is the ability to passively allow your television or online screen app to deliver the next episode, video, or content automatically, without you *doing anything*. This passive approach, as mentioned earlier in this chapter, is how streaming content providers run their systems; unless you purposely opt out of this feature, you'll be effortlessly fed content until you either turn it off or walk away. But how many times have you sat in front of your screen and allowed the next video or episode to come on and swore that this would be the last one? Everyone has certainly done this. *The problem here is that addictive behavior is facilitated by doing nothing.* Effortless addiction is perhaps the most insidious because you never even have to move off your couch.

The organizing part of your brain doesn't really like endless or unfinished things, or rather, it doesn't like to leave them endless. This is in part because you're neurologically designed to finish and complete perceptual and cognitive tasks. This concept of completion is sometimes called the Zeigarnik effect and is borrowed from the perceptual and cognitive science of how you perceive the world around you. It's quite simple. If you draw a series of numbers that reflect a pattern on a whiteboard, your brain will naturally attempt to complete the pattern; this is also true if you draw a near-circle on the board. Even if the lines do not meet, if they are close enough together, the perception will be of a circle. The reason for this principle of *closure* and *completion* comes from your brain being designed to organize and categorize as efficiently as possible — putting things in order allows expediency and predictability for living in the world. This trait has helped humans survive and allows you to create shortcuts for managing your environment.

When digital media is endless, however, your brain still tries to finish it. You want to get to the completion — to finish that process. The problem is that with a seven-season TV show, it is going to take a lot of time to get there. The Internet is never done, but your brain nevertheless tries hard to finish it.

REMEMBER

All *boundaries* in dealing with the Internet and anything streamed must come from your *conscious intention* and behavior, to go against the natural ease of access of your streaming screen.

Unpacking user experience engineering

This is the million-dollar question: How much social and behavioral engineering goes into Internet entertainment (this can include news, social media, movies, TV, shopping, video games, and more)? The answer is plenty. The Internet medium as a digital modality is designed and managed using specific algorithms that are unique to your online history, demographics, and use patterns. Your *user experience* is sculpted to sell you content those producers and providers have to offer, or if they do not offer it, they will sell your name to someone who does. The technical term for this is *user experience engineering,* which is a fancy way of saying personalized manipulation. This is hardly a nefarious endeavor. These people are not out to get you, but they *are* out to get your time and attention and make money. The question you must ask is "How much time do I want to give?"

So, what kind of brain science is going on here? Well, a lot. Behavioral psychology and neuroscience (along with social psychology and consumer science) all have input into understanding human screen behavior. Video game developers will go to elaborate lengths to test sounds, music, A-B comparison of colors, and reward contingencies to arrive at a perfect formula that will enhance your user experience. But what exactly does *enhance the user experience* mean?

REMEMBER

An *enhanced user experience* is code for an experience that produces a long use period. Whether this is a game, a TV series, or other digital media content, the idea is to get your eyes on board and to keep them there if possible. Unfortunately, your body (and life) tends to be where your eyes and attention are, so this all adds up to a heck of a lot of time on your screens.

All reinforcement and reward contingencies used by providers are well researched and based on both animal and human studies. There is over a hundred years' worth of data on how to increase specific behaviors and how to reward people in a manner that increases the likelihood of maintaining that behavior. This is science that has been experimentally proven, and all this data (as well as new research) is available to the content producers, developers, and service providers that bring you the content and experiences that you enjoy. The question is, do you *really* love it, or do you *love* it because of the *way* it is given to you?

TECHNICAL STUFF

The concepts of boundaries, stimulating content, synergistic amplification of content, reward latency, variable reinforcement, interactivity, and endless content all represent well-researched topics in behavioral and consumer science. The fields of cognitive brain science and cognitive psychology have devoted a lot of research to how to manage attention and how people process information. We have now moved from the *information age* to the *attention age,* and whoever gets to manage and control your attention has tremendous power.

Seeing the influence of social media

The integration of streaming, social media, and social influence on consumer behavior is a potent new force. The ability to utilize people (who are not celebrities) to help sell and influence purchases marks a new dawn in the world of marketing as well as entertainment. No one foresaw the use of social media and the way it has evolved over the last decade; short videos that stream on YouTube, Instagram, and TikTok capture people's attention like flies on flypaper. The use of social capital and social influence on marketing and sales provides even greater power to the Internet medium to impact people's lives and decisions. Even the news uses gamification and social influencing to keep your eyes onscreen. It's impossible to insulate yourself from this process if you use the Internet, and frankly, nearly everybody who has Internet access is affected and influenced in some way. You use the Internet not only because of what you can *do* online, but also because of what it *does to you.*

REMEMBER

Television, and to a large extent the Internet, needs your eyes onscreen to fund its existence. Anything you see streamed online or on TV (and the lines between these media have now blurred) is *funded* with your attention. You always pay with your time, and it's important to ask yourself how valuable your time is.

TEACHING YOU THAT YOU MUST SEE WHAT'S ON NEXT

Autoplay is almost as important an invention for YouTube, Netflix, Amazon Prime, Hulu, and most streaming services as the *Like* button was for Facebook. What do we mean by this? Well, consider this example: It's Thursday evening, you've had a heck of a week so far at work, and you are looking forward to sitting on the couch to start to watch the newest season of your favorite show that was released the night before. It's 9 p.m. and you turn on your smart TV and choose one of the streaming services that carries, and more than likely produces, the show. There is a whole new season of ten episodes, and you are going to watch the season opener and then get ready for bed, as you have one more weekday to get through, and you need to be at work early for a meeting.

The show was amazing, everything you hoped for. The ending was so suspenseful (and left you wanting more) that you let the credits roll while you stretched, and the next thing you know, there is a little circle that begins to turn at the bottom-right corner of your screen, telling you to hit cancel if you do not want the next episode to play in the next ten seconds. Ten, nine, eight. . .*should I just watch one more? I can probably watch one more and still get to bed at a reasonable hour.* Seven, six, five. . .*okay, what's one more episode going to do anyway? It's not like I'm going to binge the whole season tonight.*

The next thing you know, it's 4 a.m. and you have just completed seven of the ten new episodes — and you have to be up in three hours for work. What happened? All you know is that you sat down to watch a show, and instead, you watched *seven*. What happened was *autoplay*. This is a very simple but powerfully clever method of you doing nothing and it getting the content producer and service provider something very valuable — your time and attention — that translates ultimately into money. You were a victim of what most of us have experienced, probably more than once. By doing nothing, you got to *passively consume* video content; this is because your energy would have to be spent to *not* do something, as opposed to *doing* something. It is a perfect use of Newton's law — that is, an object at rest (and lying on the couch counts) tends to stay at rest unless acted upon by a force. The same also applies to an object in motion. The problem is that at 2 a.m., there are not a lot of forces hanging around to help.

Looking at Other Problems of Watching TV All the Time

The problem with television is that in some ways, it is too good. After all, where else can you tune in 24 hours a day and be pleasantly entertained or distracted — except the Internet? The issue is further complicated by the fact that the Internet and television have finally merged to a large extent. Thanks in part to streaming shows and services (many competing with cable programming), the ability to find, watch, and binge TV today is perhaps greater than ever.

In the earlier days of television, there was not much to watch, and on most stations, broadcasting ended at 1 or 2 a.m. There was no Wi-Fi, no Internet streaming, no cable — just a few television networks transmitting through the air without much competition for viewers' attention. The problem with watching TV today is that it is *always on,* with hundreds of choices, and if you add streaming, there are even more choices. The ease of access of TV integrated with the Internet is that you now have television on *steroids.*

You find out about the ease of binge watching earlier in this chapter. The following sections go over other problems and pitfalls of watching TV all the time.

Intensity is addictive

When it comes to television, *bad news* is compelling. Not that you like bad news, but there is something about scary or bad news that keeps you watching. It's likely that this is a primitive self-protection mechanism in that you need to know whether there is any potential danger; the problem is that it compels you to feel that the world is unsafe and dangerous, when in fact, it is safer today than it was 100 years ago. However, because you are constantly immersed in instant access to all the bad news happening all over the world, you feel as if danger is lurking around every corner. This is not to say that bad things do not happen, but before television, and especially before Internet-linked, cable, satellite, and streaming television, it took a while to find out.

Near-instant access means that you will hear and see everything that happens everywhere in the world, almost in real time. This is not bad or good, but it is certainly a potent force in impacting your emotions and consciousness. Being informed is important. Being saturated with bad news that leaves you feeling stressed, overwhelmed, and scared is *not.*

REMEMBER

There must be a balance in the Internet attention age. Digital screen technologies are wonderful and help you do many great things, but they also add a layer of stress (along with eating up your time). Many times, you can get caught up in the amazing things you can see, do, and hear online, but less often do you address how much time and energy all this *convenience* costs you.

TV acts as your social companion

We're lonely. In fact, we're lonelier today than we were 50 years ago. We have more square footage in our homes than ever, but at the same time, fewer close, personal friendships than ever. We consume a lot of material goods and intoxicating Internet content, but we also find that it contributes to feelings of further isolation. We often view television as a companion, with the soft drone of whatever is on as background noise, acting as a backdrop to our lives. It's not that TV is bad, but just like the Internet (which has essentially merged with TV), it's almost too good, and like chocolate ice cream, too much of a good thing can hurt you.

Television has become a place to hang out with your shows, movies, and content (all provided with autoplay, as described earlier in this chapter). You can be passively entertained for hours upon end without moving a finger. But this can really become too much. Many people may recall how appealing the thought of watching several episodes in one night was, but when they gave in to this temptation, it was usually at the expense of something else — namely sleep or a task waiting for their attention. The problem here is that pleasurable behavior (which also happens to be addictive) is provided and consumed in such completely a passive manner — essentially, you do nothing except talk into your remote. This is the path of least resistance, and changing this pattern requires active choice and movement.

One form of screen use is almost as good as another

When someone stops heavy Internet and video game use, it's not unusual for them to switch to watching huge amounts of TV. Because television is now integrated with the Internet, it is easily overused and at times can become an addiction itself. The ability to binge on TV with streaming capability makes it very easy to lose track of time. The word *stream* really describes the endless flow of content without interruption. The ability to choose from hundreds of options, and to have instant access, makes stream-based television a whole new game. Many patients seeking treatment have developed television addictions once they no longer had free access to the Internet or video games, and so they were essentially swapping addictions. It's important to try not to switch from compulsive Internet or video game use to excessive television viewing, especially when the line between TV and the Internet has essentially disappeared.

TECHNICAL STUFF

The average daily use of the Internet has now surpassed television usage, but it's hard to tell where all this will lead when distinguishing the Internet from television is becoming steadily more difficult.

It's a Choice: Screening the Stream

Because you have limited time to spend on your screens, including TV, how do you know what to watch and how much is too much? The idea really comes down to *choices*. You make choices every day in terms of how much time you spend on everything you do; the trick with screen technologies is to apply this principle of conscious choice to the seemingly harmless aspects of staring at a screen. Whether TV, the Internet, or a video game, it all eats up your time and attention, and often in a way in which you cannot appreciate what you've been doing for all those hours (and what you neglected in your life).

You must make choices, and because you cannot do everything, you need to make sure that you see your TV and Internet use as an *expendable* activity, not a *necessary* one. We're not talking about the work or school activities you do online or the show you like to watch. We're talking about all the hours you spend endlessly channel surfing or Internet scrolling, hoping to see something that gives you some hit of pleasure. Because you often cannot appreciate the passage of time when staring at a screen (see Chapter 1 in Book 7), you must make those decisions *before* you start watching.

TIP

Set limits on how much time you want to watch and stick to those limits. Think about the other valued activities you have in your life and how those hours of watching will impact your sleep, health, relationships, work, or academic performance. Your technology and screens can be wonderful additions to your life if you apply your humanity to them; left to their own devices (pun intended), your screens will slowly encroach on your essential humanity, and you will lose what is truly important. Flip to Chapter 5 in Book 7 for more tips on living a balanced life with the Internet and technology.

REMEMBER

Whether it is Internet-enabled TV, where you can stream almost anything, or old-fashioned broadcast TV, your central power is from you deciding when to turn it *on* and when to turn it *off*. You cannot wait for an external reminder to limit your use or do something else, because that reminder may never come. You must remember that all these wonderful technologies are here to *serve you*, and if you are not careful, you will end up *serving them* instead.

IN THIS CHAPTER

» **Knowing that life is too big to fit on a screen**

» **Undergoing a digital detox**

» **Watching your online time and content use**

» **Matching your values to your tech time**

» **Saying goodbye to addictive notifications and apps**

» **Taking part in real-time activities**

Chapter **5**

Adopting Self-Help Strategies

et's face it: Addictions are human problems, and they are a biological part of the human condition. Many people face an addiction, compulsion, habit, or abuse of a substance or behavior at some time during their lives. Although drugs and alcohol are the most typical addictions you hear about, many other addictive behaviors create challenges and leave many people struggling. Gambling, sex, food, and exercise are just a few, and since all addictions share the same underlying neurobiology, it isn't at all surprising that Internet, video gaming, and smartphone technologies can be addictive.

Self-help is about finding information, techniques, resources, treatment, suggestions, and support to help in the process of managing an addiction. People typically think of self-help when it comes to addictions — in part because the mental health and addictions fields have not had a stellar track record in effectively treating addictions. Over the last century, many self-help groups and organizations have provided valuable information, support, and inspiration to addicts and their loves ones.

The hard part about self-help is that it is generally left up to the addict to seek out when and if they are ready. However, many Internet addiction patients do not initially see themselves as having a problem serious enough to seek support for it. As with all addictions, friends and family are often the first to notice and to be affected by those who are addicted; these friends and family can significantly benefit from support as well.

REMEMBER

Self-help is also about anything you can do to access help, information, and support in *any* part of your life — not just limiting it to recovery from an addiction. Some of what is in this chapter is about general use and overuse of screens, as well as an addiction to Internet technology, and there are many people who overuse their screens but who may not meet the criteria for an addiction. Internet and screen problems exist on a continuum, with use, overuse, abuse, and finally progressing to an addiction.

Remembering That Life Isn't Lived on a Screen

Screen technologies are very compelling. They are fun, interesting, and rewarding to your brain. With a promise of better living through technology, there are many ways in which modern life encourages you to use the Internet and screens for everything. It's easy to get caught up in the distraction, boredom avoidance, perceived convenience, and ease of access that these digital devices provide.

But there is another side to the equation. All the fun, avoidance of boredom, and convenience comes at a price — not just the price of overuse and potential addiction, but the price of losing your humanity and valuable time. The following sections remind you of the benefits of reducing your screen time.

Recognizing that it's tough to limit tech use

It's hard to limit something that feels limitless. After all, screen tech is everywhere and it's only expanding. People have faster processors, screens on everything in their homes, 5G wireless smartphones, and abundant messages from corporate media on how *good* it is to be always connected to everything. But is it *good* for you? The Internet will soon be available from all corners of the planet, and that can be a good thing, provided there is a connection between the technology and human side of the equation.

Part of what the Internet brings is the expectation (more of a constant, subtle insistence) that we should all be on our devices all the time — but when we are, we have no time off-line. How can we rejuvenate when we work, shop, scroll, surf, and are entertained no matter where we are or what we are doing? Even the news is interspersed with humor, games, stories, ads, backlinks, and click-bait. Sometimes you may lose track of what you started to read because you fell into an Internet sinkhole and didn't even realize it. With high-speed Internet and the smartphone highway, there is no off-ramp.

REMEMBER

Saying no to something that everyone *does* and everyone *has* is hard. There is a feeling that you will somehow be left behind. Terms like FOMO (fear of missing out) and NOMOPHOBIA (fear of being detached from your mobile phone) speak to the idea that somehow, if you are not readily available with access to your screens, you will miss out on something important. Ironically, you have your eyes on your screens so much that you, in fact, miss *many* things that are important.

Striving for lower-tech (not no-tech) living

People live at a fast pace. Although many people are still not connected via high-speed Internet, Wi-Fi, and smartphones, a large percentage of the United States is. There are estimates that 81 percent of Americans have smartphones, with 96 percent owning a cellphone, and the numbers have gone up over 250 percent in a few short years, according to the Pew Research Center. Let's face it: People are wired, or rather wireless. Many people use their smartphones as their primary Internet access connection and are rarely without it, so essentially, they are never without the Internet.

The net effect of this (forgive the pun) is that you are always updating and receiving streamed input; in short, you have no downtime — ever. Although people are often online in some way, that doesn't mean they always have to be. The choice is now *internal* as opposed to *external*, not unlike food or nutrition, where you have a plethora of opportunities in terms of choosing your calories. However, people often choose foods based not on nutritional factors, but rather on taste, craving, emotions, and other reasons. At times, you may feel helpless in terms of your control over food choices, and the same may be true of your choices around Internet and screen access.

REMEMBER

Having the world at your immediate disposal and fingertips is powerful. It is also addictive and involves primitive reward circuits in the brain. This power needs to be respected for its potential impact on your life. Whether it is the desire and ability to video game, use social media, or just scroll around on your smartphone, all of it consumes your time and attention, and it can all lead to the stress of being *ever-on* — without periods of lower stimulation.

We have now become a *boredom-intolerant* culture. No one can be bored for even a moment. As an experiment, the next time you brew a pot of coffee or go into a waiting room, don't pull out your phone automatically. Just sit for a few minutes and do nothing. This almost sounds blasphemous. Do nothing? That means not be entertained by social media, TikTok, email, text, sports scores, banking, or stock trading, and not order those coffee filters that you forgot yesterday. Nothing. You may believe that this is a waste of time, but it is not. It is relearning the *value* of time. It is finding the nutritional value of *your* precious time that you've given to the mindless autopilot of your tech use.

REMEMBER

Life is lived in the gaps between tasks, not in the tasks themselves. Screens keep you busy, but not necessarily happy. The data regarding people who take a temporary or partial respite from screens unequivocally shows increased happiness scores and lower incidence of mental health issues.

REMEMBER

Lower-tech living is exactly that: It is using technology and screens for what you need to, but cutting out the extra use that is harmful. The number that seems to work is about two hours a day, give or take. Numerous studies looked at this number, and it seems that less than that is too little and more is too much. Two hours is the *Goldilocks* number, although one study found one hour to be even better for children and teens. This is even more critical if you are under 25, when the frontal cortex of your brain is not fully developed, making you both more susceptible to addiction and having less executive judgment capacity.

Decreasing your stress with less tech

Whether you are an Internet addict or an over-user of your screen tech, the issue ultimately leads to the same result: diminished time and life imbalance. More subtle effects may also be associated with being ever-connected to your screens. Besides all the physical and psychological issues, people are unable to live fully in the present moment without distraction. In a sense, not only have they become *boredom intolerant,* but they have also become *distraction dependent.*

It might seem obvious, but using less tech means that you can spend that precious time doing the things you want and need to do. You may not realize what you have lost while you blindly donated your waking hours to your smartphone, laptop, and tablet, which all clamor for your attention. Your life erodes slowly, below your conscious awareness; then you find that you spent hours a day on your smartphone and all your other addictive screen activities.

WARNING

The fact is that excess use of screen-based technologies increases your overall stress level. Some of this is due to increases in cortisol (the stress hormone), and some of it is simply the result of the amount of time that is spent. This leaves less time for everything else you must do, and that remaining time becomes compressed. When you compress life, you experience this as pressure and stress.

When they look at their screen use levels, most people are shocked to find how much time they are spending online. Even without an obvious addiction to video games, online pornography, social media, or other online activities, average users in the United States come in at 4 to 9 hours per day. Age seems to make a difference, with teens being in the highest use group. Think about this. Of the 16 waking hours we have each day, on average, approximately 25 to 50 percent of it is spent on nonproductive screen use. That includes TV, smartphones, tablets, computers, and so on. These numbers are staggering, but the data doesn't lie. Screen use is perhaps one of the few areas of your life that can be tracked, and it is one of the things you do that absorbs huge amounts of time, creating stress in its wake.

REMEMBER

All the tech you consume is a constant call to action to your nervous system; this consumption is potentially limitless, but your capacity to manage the input and handle the psychological effects of excess screen use is limited.

Disrupting Your Tech Habits with a Digital Detox

Sometimes it's necessary to limit access to an addictive behavior. Unlike most addictive substances and behaviors, screens are now so easily accessible that you may need to limit certain content and devices.

To treat an addiction, patients need to have some period of at least partial detox, where they have an opportunity to reduce some of the established reward connections in the brain, and to help re-regulate their dopamine levels. Even for someone who overuses technology, placing limits on the total time or on problem websites or apps can help provide a safety net to limit their use.

REMEMBER

The Internet and screens aren't dangerous in and of themselves; rather, they are powerful and therefore can impact your brain, your behavior, and your life.

Defining a "digital detox"

REMEMBER

A *digital detox* is exactly what it sounds like: It is the absence, or in some cases reduction, of a substance or behavior. It results in a detoxification from the overuse of that substance or behavior. In this case we're talking about screens. A detox from the Internet and screens is different from a detox from drugs or alcohol in that users experience little physiological dependence and withdrawal. They experience some withdrawal symptoms, but these are typically seen in the form of psychological adjustment to reduced dopamine, and to the re-regulation of the brain's reward system. This period can be marked with anger, frustration, irritability, anxiety, depression, a feeling of loss, and overall discomfort.

Detox allows some of the well-worn neural pathways to degrade, thus allowing new behavioral patterns to be established; it also allows for the up-regulation of down-regulated dopamine receptors in the reward centers of the brain. The goal here is to break some of the biological and psychological connections with screen use.

Whether you're an addict yourself, or you have a loved one who is, or you simply want to be less connected to your screens, you need to change patterns of behavior. The behavior change sets up your nervous system to be receptive to new, rewarding behaviors and to allow you to obtain dopamine elevations from more constructive sources.

WARNING

The use of *willpower* to manage your tech use is a bad bet. Everyone has good intentions to stop or limit behaviors, and Internet addicts and over-users will gladly promise themselves, and others, that they will change their behavior, but this change is generally short-lived. Not because they have no intention to do so, but rather because under a specific set of circumstances, willpower is not enough to prevent a habitual pattern from reoccurring.

Getting set for success

Many patients who seek consultation, parent coaching, or treatment are under 30 years old. Most of the initial requests for help come from their parents or other loved ones. This presents some unique challenges in terms of supporting (and at times insisting on) changes to the screen-use habits of the child, teen, or young adult.

REMEMBER

You cannot force anyone to do anything. Ultimately, you must clearly communicate your intentions and the appropriate consequences if they are not agreed on. Consistency, follow-through, and clear communication are necessary. It may also take good apps or software that can provide adequate blocks or limits and an IT consultation to help you structure any kind of limits at home. Most Internet addicts are incredibly resourceful when it comes to hacking through blocks, filters, or monitors placed on a device. Some Internet addicts have found old computers and old smartphones that barely work just to get some access after parents removed their main screens. Also, none of this should be attempted without an experienced mental health or addictions professional guiding you through this process. Detox, absent of a comprehensive treatment plan, typically fails; the converse is also true, that treatment, without some limits and detox, also fails.

WARNING

The Internet, smartphone, or video game addict will promise the moon when you threaten a complete or partial detox, but take care not to trust an addicted brain's promises. Note that the part of the brain that is involved with the addiction is not logical, and it only wants what it wants: to feel good. Your loved one will likely promise anything to get their screen back, but once they are reunited with their screen, the well-established pattern of addiction will quickly return.

Monitoring and Limiting Your Time and Content on Screens

Sometimes people decide to create a *dosing schedule* where they allow a more moderate amount of time online and on their devices. If there is an endless stream of potential access, the brain will want to use that time. When the resources become more limited, there is a natural adjustment to make do with what time is available. The following sections go over the basics of changing your time and content use online.

Turning off Internet access at a specified time

Time is everything when it comes to screen use, overuse, and addiction. It is the *fuel* that is used by the addiction. You cannot be a screen addict without spending a lot of time online and on your devices.

Time is the human capital that is usurped by screen technology, and it so happens that the Internet is very good at distorting your perception of time. So, what this means is that you must limit your own use of time (which is not always easy to do); if you're dealing with a loved one who is overusing or is addicted to their tech, then providing automated software or apps that limit total time consumption can be a very helpful approach.

TIP

Having these limits automated is key (ironic that we're advocating technology here) because it takes you, the parent or family member, out of the loop. In other words, the device is set to allow access only for a certain amount of time online, or it can be set to allow a certain amount of time on specific content areas such as video games, social media, or even adult sexual content. It is important to use reliable and easy-to-use software and applications; two options are Circle (https://meetcircle.com/) and Qustodio (www.qustodio.com/en/), but there are many other options as well.

It's also important to have an IT person help set this all up — or at least guide you through the process. Many parents have some IT experience and want to do it all themselves, but this often does not work well for a variety of reasons. Many complex emotions and family dynamics are involved, and if you are doing this for a child or teen, that can complicate the process of doing the technical setup. Having a parent do the setup also makes it that much easier for the addict to try to sidetrack the whole process and possibly try to manipulate changes in the treatment plan. Some parents handle it just fine, but many find the process difficult.

There is a lot of variation to each situation, so it's important to have someone who can be available for changes and adjustments, which are often necessary. If you want to find an IT person and the doctor or therapist you're working with does not have one, make sure you find one who is familiar with monitoring, blocking, and filtering programs such as the two mentioned earlier; make sure the IT person also interacts with the doctor or therapist who is coordinating the treatment plan. It is *not* a recommendation to only use software or applications to solve an addiction problem, but rather it is part of a comprehensive treatment plan to help the addict.

You can set a specific dose of Internet daily screen time, in addition to turning off all access to the Internet or specific content areas or apps. At the very least, devices, and perhaps the router itself, should be set to go off at a reasonable time and/or after a specific dose of time for the addict. Left to their own devices (another pun), all over-users, and especially addicts, can easily be lulled into a *cybercoma* and stay on way longer, and much later, than they intended.

Limiting specific content

The idea of limiting specific content becomes even more critical in cases where there is an addiction to potent content. Again, the *synergistic amplifying* effect of the Internet modality, along with addictive and stimulating content, is a perfect combination for endless use. Blocking or limiting specific content can be invaluable in helping to treat a problem, while also preserving access to needed aspects of the Internet and screen use.

People must use the Internet. Too much of their lives are integrated with their smartphone and other screens to simply avoid them altogether. There are ways to block or limit complete content categories such as video gaming, gambling, pornography, social media, YouTube, and so on. Some of these content areas can largely be eliminated, while still preserving access to the necessary aspects of Internet and smartphone use; however, this can be tricky technically, so again, you should get someone to help with the IT process.

One way you can limit content areas (websites or apps) is by creating an allowed list, called a *whitelist,* or a disallowed list, or *blacklist.* Sometimes you can combine both, depending on what you're trying to accomplish.

REMEMBER

Make sure that whatever approach you take with blocking, monitoring, or filtering, you do *not* give the addicted person *administrative privileges* for their devices; otherwise, they will be able to delete whatever software or app you install.

These issues can also become more complicated if your child is going to a boarding school or college, as you will have potentially fewer options; sometimes you may need to connect your IT person with the IT department at the school to coordinate planning.

REMEMBER

You'll likely have to tweak and adjust all these Internet blocks, limits, and filters several times. Sometimes they glitch, and often you'll need to adjust settings based on changing needs or other issues, such as equipment changes.

At times you may need more data to understand what is going on with your screen use or that of your child or loved one. In such cases, you may simply elect to monitor the time and content to ascertain where the problems are. Sometimes this step is used to collect information to help structure blocking and filtering, and sometimes it can be used to help educate the user or addict on how much time they are in fact spending and how they are using that time.

Establishing Values-Based Tech Use

Of all the suggestions in this book, this one may ultimately prove the most useful. It may be harder to implement for a loved one, but in the bigger picture, this is where you must go to survive ever-encroaching screen tech in your life.

Values-based use is simply that. As you find out in this section, it is deciding how and when to use your screens (especially Internet-enabled devices) based on what your life goals and values are. The goal is to fit the screen technology around what you hold to be most important, as opposed to fitting in what is most important as an afterthought to your technology use. The reason is simple: If you use the latter approach, you'll never get to the most valued and important parts of your life. Internet technologies simply eat way too much time, and you often unconsciously allow such technology to dictate how you spend your time.

Introducing a values map

A *values map* is two things: a diagram that depicts how and where you spend your time, and a map that marks out your values. Unfortunately, they are often not aligned. The idea is to create a map that represents how you *currently* spend your time, and how you would *ideally* like to spend your time.

You need to see your technology from the perspective of how it can enhance your life, and not just because it is another new cool app, program, or website. You may have many apps that you never use, and tons of junk email that you do not have time to get rid of. All of this consumes mental and physical energy, and even if a new app does something great, you need to ask whether it is good enough to justify the time it uses (including installing, maintaining, and learning it) and whether it takes away from other parts of balanced living.

A values map is based on the idea that you have limited time and limited attentional energy. You simply cannot manage numerous streams of information and content, so you must set *attentional boundaries.* That is a mouthful, but what you need to do with your screen time is what you do when you go through your junk mail: *get rid of what you do not want or really need.* By *really need*, we mean what will enhance your life, not simply be sort of fun or interesting. Be picky and do not let your time and attention be wasted without some scrutiny.

REMEMBER

Do not lie to yourself. And if it is a child or loved one who is overusing or is an addict, then try to help them to be honest with themselves. Mind you, you cannot make anyone see or do anything that they are not ready or willing to see or do. But that does not mean you cannot help structure life at home in a way that helps support a healthier and sustainable relationship with screens and the Internet.

Deciding where your eyes go

REMEMBER

By thinking about what is truly important to you — health, exercise, friendships, marriage or primary relationship, work, religious or spiritual activities, hobbies, travel, and so on — you can see what is needed to get these things done. The idea is not to use leftover time to live your life, but rather to use leftover time for entertainment, boredom management, avoidance of tasks, a dopamine hit, or just fun. Many things are fun, but they are not always as time-distorting as screens. You must decide where your eyes go. Don't let your eyes decide where you go.

A values map isn't actually a map; rather, it's a piece of paper where you track your thoughts and considerations (along with a conclusion and plan). It's called a map because it can help guide you through the process of making important choices. For example, if your main value is to stay connected to family and friends, do you keep Facebook and delete Twitter and other social media apps to focus on just one? Or do you delete all social media and focus on using FaceTime, Zoom, Skype, and so on to make direct calls and chats? The idea is to preferably use the most direct and efficient means to accomplish your goal to be connected to your friends and family.

The problem with social media is that it is a circuitous route to get to the desired goal of connection — and it is filled with ads, detours, distractions, and time-wasting entertainment. You end up spending your precious time watching cat videos on Facebook or Instagram. If you're under 30, phone calling is less of a thing, but there really is no better way to connect (other than in person) with perhaps the exception of FaceTime, Zoom, or another video platform. Text your friend or loved one and set up a time to really connect, and save the social media for some limited entertainment if you must.

It is dangerous when it is so easy to waste several hours a day on your smartphone or on a video game. The problem with screens is that often you cannot easily manage time while you're on them, and it is this psychoactive and time-distorting power of screens that you need to address — *otherwise, a pastime will become all your time.* Values-based tech use acknowledges your limited time and energy; it also acknowledges the addictive allure of the Internet and your screens, and it assumes that life is what happens (at least much of the time) when you are *not* on your screen.

REMEMBER

Here's a phrase to consider: *Today is your future's past.* Sounds morbid, but it can be instructive. Imagine how you would feel if you had very limited time left. What would you miss? What would you wish you had done more of? What would you want to say to certain people, and what websites, apps, games, or social media accounts would you want to log onto? Would you want to be posting on Facebook with limited time here on earth? Again, not to be morose, but *you do have limited time left.* We all do. Don't act like you have unlimited time such that you waste huge amounts of it online — yes, *waste.* To paraphrase Andy Dufresne in *The Shawshank Redemption*, you either "get busy living, or get busy dying" — there is nothing in between. Screens do not care if you are on them, so you must take charge of them — otherwise, they will take charge of you.

Removing Notifications and Addictive Apps

Sometimes it is necessary to remove an app, program, website, or notification. It is far easier to avoid overuse or addictive behavior if you do not have the most tempting lures in front of your face. If you are an alcoholic or watching what you eat, you probably do not want beer in the fridge or a box of chocolates in the cupboard. The idea is to remove the most tempting, problematic, and triggering components from your smartphone, computer, tablet, or another screen device. This is especially true of video games, social media sites, and even news sites that are purposely designed and gamified to keep you onscreen. This also goes for notifications, which are repeated invitations to engage in online behavior.

Knowing that notifications invite you to waste time

Notifications are a touchy subject. They can be a real problem on your smartphone because they act like the crack cocaine of smartphone apps; app developers and wireless providers are always asking you about notifications because they know this is a gateway to getting you onscreen. They know that if you receive a notification, you are more likely to use the app, thus keeping your eyes onscreen and perpetuating the addictive cycle and making money off you. Notifications trigger your brain's reward center and thus kindle the dopamine innervation cycle.

REMEMBER

The problem is that everything you have and do on your phone has a notification potential unless you turn them off or remove the app all together.

Getting rid of apps, websites, and software

Uninstalling apps can be complicated in that not only do you have to delete the app or program (or block a website), but you also must block the ability to download and reinstall it. It does you (or your loved one) no good to get rid of something on the smartphone or another device if you can just have it reappear from the cloud. It must be deleted completely, and ideally a block should be set up that will prevent the app or program from being reinstalled. This is more easily done on a smartphone or tablet, where you can easily set up a block to prevent the downloading of new apps; this can also be done on a computer, but it requires some external software or setting to accomplish this. An IT professional can help you with this.

Do not assume that if you delete something addictive, either you or your loved one will not reinstall it in short order. Unless you block the reinstall feature, it's highly likely that your willpower (or your loved one's) will quickly crumble, and back it will come to your smartphone or other screen devices.

Some blocking or monitoring software can notify whoever is keeping tabs on the software (the IT person, a parent, or the doctor or therapist who is directing the treatment) that there was an attempt to turn off the blocks or filters, or an attempt to reinstall something that was removed or turned off. This keeps everyone honest, and it is human nature (especially if a person is addicted) to push limits and to relapse. Relapse is a very normal part of addiction treatment, and it's best to assume that this will occur and to take appropriate steps.

If you or your loved one are addicted, then it may be necessary to block the ability to download new or previous apps. Sometimes you can give the smartphone password to a friend or family member who can manage the blocks that are set up on the phone's operating system. Sometimes you may need other external software that is mentioned earlier, in which case an IT person would be helpful.

Filling Your Life with Real-Time Activities

Nature abhors a vacuum, and the same may be said for your screen use. If you stop addicted or heavy screen use, you need things to replace the dopamine hit you used to get and to fill the physical time gaps that are left open. A relapse to previous levels and pattern use is certain to occur if you do not help yourself or the addicted person to create a *real-time living plan.* This section can help.

Even if you can break the addictive cycle, there is still a need to quickly fill time with activities and behaviors that can help provide some of the dopaminergic innervation previously experienced from screen use. A window exists where the brain is looking for something that fits in that space. Your brain loves to organize, categorize, and make sense of your world — the idea is to give it something to fit into that empty hole.

Left to its own devices (there is that pun again), the brain will look either to relapse or to find substitute stimulation to replace what was lost. The idea is to provide a reasonably benign substitute.

Watching hours of TV is a common activity that occurs when an addict stops excessive video gaming or other screen behaviors such as YouTube, social media, or even watching pornography. Switching from Internet behavior to watching hours of television is not a productive change, but sometimes this is allowed on a temporary basis as an interim step. However, a change needs to be made to decrease TV use in short order, and the addicted person should develop a list of 100 things that can be fun (and provide some stimulation), but that do not involve a screen of any type.

If you ask someone to write a list of 100 things that could be fun or interesting, they may initially say that there aren't 100 things on the planet that you can do without a screen. Take comfort that there has never been anyone who was ultimately unable to do this, although at times it took a few days of thought. It is important to note that you must do the *Real-Time 100* after you have had some detox (introduced earlier in this chapter); otherwise, there will be little to no motivation (remember, reward deficiency syndrome) to engage in developing the list, let alone doing any of the tasks.

REMEMBER

The idea is to create a list of 100 activities, behaviors, or tasks that you can easily do without involving a screen. (Figure 5-1 gets you started on your list; feel free to make copies of this figure and renumber the lines as you reach 100. Or, you can get out a pen and paper and make your list the good old-fashioned way.) Initially, you may feel there are not 100 things you can possibly do without a screen, but it just takes a little time to figure it out. The items should be relatively simple and easily doable. In other words, they should be things you can realistically do now, not in the future. You should also be able to do them with minimal equipment or supplies, although some basic materials are okay.

TIP

Some tasks that people have used include hiking, listening to music, calling a friend, drawing, playing a sport of any kind, building something, taking music lessons or playing an instrument that you may already know, being outside in some way, flying a drone or model rocket, reading a book or magazine (preferably the paper kind), doing a puzzle, making a model of some kind, exercising, cooking a meal, teaching something you know to someone, going out for coffee or a snack, watching a movie with a friend or family member (yes, it's okay if you're doing it as part of a social experience), helping out a friend, and growing something.

Real-Time 100 Living Plan

Instructions: The idea is to create a list of 100 activities, behaviors, or tasks you can easily do without involving a screen. Initially, you may feel there are not 100 things you can possibly do without a screen, but I have found that it just takes a little time to come up with them. The items should be relatively simple and easily doable. In other words, they should be things you can do now realistically, not in the future. You should also be able to do them with minimal equipment or supplies, although some basic materials are okay.

Name: _____ Date: _____

DOB: _____

1. _____
2. _____
3. _____
4. _____
5. _____
6. _____
7. _____
8. _____
9. _____
10. _____
11. _____
12. _____
13. _____
14. _____
15. _____
16. _____
17. _____
18. _____
19. _____
20. _____

FIGURE 5-1: With the Real-Time 100, you make a list of 100 activities that don't involve a screen. This sheet can help you get started.

Index

A

abuse, negatively affecting development of stress responses, 177

Acceptance and Commitment Therapy (ACT), 15

Acceptance and Commitment Therapy (Hayes), 110

Active Isolated Stretching (AIS), 275, 277

Adams, Juliet, 70

adaptive coping, 194–195

adaptive habits, 179

addiction, junk food, 325–326

addiction, to technology

  addictive platforms

    overview, 492

    social media, 492–493

    streaming audio and video, 493

    video games, 493–494

  conditioning, 502, 503

  defined, 488–489

  dopaminergic factors of

    broadcast intoxication, 506

    content, 502–506

    dynamic interaction, 510

    ease of access, 501

    illusion of productivity, 502

    lack of boundaries, 506–507

    multi-tasking, 507

    overview, 499–500

    time distortion, 501–502

    variable ratio reinforcement, 509–510

  overview, 487–488

  psychology of, 508–509

  recovering from, 496–497, 499–500

  science behind, 489–490

  self-help for

    creating dosing schedules for, 539–541

    creating real-time living plans, 545–547

    digital detoxing, 537–539

    establishing values-based tech use, 541

    limiting use of technology, 534–537

    removing notifications, 544–545

    uninstalling addictive apps, 544–545

  social interactions on, 507–508

  social media

    overview, 511–512

    social network, 512–513

    social validation looping, 514–515

    undeveloped emotional qualities due to, 517–518

    variable reinforcement, 515–516

  symptoms of, 494–496

  technology encouraging, 491

  uninstalling addictive apps, 544–545

  user experience engineering contributing to, 527–528

  watching television

    disadvantages of, 529–531

    limiting amount of time spent, 532

    overview, 523–524

    by streaming, 524–529

additives, health dangers of, 322–324

adenosine triphosphate (ATP), 367

adequate intake (AI), 363

aerobic exercise

  checking pulse, 252–253

  comparing, 244

  cooling down, 246

  measuring heart-rate, 248–252

  monitoring level of intensity during, 246–248

  overview, 242–243

  warming up, 245–246

agape love, defined, 135

AI (adequate intake), 363

AIS (Active Isolated Stretching), 275, 277

alcohol, avoiding, 424

Alidina, Shamash, 70

all-cause mortality, 366

allostasis, 188

amino acids, 355

anaerobic exercise
checking pulse, 252–253
comparing, 244
cooling down, 246
measuring heart-rate, 248–252
monitoring level of intensity during, 246–248
overview, 242–243
warming up, 245–246

anaerobic threshold, 250

anger, as cause for procrastination, 441

antibiotics, in foods, 348

anticipation factor, in technology, 504–505

anticipatory anxiety, when reducing workplace stress, 470

Anusara yoga (Power Yoga), 290

appetite, 377

appetitive tastes, 336

apps, uninstalling, 544–545

artificial fat substitutes, avoiding, 333

artificial ingredients, 348–351

artificial mouthfeel, 327

artificial sweeteners, avoiding, 333

aspartame, 348–349

AT (autogenic training), easing bodily tension with, 417–418

ATP (adenosine triphosphate), 367

attention, improving with mindfulness, 52–53

attentional boundaries, setting for technology, 542

attention-shifting, 507

attitudes, for practicing self-compassion, 113–115

autogenic training (AT), easing bodily tension with, 417–418

autonomic nervous functions, 417

autoplay (effortless starting), on streaming, 526–529

auto-relaxation technique, 471–472

availability, of technology, 501

awareness
bodily, gaining through mindfulness, 20–21
mindful, 30–31
to time-management
activities to spend more and less time on, 428–429
with cues, 429–430
overview, 426
with prompts, 429–430
by self-examining, 430–431
by tracking, 427–428

B

back expansion stretch, 281–282

back pain, reducing by stretching, 274

backsliding, when clean eating, 342–344

barefoot running, 259

B-complex vitamins, 364–365

behavior
changing through mindfulness, 33
motivated by emotions, 212

behavioral addictions
addictive platforms encouraging
overview, 492
social media, 492–493
streaming audio and video, 493
video games, 493–494
binging television
disadvantages of, 529–531
limiting amount of time spent, 532
overview, 523–524
by streaming, 524–529
conditioning, 502, 503
defined, 488–489
dopaminergic factors of
broadcast intoxication, 506
content, 502–506
dynamic interaction, 510
ease of access, 501
illusion of productivity, 502
lack of boundaries, 506–507

multi-tasking, 507
overview, 499–500
time distortion, 501–502
variable ratio reinforcement, 509–510
overview, 487–488
psychology of, 508–509
recovering from, 496–497, 499–500
science behind, 489–490
self-help for
creating dosing schedules for, 539–541
creating real-time living plans, 545–547
digital detoxing, 537–539
establishing values-based tech use, 541
limiting use of technology, 534–537
removing notifications, 544–545
uninstalling addictive apps, 544–545
social interactions on, 507–508
to social media
overview, 511–512
social network, 512–513
social validation looping, 514–515
undeveloped emotional qualities due to, 517–518
variable reinforcement, 515–516
symptoms of, 494–496
technology encouraging, 491
being mode of mind
description of, 49–50
encouraging, 54–55
focusing on present moments, 58–60
managing emotions with, 56–57
practice exercises for, 57–58
belly-button balloon breathing, 410–411
beriberi, defined, 365
Bikram yoga, 291
binging, on television, 524–525
bitter taste, 336
blood sugar, balancing to reduce workplace stress, 480–482
blood vessels, effect of stress response on, 189
bodily awareness, gaining through mindfulness, 20–21

bodily tension, easing
with AT, 417–418
bringing awareness to, 405
with massage, 420–422
overview, 403
with progressive relaxation method, 413–416
scanning exercise for, 405, 406–411
by stretching, 419
symptoms of, 403–404
techniques for, 422–424
body sculpting classes, 307–308
boot camp classes, 308
boredom-intolerance, 536
boundaries, for technology
attentional, 542
lack of, 506–507
setting, 234
boxing classes, 308–309
brain, effect of stress response on, 190
breakfast, managing stress by habitually eating, 385, 471
breaks, scheduling, 435
broadcast intoxication, when using technology, 506, 519–520
Buddhism, Four Noble Truths of, 118–120
business travel, when reducing workplace stress, 472–473
butterfly stretch, 286–287

C

caffeine, reducing stress by lowering intake of, 349, 481
calcium, 367
calories, in excess, 351–354
carbohydrates
comparing complex to simple, 357–358
in excess, 352
as macronutrients, 347
cardio-machine classes, 310–311
cardiovascular exercise, 243–244
cardiovascular system, effect of stress response on, 189

Cat Pose yoga position, 298

catalogs, unsubscribing from, 459

Caught in the Net (Young), 497

challenges, embracing, 206

checklist, for time-management, 425

chemicals, in foods, 323–324

cherry-picker stretch, easing bodily tension with, 474

chest expansion stretch, 280–281

childhood experiences, determining factors of resilience, 177–178

Child's Pose yoga position, 296–297

chloride, 368

chores, implementing mindfulness when doing, 84–88

chromium, 340, 369

chronic inflammation, due to stress, 398–399

chronically tense muscles, caused by stress, 398

circuit training classes, 308

classes, exercise
  accepting correction during, 305
  live instructors during, 304–305
  overview, 303
  signing up, 304
  types of, 306–311
  virtual, 311–313
  yoga, 292–293

clean eating
  applying to lifestyle
    backsliding, 342–344
    feelings of deprivation, 341–342
    managing cravings, 339–341
    overview, 331–332
    principles of, 333–338
  benefits of
    general health, 326–328
    longevity, 329
    overview, 326
    weight loss and disease prevention, 328–329
  comparing processed to whole foods, 319–320
  dangers in processed foods
    additives, 322–324
    junk food addiction, 325–326
    label claims, 324–325
    overview, 322
    preservatives, 322–324
  improving appearance with, 335
  incorporating into daily routines, 386
  nutritional needs met by
    artificial ingredients, 348–351
    digestive process, 346–347
    digestive system, 346
    excess calories, 351–354
    fiber, 371–373
    macronutrients, 347–348, 356–366
    micronutrients, 355
    minerals, 366–370
    overview, 345
    vitamins, 362–366
    water intake, 373
  overview, 318–319
  six degrees of, 320–321

clothing, for yoga, 293

clutter roadmap, creating, 452–453

cognitive reappraisal, 218–219

collagen, 364

color additives, 323

commitment, developing mental toughness with, 205

common humanity
  avoiding perfectionism, 144–145
  core values of
    determining experiences through, 162–163
    dissatisfaction when unidentified, 163
    finding meaning through, 161–162
    identifying, 166
    implementing changes based off, 166–167
    importance of hardships in building, 168–171
    overview, 159–160
    practice exercises for, 163–166
  cultivating lovingkindness, 149–150
  developing self-worth, 142–144
  diversity in, 141–142
  interdependency
    challenges of, 137–141
    importance of, 130–134
    love contributing to survival, 134–137

overview, 129–130

practice exercises for, 145–148

practicing lovingkindness, 152–158

pursuing happiness, 150–151

in self-compassion, 98–99

commuting, reducing workplace stress, 471–472

complementary proteins, 357

complete proteins, 356–357

complex carbohydrates, 358–359

compromised immune system, caused by stress, 400

conditioning, for addictions to technology, 502, 503

confidence, developing mental toughness with, 207

conscious choice, increasing resilience with, 228

consignment, 455

content delivered by technology

content intoxication, 503

infotainment, 504–505

instant gratification, 504–505

interactivity in, 503–504

overview, 502

variability in, 503–504

content intoxication, 503

control, developing mental toughness with, 203–204

Control, Commitment, Challenge, Confidence (4Cs), 202–203

cooling down, after exercise, 246

coping habits, determining factors of resilience, 179

coping types, emotions influencing, 193–195, 213–214

copper, 369

core values, of common humanity

determining experiences through, 162–163

dissatisfaction when unidentified, 163

finding meaning through, 161–162

identifying, 166

implementing changes based off, 166–167

importance of hardships in building, 168–171

overview, 159–160

practice exercises for, 163–166

coronavirus pandemic, stress caused by, 390–391

counter-social aspects of social media

broadcast intoxication, 519–520

cyberbullying, 520–521

cyberstalking, 521

overview, 519

trolling, 521

cover crops, 370

cravings, managing, 339–341

cross-country skiing, 266–267

Culp, Stephanie, 462

cultural obstacles faced when identifying core values, 165

culture, determining factors of resilience, 178

cyberbullying, 520–521

cyberstalking, 521

cycling, as outdoor exercise, 261–263

D

dance-based workouts, 309–310

de-cluttering

attitude toward, 453–454

avoiding discouragement, 454

creating clutter roadmaps for, 452–453

excuses for avoiding, 450–452

finding motivation for, 452

gaining momentum when, 453

overview, 450

techniques for, 454–456

deep-muscle relaxation, 413–414

delayed gratification, 205

delegating, 266, 443–445

deprivation, managing feelings of, 341–342

desire, motivated by stress, 188

diabetes, 353

diaphragm, breathing through, 407, 408

diet. *See* clean eating

dietary reference intakes (DRI), 363

digestive process, 346–347

digestive system, 346

digital detoxing, 537–539

digital documents, organizing, 461–462

digital drug delivery, 502, 505

digital footprint, 496

disapproval, procrastinating from fear of, 441

discomfort, when practicing self-compassion, 110–112

discouragement, avoiding when de-cluttering, 454

Discovering Our Core Values exercise, 191

disease, linked to stress, 397–401

disease prevention, clean eating contributing to, 328–329

disorganization, identifying, 449–450

dissociation, when using technology, 491

distraction dependence, 536

distractions, minimizing, 436–440

disturbed sexual performance, due to stress, 401

diuretics, 349

diversity, in common humanity, 141–142

diverticulitis, 372

documents, organizing, 458, 460–461

doing mode of mind, 47–49

dopamine hits, 504

dopaminergic factors of technology
  broadcast intoxication, 506
  content, 502–506
  dynamic interaction, 510
  ease of access, 501
  illusion of productivity, 502
  lack of boundaries, 506–507
  multi-tasking, 507
  overview, 499–500
  time distortion, 501–502
  variable ratio reinforcement, 509–510

dosing schedules, creating, 539–541

double calf stretch, 284–285

Downward-Facing Dog yoga position, 294–295

DRI (dietary reference intakes), 363

driving, implementing mindfulness when, 83–84

Dweck, Carol, 313

dynamic interaction, when using technology, 510

E

EAR (estimated average requirement), 363

ease of access, to technology, 501

eating. *See* clean eating

Eating Clean (Nader), 332

economy, as causing stress, 391

effortless starting (autoplay), on streaming, 526–529

eicosanoids, 361

80/20 rule, 436

electronic documents, organizing, 463–464

electronics, minimizing distractions from, 436–437

email, organizing, 464–465

emotional eating, avoiding by practicing mindfulness, 84–89

Emotional Intelligence (Goleman), 25

emotions
  managing with mindfulness, 27–28
  negative, healing, 235
  regulating
    with cognitive reappraisal, 218–219
    by evaluating, 214–215
    by increasing feelings of love, 220
    by increasing self-awareness, 219
    influence on coping, 213–214
    influence on perception, 213–214
    options for, 215–217
    overview, 211
    with positive detachment, 218–219
    purposes of, 211–212
    relaxation techniques for stress responses, 217–218
  support systems for, 455

empathy, as undeveloped on social media, 517–518

employee assistance programs, reducing workplace stress with, 483

encrypted documents, 461

endless choice, in streaming, 525–526

endorphins, 380

enhanced user experience, as contributing to addictions to technology, 528 equipment, for yoga, 293

ergonomics, when reducing workplace stress, 478–479

essential amino acids, 356

estimated average requirement (EAR), 363

excitotoxins, in foods, 350

exercise
  as act of self-care, 233–234
  cardiovascular types of, 243–244
  classes for
    accepting correction during, 305
    live instructors during, 304–305
    overview, 303
    signing up, 304
    types of, 306–311
    virtually, 311–313
  comparing aerobic and anaerobic forms of
    checking pulse, 252–253
    comparing, 244
    cooling down, 246
    measuring heart-rate, 248–252
    monitoring level of intensity during, 246–248
    overview, 242–243
    warming up, 245–246
  cross-country skiing, 266
  involving flow, 53
  outdoor
    cycling, 261–263
    overview, 255
    running, 258–261
    walking, 256–258
    water aerobics, 263–267
  practicing mindfulness during, 67–68
  reducing stress through, 471
  static stretching
    overview, 278
    routine for, 279–287
    rules of, 278–279
  stretching
    benefits of, 273–276
    overview, 269–270
    techniques for, 276–278

for weight loss, 334
weight training, 270–273
yoga
  classes for, 292–293
  clothing for, 293
  equipment for, 293
  intensity of, 290
  overview, 289
  routine for, 294–301
  styles of, 290–291
  tips for beginners, 293–294

external obstacles faced when identifying core values, 165

extinction resistance, 515

F

failure, procrastinating from fear of, 441

fast food, avoiding, 383–384

fat-free mass, 273

fatigue, caused by stress, 421

fats
  avoiding artificial substitutes for, 333
  comparing types of, 358–362
  in excess, 352
  as macronutrients, 348

fat-soluble vitamins, 365–366

fatty acids, 360–362

Fearless Heart, A (Jinpa), 145

feedback loops, 190–192

feminine side, to self-compassion, 102

fertilizers, 370

fiber, 371–373

fight-or-flight response, 189–190

files, organizing, 460

first noble truth, 118–119

fitness bands, checking pulse on, 253

Fitness Walking For Dummies (Neporent), 257

fixed mindset, growth mindset versus, 201–202

flexible attention, developing with meditation, 10

flow state, 52–53

focus, improving with mindfulness, 13–14

Focus (Goleman), 25

folders, organizing, 460

food. *See* clean eating

food addiction, 340

food journals, 386

formal meditation, 10

fortified foods, 324

Forward Bend yoga position, 295–296

Four Noble Truths, The, 118–120

4Cs (Control, Commitment, Challenge, Confidence), 202–203

fourth noble truth, 120

free glutamic acid, in foods, 350

free radicals, 355

Future Shock (Toffler), 390

G

gaming disorder, 500

gastric emptying, 381

gastrointestinal (GI) tract, effect of stress on, 189, 399–400

Generally Recognized as Safe (GRAS) list, 322, 323

genetics, determining factors of resilience, 177

Germer, Chris, 104

ghrelin, 350

GI (gastrointestinal) tract, effect of stress on, 189, 399–400

glutamic acid salts, 336

G-protein receptors, 336

GRAS (Generally Recognized as Safe) list, 322, 323

gratification, delaying, 205

gratitude, as act of self-care, 235

grazing, 384–386

growth mindset, fixed mindset versus, 201–202

gustducin protein, 336

gyms, reducing workplace stress with, 482

H

happiness, pursuing, 150–151

hassles, causing stress, 395–396

Hatha yoga, 291

Hayes, Stephen, 110

HCl (hydrochloric acid), 347

head colds, caused by stress, 401

headaches, caused by stress, 401

headphones, avoiding interruptions by wearing, 437

health clubs, reducing workplace stress with, 482

healthy diet, as act of self-care, 233

healthy foods, choosing. *See also* clean eating
  avoiding fast food, 383–384
  grazing, 384–386
  overview, 381–382
  when packaged, 382–383

heart disease, caused by stress, 398–399

heart-rate, measuring, 248–252

heart-rate monitor, tracking heart rates with, 248–249

herbicides, 370

high-fructose corn syrup (HFCS), dangers of, 333, 350

high-impact classes, 306–307

high-intensity interval training (HIIT), 306

hip stretch, 285–286

hobbies, involving flow, 53

home-life, causing stress, 392–393

homeostasis, 188

hopelessness, overcoming, 184

hormones, in foods, 350

humanity. *See* common humanity

humor, determining factors of resilience, 180

hunger cues
  choosing healthy foods
    avoiding fast food, 383–384
    grazing, 384–386
    overview, 381–382
    packaged foods, 382–383
  overview, 375
  recognizing, 376

hybrid bikes, 259

hydrochloric acid (HCl), 347

hydrogenation, 343

hypereating, 380

I

immediate feedback, 53

immune system

  effect of stress response on, 189

  strengthening by reducing stress through meditation, 11–12, 21–22

imposter syndrome, 138

incomplete proteins, 356–357

inflammation, due to stress, 398–399

informal meditation, 10

infotainment, from technology, 503, 504–505

ingredient labels, 382

insoluble fiber, 371

instant access, with streaming, 526

instant gratification, from technology, 504–505

Integral yoga, 291

intensity level, monitoring during exercise, 246–248, 290

intentions, for practicing mindfulness, 41–42

interactivity, of technology, 503–504

interdependency, in common humanity

  challenges of, 137–141

  importance of, 130–134

  love contributing to survival, 134–137

internal obstacles faced when identifying core values, 165

internet addiction

  addictive platforms

    overview, 492

    social media, 492–493

    streaming audio and video, 493

    video games, 493–494

  binging television

    disadvantages of, 529–531

    limiting amount of time spent, 532

    overview, 523–524

    by streaming, 524–529

  conditioning, 502, 503

  defined, 488–489

  dopaminergic factors of

    broadcast intoxication, 506

    content, 502–506

    dynamic interaction, 510

    ease of access, 501

    illusion of productivity, 502

    lack of boundaries, 506–507

    multi-tasking, 507

    overview, 499–500

    time distortion, 501–502

    variable ratio reinforcement, 509–510

  overview, 487–488

  psychology of, 508–509

  recovering from, 496–497, 499–500

  science behind, 489–490

  self-help for

    creating dosing schedules for, 539–541

    creating real-time living plans, 545–547

    digital detoxing, 537–539

    establishing values-based technology use, 541

    limiting use of technology, 534–537

    removing notifications, 544–545

    uninstalling addictive apps, 544–545

  social interactions, 507–508

  social media

    overview, 511–512

    social network, 512–513

    social validation looping, 514–515

    undeveloped emotional qualities due to, 517–518

    variable reinforcement, 515–516

  symptoms of, 494–496

  technology encouraging, 491

  uninstalling addictive apps, 544–545

  user experience engineering contributing to, 527–528

interruptions, wearing headphones to avoid, 437

intuition, improving with mindfulness, 24

iodine, 369

iron, 368

Iyengar yoga, 291

J

Jinpa, Thupten, 145

junk food addiction, health dangers of, 325–326

junk mail, organizing, 458–459

Just Like Me meditation, 145–147

K

Karvonen method, for finding target heart rates, 251

ketosis, 352

kettlebells classes, 307–308

Kripalu yoga, 291

Kundalini yoga, 291

L

label claims (marketing hype), health dangers of, 324–325

lap swimming, 264

large intestine, role in digestive process, 347

LDT (low discomfort tolerance), as cause for procrastination, 441

learned helplessness, overcoming, 182–183

leg lift, easing bodily tension with, 475

leg-lift stretch, 419

lipolysis, 352

live instructors, during exercise classes, 304–305

Lockett, Katherine, 70

longevity, clean eating contributing to, 329

looking deeply, defined, 59

love

accepting as act of self-care, 237–239

contributing to survival, 134–137

regulating emotions by increasing feelings of, 220

lovingkindness

cultivating, 149–150

meditation for, 72

practicing, 152–158

low discomfort tolerance (LDT), as cause for procrastination, 441

low-impact classes, 306–307

ludus, defined, 135

M

macronutrients

carbohydrates, 347–348, 357–358

complete and incomplete proteins, 356–357

in excess, 351–354

fats, 358–362

overview, 356

magnesium, 367

Maier, Steven, 183

mailing lists, unsubscribing from, 458

maladaptive coping, 194

maladaptive habits, 179

mammalian caregiving system, for self-compassion, 103–105

manganese, 369–370

mania, defined, 135

Man's Search for Meaning (Frankl), 29

marketing hype (label claims), health dangers of, 324–325

martial-arts classes, 308–309

masculine side, to self-compassion, 100–102

massage, easing bodily tension with, 420–422

master to-do list, 431–432

maximum heart rate, 250

MBSR (mindfulness-based stress reduction), 68

meditation

for developing mindfulness, 9–10

Just Like Me exercise for, 145–147

for lovingkindness, 72

metta type of, 72

mini sessions of, 75–76

strengthening immune system by reducing stress through, 21–22

mental clarity, developing, 208–209

mental focus, improving with mindfulness, 25–27

mental toughness, developing

committing to change, 205

confidence, 207

embracing challenges, 206

overview, 202–203

sense of control, 203–204

metabolic conditioning, 234

metabolic system, effect of stress response on, 190

metta meditation, practicing, 72

micronutrients, 355

microvilli, 347

mind
  effect of stress response on, 190
  quieting, 234–235

mind-body exercise, 289

mindful awareness, 30–31

mindful flow, psychology of, 52–53

Mindful Path to Self-Compassion, The (Germer), 104

Mindful Self-Compassion (MSC) program, 94–95, 96, 105–108

mindful visualization exercise, 43–44

mindfulness
  accepting present-moment experiences by developing
    gaining wisdom with, 14–15
    improving focus with, 13–14
    overview, 10–11
    personal discovery through, 15–17
    reducing stress, 11–12
    relaxation through, 12–13
  avoiding emotional eating by, 84–89
  being mode of
    description of, 49–50
    encouraging, 54–55
    focusing on present moments, 58–60
    managing emotions with, 56–57
    practice exercises for, 57–58
  benefits of
    bodily awareness, 20–21
    connecting with physical senses, 24–25
    improving immune system, 21–22
    improving mental focus, 25–27
    making intuitive decisions, 24
    managing emotions, 27–28
    overview, 19
    reducing pain, 22

    re-focusing thoughts, 22–23
    relaxation, 20
    self-discovery, 29–31
    spirituality, 28–29
  building healthy relationship with yourself by implementing, 70–72
  combining modes of, 50–52
  doing mode of, 47–49
  establishing as daily habit
    choosing time of day for, 39–41
    clarifying intentions for, 41–42
    exercises for developing visions for, 44–46
    gradually, 35–36
    learning to change behavior, 33
    mindful visualization exercise for, 43–44
    overview, 33
    planning for, 34–35
    practice exercise for, 36–39
    sentence-completion exercises for, 44
  improving work–life balance with, 70
  meditation for, 9–10
  origins of, 8–9
  overview, 7
  practice exercises for, 17, 62–66
  practicing during physical exercise, 67–68
  preparing for sleep with, 68–69
  psychology of mindful flow in, 52–53
  on public transport, 84–85
  in self-compassion, 98
  when doing chores, 84–88
  when driving, 83–84
  when walking, 82–83
  at work
    avoiding multi-tasking, 81
    beginning with exercises, 74–75
    creative problem solving, 78
    mini meditations, 75–76
    overview, 74
    practicing mindful working, 79–80
    responding versus reacting, 76–78

Mindfulness at Work For Dummies (Alidina & Adams), 70

mindfulness-based stress reduction (MBSR), 68

Mindset (Dweck), 312–313

mindset, of resilience

  developing mental toughness, 202–207

  fixed versus growth, 201–202

  overview, 199–201

minerals, 366–370

mini meals. *See* grazing

mixed tocopherols (vitamin E), 366

Modified Sage Twist yoga position, 297–298

molybdenum, 370

monosodium glutamate (MSG), in foods, 350

monounsaturated fats, 360

mood, effect of stress response on, 190

motivation, for de-cluttering, 452

mouthfeel, 327, 335

MSC (Mindful Self-Compassion) program, 94–95, 96, 105–108

MSG (monosodium glutamate), in foods, 350

MTQ48 Psychometric Tool, 202–203

multi-tasking, when using technology, 507

Mumford, Jeni, 70

muscle imbalances, correcting by stretching, 274

muscles, effect of stress response on, 189, 398

music, reducing stress with, 477

myofascial release, 278

N

Nader, Ralph, 332

neck stretch, 280

Neff, Kristin, 96

negative behaviors, overcoming

  hopelessness, 184

  learned helplessness, 182–183

  overview, 180–181

  victim mentality, 181–182, 185

negative emotions, healing as act of self-care, 235

negative feedback loop, 191–192

Neporent, Liz, 257

net effect, 493

nitrates, in foods, 350

nitrites, in foods, 350

nitrosamines, in foods, 350

noise, minimizing distractions from, 437–438

noise-canceling headphones, avoiding interruptions by wearing, 437

notifications, uninstalling, 544–545

nutrient deficiencies, 343

nutrition provided by clean eating

  artificial ingredients, 348–351

  digestive process, 346–347

  digestive system, 346

  excess calories, 351–354

  fiber, 371–373

  macronutrients

    carbohydrates, 347–348, 357–358

    complete and incomplete proteins, 356–357

    in excess, 351–354

    fats, 358–362

    overview, 356

  micronutrients, 355

  minerals, 366–370

  overview, 345

  vitamins, 362–366

  water intake, 373

O

olestra, in foods, 351

omega-3 fats, 360–362

omega-6 fats, 360–362

online resources

  Cheat Sheet link, 2

  Circle website, 539

  Future Me website, 45

  Kristin Neff's website, 96

  link to self-compassion test, 96

  Qustodio website, 539

  showing recommended portion sizes, 334

  for unsubscribing from catalogs, 459

  for unsubscribing from mailing lists, 459

online workout subscriptions, 312–313

organization, reducing stress with

creating system for
  digital documents, 461–462
  documents, 458, 460–461
  electronically, 463–464
  email, 464–465
  files and folders, 460
  junk mail, 458–459
  overview, 459
de-cluttering, 450–456
delegating, 266
guidelines for, 456–457
identifying personal disorganization, 449–450
maintaining, 465–466
overview, 447
strategies for, 448–449
for workplaces, 477
osteoporosis, strength training to avoid, 271
outdoor exercise
  cycling, 261–263
  overview, 255
  running, 258–261
  walking, 256–258
  water aerobics, 263–267
Overworked American, The (Schor), 393
oxytocin, 220

P

packaged foods, choosing healthy options for, 382–383
pain, reducing with mindfulness, 22
parasympathetic nervous system, 190, 417
Pareto principle, 436
password-management systems, 461–462
PDCAAS (Protein Digestibility Corrected Amino Acid Score), 356
pec stretch, easing bodily tension with, 475
pellagra, 365
people, minimizing distractions from, 437
pepsin, 347
perceived exertion method, 247–248
perception, emotions influencing, 213–214
perfectionism, overcoming, 144–145, 440–441

personal needs, providing for as act of self-compassion, 102
pesticides, 370
phenotypes, 177
philautia, defined, 135
philia, defined, 135
phosphorus, 367
physical exercise
  as act of self-care, 233–234
  cardiovascular types of, 243–244
  classes for
    accepting correction during, 305
    live instructors during, 304–305
    overview, 303
    signing up, 304
    types of, 306–311
    virtually, 311–313
  comparing aerobic and anaerobic forms of
    checking pulse, 252–253
    comparing, 244
    cooling down, 246
    measuring heart-rate, 248–252
    monitoring level of intensity during, 246–248
    overview, 242–243
    warming up, 245–246
  cross-country skiing, 266
  involving flow, 53
  outdoor
    cycling, 261–263
    overview, 255
    running, 258–261
    walking, 256–258
    water aerobics, 263–267
  practicing mindfulness during, 67–68
  reducing stress through, 471
  static stretching
    overview, 278
    routine for, 279–287
    rules of, 278–279
  stretching
    benefits of, 273–276
    overview, 269–270
    techniques for, 276–278

physical exercise *(continued)*
  for weight loss, 334
  weight training, 270–273
  yoga
    classes for, 292–293
    equipment and clothing for, 293
    intensity of, 290
    overview, 289
    routine for, 294–301
    styles of, 290–291
    tips for beginners, 293–294
physical pain, mindfulness reducing, 22
physical signs of stress, 397
physiological hunger, 376
physiology, emotions influencing, 212
pica, 343
platforms with addictive qualities
  overview, 492
  social media, 492–493
  streaming audio and video, 493
  video games, 493–494
PNF (proprioceptive neuromuscular facilitation)
    stretching, 277
politics, causing stress, 391
polyunsaturated fats, 360
portion control, 334, 378
positive change, influencing, 195–197
positive detachment, 218–219
positive expectations, maintaining, 192–193
positive feedback loop, 190–191
positive social reinforcer, 528
post-traumatic growth, 169
posture
  maintaining by stretching, 274
  reducing physical stress by improving, 411, 479
  for walking, 257
potassium, 367–368
Power Yoga (Anusara yoga), 290
practice exercises
  for being mode, 56–57
  breathing space exercise, 62–66
  for common humanity, 145–148

for developing visions for mindfulness, 44–46
Discovering Our Core Values, 191
for establishing mindfulness as daily habit,
    36–39, 44
for identifying core values, 163–166
for mindful visualization, 43–44
for mindfulness, 59–60
for practicing self-compassion, 116–117
pragma, defined, 135
present-moment experiences, accepting by
    developing mindfulness
  gaining wisdom with, 14–15
  improving focus with, 13–14
  overview, 10–11
  personal discovery through, 15–17
  reducing stress, 11–12
  relaxation through, 12–13
preservatives, health dangers of, 322–324
prior-sanctioned substances, 323
process addictions. *See* behavioral addictions
processed foods
  comparing whole foods to, 319–320
  dangers in
    additives, 322–324
    junk food addiction, 325–326
    label claims, 324–325
    overview, 322
    preservatives, 322–324
procrastination, overcoming, 441–443
professional help, for recovering from internet
    addiction, 497
progressive relaxation method, easing bodily
    tension with, 413–416
proprioceptive neuromuscular facilitation (PNF)
    stretching, 277
Protein Digestibility Corrected Amino Acid Score
    (PDCAAS), 356
proteins
  complete and incomplete, 356–357
  in excess, 352
  as macronutrients, 348
pseudo-hormones, in foods, 350
psychological hunger, 377

psychological obstacles to time-management, 440–443

psychological outlook, determining factors of resilience, 178

psychological pain, mindfulness reducing, 22

psychology
  of addiction to technology, 508–509
  of mindful flow, 52–53

public transport, implementing mindfulness when using, 84–85

pulse, checking, 252–253

pupils, effect of stress response on, 189

Q

qualities, identifying, 229–230

quieting mind, 234–235

R

RDA (recommended daily allowance), 363

reading, in flow, 53

real-time living plans, creating, 545–547

rebound reflex, 277

receptiveness to self-compassion, 121–124

recommended daily allowance (RDA), 363

reflected self-esteem, 515

relaxation, through mindfulness, 12–13, 20

relaxation techniques, for stress responses, 217–218

reproductive system, effect of stress response on, 189

resentment, as cause for procrastination, 441

resilience
  determining factors of, 176–180
  developing, 175–176
  increasing with self-worth
    accepting personal uniqueness, 230–231
    celebrating yourself, 229
    conscious choice, 228
    identifying your strengths, abilities, and qualities, 229–230
    overview, 221–222
    by practicing self-awareness, 227–228
    self-criticism as opportunity for reflection, 224–225
    self-value inventory checklist, 225–227
    showing self-love, 232
    taking care of you, 233–239
    traits displayed in, 223–224
  mental clarity contributing to, 208–209
  mindset of
    developing mental toughness, 202–207
    fixed versus growth, 201–202
    overview, 199–201
  overcoming negative behaviors by developing
    hopelessness, 184
    learned helplessness, 182–183
    overview, 180–181
    victim mentality, 181–182, 185
  stress affecting
    coping types, 193–195
    desire motivated by, 188
    influencing positive change, 195–197
    maintaining positive expectations, 192–193
    overview, 187
    stress responses, 189–192

resistance training, 234

respiratory system, effect of stress response on, 189

resting, as act of self-care, 236–237

resting heart rate, 249

routines
  incorporating clean eating into, 386
  for yoga
    Cat Pose, 298
    Child's Pose, 296–297
    Downward-Facing Dog, 294–295
    Forward Bend, 295–296
    Modified Sage Twist, 297–298
    overview, 294
    Sun Salutation, 300–301
    Triangle Pose, 299

running, as outdoor exercise, 258–261

S

salt, lowering intake of, 338

salty taste, 336

satiety, 379–381

saturated fats, 360

scanning exercise, for easing bodily tension, 406–411

schemas, 114

Schor, Juliet, 393

screen addiction

  addictive platforms

    overview, 492

    social media, 492–493

    streaming audio and video, 493

    video games, 493–494

  conditioning, 502, 503

  defined, 488–489

  dopaminergic factors of

    broadcast intoxication, 506

    content, 502–506

    dynamic interaction, 510

    ease of access, 501

    illusion of productivity, 502

    lack of boundaries, 506–507

    multi-tasking, 507

    overview, 499–500

    time distortion, 501–502

    variable ratio reinforcement, 509–510

  overview, 487–488

  psychology of, 508–509

  recovering from, 496–497, 499–500

  science behind, 489–490

  self-help for

    creating dosing schedules for, 539–541

    creating real-time living plans, 545–547

    digital detoxing, 537–539

    establishing values-based tech use, 541

    limiting use of technology, 534–537

    removing notifications, 544–545

    uninstalling addictive apps, 544–545

  social interactions on, 507–508

  social media

    overview, 511–512

    social network, 512–513

    social validation looping, 514–515

    undeveloped emotional qualities due to, 517–518

    variable reinforcement, 515–516

  symptoms of, 494–496

  technology encouraging, 491

  uninstalling addictive apps, 544–545

  user experience engineering contributing to, 527–528

  watching television

    disadvantages of, 529–531

    limiting amount of time spent, 532

    overview, 523–524

    by streaming, 524–529

second noble truth, 119

selenium, 370

self-awareness

  increasing resilience with, 227–228

  regulating emotions by increasing, 219

self-comparison, due to social media, 515–516

self-compassion

  balancing self-kindness when practicing, 99–100

  benefits of, 96–97

  break practice exercise for, 106–108

  challenges of

    attitudes towards, 113–115

    feeling discomfort, 110–112

    learning slowly, 116

    overview, 109–110

    practice exercise for, 116–117

  checking in with your personal needs, 102

  customizing

    developing self-worth, 126–127

    level of tolerance for, 124–126

    overview, 120–121

    tracking receptiveness to, 121–124

  defined, 97–98

  mammalian caregiving system for, 103–105

  masculine and feminine sides to, 100–102

  MSC program for, 105–108

MSC program's guided reflection for, 94–95
overview, 93–94
role of common humanity in, 98–99
role of mindfulness in, 98
taught in The Four Noble Truths
   first noble truth, 118–119
   fourth noble truth, 120
   second noble truth, 119
   third noble truth, 119–120
self-criticism, 71, 224–225
self-discovery, through mindfulness, 15–17, 29–31
self-esteem, undeveloped on social media, 517–518
self-help, for recovering from internet addiction
  resources for, 497
  strategies for
   creating dosing schedules for, 539–541
   creating real-time living plans, 545–547
   digital detoxing, 537–539
   establishing values-based technology use, 541
   limiting use of technology, 534–537
   removing notifications, 544–545
   uninstalling addictive apps, 544–545
selfies, validation through, 516
self-kindness, balancing when practicing self-compassion, 99–100
self-love, increasing resilience with, 232
self-mastery, 176
self-value inventory checklist, 225–227
self-worth
  developing for common humanity, 142–144
  increasing resilience with
   accepting personal uniqueness, 230–231
   celebrating yourself, 229
   conscious choice, 228
   identifying your strengths and weaknesses, 229–230
   overview, 221–222
   by practicing self-awareness, 227–228
   self-value inventory checklist, 225–227
   showing self-love, 232
   taking care of you, 233–239

traits displayed with, 223–224
using self-criticism as an opportunity for reflection, 224–225
practicing, 126–127
Seligman, Martin, 183
senses, connecting through mindfulness to, 24–25
sensory overload, 339
sentence-completion exercises, 44
serving sizes, 378
sexual harassment, as causing stress in workplaces, 393
sexual performance, disturbed due to stress, 401
shaking, to relieve tension, 423
showing self-love, 232
simple carbohydrates, 358–359
Sivananda yoga, 291
sleep
  implementing mindfulness to prepare for, 68–69
  lowering stress through, 470–471
slow learning, when practicing self-compassion, 116
small intestine, role in digestive process, 347
smartwatches, checking pulse on, 253
snowshoeing, 266–267
social interactions, on technology, 507–508
social media
  addictive quality of
   defined, 492–493
   overview, 511–512
   social network, 512–513
   social validation looping, 514–515
   undeveloped empathy and self-esteem, 517–518
   variable reinforcement, 515–516
  counter-social aspects of
   broadcast intoxication, 519–520
   cyberbullying, 520–521
   cyberstalking, 521
   overview, 519
   trolling, 521
  influence on television, 528–529
  superficial aspects of, 517
  taking breaks from, 522

social network, 512–513

social support, determining factors of resilience, 179

social validation, 528

social validation looping, 514–515, 522

sodium, 367–368

software, uninstalling, 544–545

soluble fiber, 371

soothing touch, from mammalian caregiving system, 103–104

sour taste, 336

specialty classes, 311

spirit lines, 144

spirituality, 28–29, 180

standing hamstring stretch, 282–283

standing quad stretch, 283–284

static stretching
  defined, 276–277
  overview, 278
  routine for
    back expansion, 281–282
    butterfly stretch, 286–287
    chest expansion, 280–281
    double calf stretch, 284–285
    hip stretch, 285–286
    neck stretch, 280
    overview, 279
    standing hamstring stretch, 282–283
    standing quad stretch, 283–284
  rules of, 278–279

storge, defined, 135

strategies
  for organization, 448–449
  for reducing workplace stress, 473–474
  for self-help
    creating dosing schedules for, 539–541
    creating real-time living plans, 545–547
    digital detoxing, 537–539
    establishing values-based technology use, 541
    limiting use of technology, 534–537
    removing notifications, 544–545
    uninstalling addictive apps, 544–545

streaming
  audio, 493
  autoplay option on, 526–528
  binging, 524–525
  designed with user experience engineering, 527–528
  endless choice in, 525–526
  influence of social media on, 528–529
  instant access with, 526
  overview, 524–525
  video, 493
  virtual workouts on, 312–313

strengths, identifying, 229–230

stress
  affecting resilience
    coping types, 193–195
    desire motivated by, 188
    influencing positive change, 195–197
    maintaining positive expectations, 192–193
    overview, 187
    stress responses, 189–192
  breathing techniques for reducing, 406–412
  causes of
    coronavirus pandemic, 390–391
    economy, 391
    hassles, 395–396
    home-life, 392–393
    overview, 389–390
    politics, 391
    technology, 393–394
    work-life, 391
  desire motivated by, 188
  disease linked to
    chronically tense muscles, 398
    compromised immune system, 400
    gastrointestinal issues, 399–400
    head colds, 401
    headaches, 401
    heart disease, 398–399
    overview, 397–398

easing bodily tension
  with AT, 417–418
  bringing awareness to, 405
  with massage, 420–422
  overview, 403
  with progressive relaxation method, 413–416
  scanning exercise for, 406–411
  by stretching, 419
  symptoms of, 403–404
  techniques for, 422–424
overeating due to, 378
physical signs of, 397
reducing with mindfulness, 11–12
reducing with organization
  creating system for, 459, 460, 460–461, 461–462, 463–464, 464–465
  by de-cluttering, 450–456
  documents, 458
  guidelines for, 456–457
  identifying personal disorganization, 449–450
  junk mail, 458–459
  maintaining, 465–466
  organizational strategies for, 448–449
  overview, 447
taking vacations to reduce, 484
stress responses
  fight-or-flight, 189–190
  negative feedback loop, 191–192
  overview, 189
  positive feedback loop, 190–191
  quieting, 196
  relaxation techniques for, 217–218
  supporting, 197
stress-related fatigue, 421
stretch reflex, 277
stretching
  benefits of, 273–276
  easing bodily tension by, 419, 474–476
  overview, 269–270

static type of
  overview, 278
  routine for, 279–287
  rules of, 278–279
  techniques for, 276–278
Successful Time Management For Dummies (Zeller), 425
Sun Salutation yoga position, 300–301
support
  emotional, 234, 455
  for recovering from addiction, 497
suppression expression, 218
survival, love contributing to, 134–137
sweet taste, 336
swimming, as outdoor exercise, 263–267
synergistic amplification, 502, 540

T

taking care of you
  accepting love, 237–239
  by eating healthy diet, 233
  with exercise, 233–234
  gratitude, 235
  healing negative emotions, 235
  quieting mind, 234–235
  receiving emotional support, 234
  resting, 236–237
target heart-rate zone, 250–252
tasks, delegating, 443–445
Tech Stress Syndrome, 525
technology, stress caused by, 393–394
technology addiction
  addictive platforms
    overview, 492
    social media, 492–493
    streaming audio and video, 493
    video games, 493–494
  conditioning, 502, 503
  defined, 488–489

technology addiction *(continued)*
  dopaminergic factors of
    broadcast intoxication, 506
    content, 502–506
    dynamic interaction, 510
    ease of access, 501
    illusion of productivity, 502
    lack of boundaries, 506–507
    multi-tasking, 507
    overview, 499–500
    time distortion, 501–502
    variable ratio reinforcement, 509–510
  enhanced user experience contributing to, 528
  overview, 487–488
  psychology of, 508–509
  recovering from, 496–497, 499–500
  science behind, 489–490
  self-help for
    creating dosing schedules for, 539–541
    creating real-time living plans, 545–547
    digital detoxing, 537–539
    establishing values-based tech use, 541
    limiting use of technology, 534–537
    removing notifications, 544–545
    uninstalling addictive apps, 544–545
  social interactions on, 507–508
  social media
    overview, 511–512
    social network, 512–513
    social validation looping, 514–515
    undeveloped emotional qualities due to, 517–518
    variable reinforcement, 515–516
  symptoms of, 494–496
  technology encouraging, 491
  uninstalling addictive apps, 544–545
  user experience engineering contributing to, 527–528
  watching television
    disadvantages of, 529–531
    limiting amount of time spent, 532
    overview, 523–524
    by streaming, 524–529

television
  addictive qualities of
    disadvantages of, 529–531
    limiting amount of time spent, 532
    overview, 523–524
    by streaming, 524–529
  binging, 524–525
  minimizing distractions from, 439
tension, reducing
  with AT, 417–418
  bringing awareness to, 405
  with massage, 420–422
  overview, 403
  with progressive relaxation method, 413–416
  scanning exercise for, 405, 406–411
  by shaking, 423
  by stretching, 419
  symptoms of, 403–404
  techniques for, 422–424
thinking patterns, emotions activating, 212
third noble truth, 119–120
thirst cues, 378–379
thoughts, re-focusing with mindfulness, 22–23
time distortion, when using technology, 501–502
time-management
  bringing awareness to
    activities to spend more and less time on, 428–429
    with cues and prompts, 429–430
    overview, 426
    by self-examining, 430–431
    by tracking, 427–428
  checklist for, 425
  creating to-do lists for
    master to-do list, 431–432
    overview, 431
    tips for, 434–436
    will-do-later list, 434
    will-do-today list, 432–433
  by delegating tasks, 443–445
  minimizing distractions, 436–440
  overview, 425
  by paying for services to be done, 445–446

psychological obstacles to, 440–443

to reduce workplace stress, 480

for technology, 498

to-do lists

master to-do list, 431–432

overview, 431

tips for, 434–436

will-do-later list, 434

will-do-today list, 432–433

Toffler, Alvin, 390

tolerable upper levels (UL), 363

tolerance, for self-compassion, 124–126

tones, from mammalian caregiving system, 104–105

traits, displayed in self-worth, 223–224

trans fats, dangers of, 333, 351

trauma, negatively affecting development of stress responses, 169, 177

Triage Method of Clutter Control, 454

Triangle Pose yoga position, 299

trolling, 521

twist stretch, 419

U

UL (tolerable upper levels), 363

ulcers, caused by stress, 400

umami taste, 336

uniqueness, accepting, 230–231

upper-back stretch, easing bodily tension with, 475–476

user experience engineering, contributing to addictions to technology, 527–528

V

vacation, reducing stress with, 484

values map, creating, 542–543

values-based tech use, establishing, 541

variability, of technology, 503–504

variable ratio reinforcement, when using technology, 502, 509–510

variable reinforcement, 515–516

victim mentality, overcoming, 181–182, 185

video games, addictive quality of, 493–494

villi, defined, 347

Vinyasa yoga, 291

virtual exercise classes, 311–313

visual resting spots, reducing stress with, 477–478

vitamin A, 365

vitamin C, 364

vitamin D, 365–366

vitamin E (mixed tocopherols), 366

vitamin K1, 366

vitamin K2, 366

vitamins, 362–366

W

walking, as exercise, 82–83, 256–258

warming up, for exercise, 245–246

water aerobics, as exercise, 263–267

water intake, 373

water-soluble vitamins, 364–365

weaknesses, identifying, 229–230

websites

Circle, 539

Future Me, 45

Kristin Neff's, 96

Qustodio, 539

uninstalling, 544–545

weight gain, from excess calories, 351–353

weight loss, clean eating contributing to, 328–329

weight training, 270–273

white-noise machines, avoiding distractions with, 438

whole foods, comparing processed foods to, 319–320

will-do-later list, 434

will-do-today list, 432–433

wisdom, gaining through mindfulness, 14–15

work, implementing mindfulness at. *See also* workplace stress

avoiding multi-tasking, 81

beginning with exercises, 74–75

creative problem solving, 78

mini meditations, 75–76

overview, 74

practicing mindful working, 79–80

responding versus reacting, 76–78

work-life, improving with mindfulness, 70, 391

Work/Life Balance For Dummies (Lockett & Mumford), 70

workplace stress. *See also* work, implementing mindfulness at

checklist for identifying sources of, 468–469

reducing

anticipatory anxiety, 470

business travel, 472–473

commuting, 471–472

with company services offered, 482–484

creating relaxing workspace for, 476–482

overview, 469–470

strategies for, 473–474

stretching to ease bodily tension, 474–476

tips for, 470–471

signs of, 467–468

workspace, creating relaxing atmosphere for

balancing blood sugar, 480–482

ergonomics, 478–479

options for, 477–478

by organizing, 477

overview, 476

time-management, 480

writing, in flow, 53

Y

yawning, reducing stress by, 412

Yerkes-Dodson Law, 124

yoga

classes for, 292–293

equipment and clothing for, 293

intensity of, 290

overview, 289

reducing stress by practicing, 424

routine for

Cat Pose, 298

Child's Pose, 296–297

Downward-Facing Dog, 294–295

Forward Bend, 295–296

Modified Sage Twist, 297–298

overview, 294

Sun Salutation, 300–301

Triangle Pose, 299

styles of, 290–291

tips for beginners, 293–294

Z

Zen breathing, 408–409

zinc, 368

About the Authors

Shamash Alidina has been teaching mindfulness since 1998. He formally trained for three years at Bangor University's Centre for Mindfulness in Wales. He also holds a master's degree in Chemical Engineering and a master's degree in Education. He runs his own successful training organization, *ShamashAlidina.com*, to introduce mindfulness to the general public, give talks, workshops, coaching, as well as offer fully online mindfulness teacher training. He has taught mindfulness all over the world, including the USA, Australia, New Zealand, the Middle East, and Europe. Shamash is also cofounder of the world's first Museum of Happiness in London. He is the author of *Mindfulness For Dummies.*

Allen Elkin, PhD, is a clinical psychologist, a certified sex therapist, and the director of the Stress Management & Counseling Center in New York City. Nationally known for his expertise in the field of stress and emotional disorders, he has appeared frequently on *Today, Good Morning America,* and *Good Day New York,* as well as programs on PBS, CNN, FNN, Fox 5, and National Public Radio. He has been quoted in *The New York Times, The Wall Street Journal, The Washington Post, Newsweek, Men's Health, Fitness, Cosmopolitan, Glamour, Redbook, Woman's Day, Self, Mademoiselle, McCall's, Parents,* and other publications. Dr. Elkin holds workshops and presentations for professional organizations and corporations, including the American Society of Contemporary Medicine, Surgery, and Ophthalmology; the U.S. Drug Enforcement Administration; Morgan Stanley; IBM; PepsiCo; and the New York Stock Exchange. He is the author of *Stress Management For Dummies.*

Dr. David Greenfield is the founder and clinical director of The Center for Internet and Technology Addiction and former Assistant Clinical Professor of Psychiatry at the University of Connecticut, School of Medicine, where he taught courses on Internet Addiction as well as Sexual Medicine and supervised residents in psychiatry. He is also the consulting medical director at the Greenfield Pathway for Video Game and Technology Addiction at Lifeskills South Florida. Dr. Greenfield is a leading authority on Internet and technology addiction, and the author of numerous articles and book chapters as well as the book *Virtual Addiction,* which in 1999 rang an early warning regarding the world's growing Internet addiction problem. His recent work is focused on the neurobiology and treatment of compulsive Internet, smartphone, and screen use. He is credited with popularizing the variable reinforcement, or *slot machine,* model of behavioral addictions and the dopamine–behavioral addiction connection. He is the author of *Overcoming Internet Addiction For Dummies.*

Dr. Steven Hickman has been a practitioner and teacher of mindfulness and self-compassion for over 20 years. As a licensed clinical psychologist and associate clinical professor in the UC San Diego School of Medicine, Steven first began practicing mindfulness as part of his training to become a Mindfulness-Based Stress Reduction (MBSR) program teacher. He taught that program for 15 years, during which time he established the UC San Diego Center for Mindfulness and its Mindfulness-Based Professional Training Institute. That center (and Dr. Hickman) has become a world leader in the field of teachers of mindfulness- and compassion-based programs. In 2018 he became the executive director of the nonprofit Center for Mindful Self-Compassion, dedicated to creating a more compassionate world through the dissemination of self-compassion practice worldwide in many forms. Steve is now retired from UC San Diego but still serves as the founding director of the Center for Mindfulness there as it continues to grow and thrive as a world leader in the field. He is the author of *Self-Compassion For Dummies.*

Linda Larsen is an author and journalist who has written more than 30 books, many of which are about food and nutrition. She earned a BA degree in Biology from St. Olaf College and a BS with High Distinction in Food Science and Nutrition from the University of Minnesota. Linda worked for the Pillsbury Company for many years, creating and testing recipes. She was a member of the Pillsbury Bake-Off staff five times, acting as Manager of the Search Team and working in the test kitchens. She is the editor of Food Poisoning Bulletin, a Google News site, which reports on outbreaks, food safety issues, and food recalls. She is the coauthor of *Eating Clean For Dummies.*

Liz Neporent is a columnist and blogger for AOL Health and That's Fit, as well as a regular contributor to many other websites, publications, and media outlets. She cowrote *The Winner's Brain* with authors Jeff Brown and Mark Fenske. Liz brings a strong science background, fitness authority, and sense of fun to all her work. She holds a master's degree in exercise physiology from New York University and is certified by the American Council on Exercise, where she served on the board of directors for six years and now serves on the emeritus board and as a national spokesperson. She's a health consultant to Harvard Medical School in the publications division and is president of Wellness 360, a New York City-based wellness management and consulting company. She is the coauthor of *Fitness For Dummies.*

Suzanne Schlosberg is a fitness, health, and parenting writer known for her humorous approach to lifestyle topics. A former senior editor of *Shape* magazine, she is the author or coauthor of ten books, including *Weight Training For Dummies, The Ultimate Workout Log, The Ultimate Diet Log, The Good Neighbor Cookbook,* and *The Active Woman's Pregnancy Log.* Her articles can be found on the websites of *Fit Pregnancy, Ladies' Home Journal, More, Parents,* and *Parenting,* among others. She is the coauthor of *Fitness For Dummies.*

Eva Selhub, MD — or Dr. Eva, as her clients like to call her — has, for over 25 years, been practicing and teaching mind body medicine and methods to tap into our innate human ability to be resilient. She is the founder of Resilience Experts, LLC, a company that provides inspirational and informative coaching and consulting specializing in helping individuals and corporations alike achieve optimal wellness, resilience, innovation, and leadership. Dr. Eva's goal: to keep people out of the hospitals and fully engaged and thriving in life, even in the face of adversity! Dr. Eva is an internationally recognized expert, physician, speaker, executive leadership and performance coach, and consultant in the fields of stress, resilience, integrative medicine, and working with the natural environment to achieve maximum health and wellbeing. As an author, a speaker, and a coach, she uses her powerful gift to translate complex information into practical and usable knowledge that any individual can access. She is the author of *Resilience For Dummies.*

Dr. Jonathan Wright, a Harvard University and University of Michigan graduate, is a fore-runner in research and application of natural treatments for healthy aging and illness. Along with Alan Gaby, MD, he has since 1976 accumulated a file of over 50,000 research papers about diet, vitamins, minerals, botanicals, and other natural substances from which he has developed all-natural treatments for health problems. Since 1983, Drs. Wright and Gaby have regularly taught seminars about these methods to tens of thousands of physicians in the United States and overseas. Dr. Wright founded the Tahoma Clinic (1973), Meridian Valley Laboratory (1976), and the Tahoma Clinic Foundation (1996). He authors *Nutrition and Healing,* a monthly newsletter emphasizing nutritional medicine that reaches over 100,000 in the United States and another 7,000 or more worldwide. He is the coauthor of *Eating Clean For Dummies.*

Publisher's Acknowledgments

Associate Editor: Zoe Slaughter

Compilation Editor: Georgette Beatty

Project Manager: Rebecca Senninger

Production Editor: Mohammed Zafar Ali

Cover Image: © WAYHOME studio/Shutterstock